Hippocrates Revisited

HIPPOCRATES REVISITED

A Search for Meaning

Editor

ROGER J. BULGER, MD

Executive Officer
Institute of Medicine of the
National Academy of Sciences
Professor of Medicine
The George Washington University School of Medicine

MEDCOM PRESS

MEDCOM
Production Staff

Publishers
Robert E. Fuisz, MD
Richard C. Fuisz, MD

Editor in Chief
David P. Lauler, MD

Executive Editor
Robert B. Wilson

Managing Editor
Ruth A. Rosenblum

Executive Art Director
Gary N. Olivo

Executive Film Producer
Alfred R. Kelman

Director of Medical Affairs
Virginia A. Malfitan, MD

Director of Dental Affairs
Stephen J. Moss, DDS, MS

Medical Consultant
Peter Philander, MB, ChB

Project Editorial Director
Norma Frankel

Editors
Susan Davis
Ann Holmes

Production Manager
Joan Milarsky

Production Director
George Nickford

Production Assistant
William K. Costigan

Art Director
Wayne Peterson

Photo Editor
Cathie Furbush

Photo Research
Janet Kinzie

Technical Research
Deborah Graham

Copy Chief
Peter Parks

Copy Editors
Marion Lazos
Martha L. Moffett
Mary Bozeman Raines
Selma Ramsey
Elena Rosti
Susan Turner Rubin

Editorial Coordinator
Doris Einhorn

Editorial Assistant
Ellen Taub

MEDC⊕M®
World leader in multimedia health education programs
2 Hammarskjöld Plaza, New York, N. Y. 10017
(212) 832–1400
MEDCOM Press. Copyright © 1973 by MEDCOM, Inc.

Library of Congress Cataloging in Publication Data

Bulger, Roger J   1933–
   Hippocrates revisited.

   1. Medical care—United States. 2. Medical ethics—United States. I. Title. [DNLM: 1. Ethics, Medical. 2. Hippocratic oath. 3. Medicine—U. S. WB 50 AAL B9h 1973]
RA395.A3B85   174'.22   72–7611

Dedication

*To my wife, children, parents, and brother.
All have demonstrated consistently to me how a
person's family can be the most cherished element
of his life, an element that is not unrelated to
some major themes in this book.*

Contents

III. THE CRACKED IMAGE: REALISTIC MOTIVATIONS AND REWARDS

IV. SOME PHILOSOPHICAL AND ETHICAL CONSIDERATIONS

V. ON PASSING THE TORCH

Contributors

Lawrence K. Altman, MD
Clinical Assistant Professor,
New York University Medical School;
Staff Medical Correspondent, The New York Times,
New York, New York

Herrman L. Blumgart, MD
Professor of Medicine, Emeritus;
Consultant, Medical Area Health Service,
Harvard University,
Cambridge, Massachusetts

Roger J. Bulger, MD
Executive Officer,
Institute of Medicine of the National Academy of Sciences;
Professor of Medicine,
The George Washington University School of Medicine,
Washington, DC

Martin Cherkasky, MD
Director, Montefiore Hospital and Medical Center;
Atran Professor of Social Medicine,
Department of Community Health and Associate Dean for Community Affairs,
Albert Einstein College of Medicine of Yeshiva University,
Bronx, New York

J. Russell Elkinton, MD
Emeritus Professor of Medicine,
The University of Pennsylvania School of Medicine,
Philadelphia, Pennsylvania

Erik H. Erikson
Professor Emeritus of Human Development,
Harvard University,
Cambridge, Massachusetts

Lawrence D. Grouse
Senior Medical Student,
University of Washington School of Medicine,
Seattle, Washington

Michael J. Halberstam, MD
Private Practice of Internal Medicine,
Washington, DC

Tinsley R. Harrison, MD
Distinguished Emeritus Professor of Medicine,
University of Alabama School of Medicine,
Birmingham, Alabama

Louis Lasagna, MD
Chairman of the Department and Professor of Pharmacology and Toxicology;
Professor of Medicine,
The University of Rochester School of Medicine and Dentistry,
Rochester, New York

Joshua Lederberg, PhD, MD
Chairman, Department of Genetics;
Professor, Genetics and Biology;
Director, Kennedy Laboratories for Molecular Medicine,
Stanford University School of Medicine,
Palo Alto, California

John H. Leversee, MD
Chairman, Department of General Practice and Chief of Staff,
Overlake Memorial Hospital,
Bellevue, Washington

John J. McDermott, PhD
Professor of Philosophy,
Queens College;
Member of the Philosophy Doctoral Faculty,
The City University of New York,
Flushing, New York

Richard M. Magraw, MD
Deputy Executive Dean,
University of Illinois College of Medicine,
Urbana, Illinois

Leonard K. Nash, PhD
Professor and Chairman,
Department of Chemistry,
Harvard University,
Cambridge, Massachusetts

Francis Weld Peabody, MD (1881–1927)
Professor of Medicine,
Harvard Medical School,
Boston, Massachusetts

Edmund D. Pellegrino, MD
Professor of Medicine and Vice President for the Health Sciences;
Director of the Health Sciences Center,
State University of New York at Stony Brook,
Stony Brook, New York

Dickinson W. Richards, MD
Lambert Professor Emeritus of Medicine,
Columbia University College of Physicians and Surgeons,
New York, New York

Eugene A. Stead, Jr., MD
Florence McAlister Professor of Medicine,
Duke University Medical Center,
Durham, North Carolina

Philip A. Tumulty, MD
Professor of Medicine,
The Johns Hopkins University School of Medicine,
Baltimore, Maryland

Ralph G. Victor, MD
Director of Mental Health Services,
Fresno Community Hospital,
Fresno, California

Preface

This volume is a collection of essays dealing with the profession of medicine at personal, philosophic, and ethical levels. For many years as I progressed through pre- and postdoctoral training, I felt the void I hope this book will at least begin to fill. I believe this void has been sensed by most of my contemporaries and is experienced even more keenly and universally by today's students. The need for inspiration and encouragement is not a sign of weakness or instability; all too often it seems that conversation of this sort has been lacking, particularly in medical schools.

The goals of this book are stated in the Introduction. Written in the summer of 1968, the Introduction was first sent to potential contributors of the proposed volume in the spring of 1969. This book represents the responses of the contributing essayists to that Introduction. Because the essays vary in subject matter, it may interest the reader to view the Introduction intact, so that the reader may reflect on the variety of responses that the original query elicited. Of course, the contributions that are reprinted from other sources are exceptions to this, as is the essay on auto-experimentation by Dr. Larry Altman.

I chose to group the essays into rather arbitrary categories. I emphasize this point as a warning to the reader to approach each essay with an open mind and with an awareness that none of the essays fits neatly or completely into the classifications superimposed after the fact by the editor.

If the authors could respond so variably to a single request for a revisitation to Hippocrates, one can anticipate a still greater variety of responses to each of the essays by each reader. After long reflection, I conclude that there is a unity in these attempts. My only hope is that the reader will learn as much from the contents of this book as I have. Putting this effort together has been a most rewarding experience.

Roger J. Bulger, MD
Washington, DC

Hippocrates Revisited

Part I
Setting the Stage

Wherever there is lost the consciousness that every man is an object of concern for us just because he is a man, civilization and morals are shaken, and the advance to fully developed inhumanity is only a question of time.

Albert Schweitzer, 1923

Chapter 1
Introduction
Roger J. Bulger, MD

It may seem extraordinary that in all the time that has elapsed since the days of Hippocrates, history has been unable to produce a statement to supersede his guidelines for medical behavior.

Life is short,
The art long,
Opportunity fleeting,
Experiment treacherous
Judgment difficult.
       Hippocrates: *Aphorisms I*

I will look upon him who shall have taught me this art even as one of my parents. I will share my substance with him, and I will supply his necessities, if he be in need. I will regard his offspring even as my own brethren and I will teach them this art, if they would learn it without fee or covenant. I will impart this art by precept, by lecture and by every mode of teaching, not only to my own sons but to sons of him who has taught me, and to disciples bound by covenant

Editor's Note: Before joining the Institute of Medicine of the National Academy of Sciences, Dr. Bulger taught internal medicine and was active in clinical investigation. His most recent full-time academic appointment was as professor in the Department of Community Health Sciences at Duke University Medical Center.

and oath, according to the law of medicine.

The regimen I adopt shall be for the benefit of my patients according to my ability and judgment, and not for their hurt or for any wrong. I will give no deadly drug to any, though it be asked of me, nor will I counsel such, and especially I will not aid a woman to procure abortion. Whatsoever house I enter, there will I go for the benefit of the sick, refraining from all wrongdoing or corruption, and especially from any act of seduction of male or female, of bond or free. Whatsoever things I see or hear concerning the life of men, in my attendance on the sick or even apart therefrom, which ought not to be noised abroad, I will keep silence thereon, counting such things to be as sacred secrets.
       Hippocrates: *Physicians Oath*

THE OATH TODAY

These famous quotations of Hippocrates yield, upon careful perusal, much wisdom, even for modern-day physicians. On the other hand, it is clear that the Hippocratic Oath contains some statements that are not, in fact, in agreement with what many, if not most, highly motivated and sincere twentieth-century physicians would hold. It may seem extraordinary that in all the time that has elapsed since the days of Hippocrates, history has been unable to produce a statement to supersede his guidelines for medical behavior. The need for such a document seems great, particularly in our own times, when social evolution and revolution are extending into the areas of the provision of health care, when the immense accomplishments of research are producing moral and ethical problems of great magnitude and immediacy, when youthful disenchantment and rebellion at the status quo and anything that can be labeled ''establishment'' at last have permeated (thank goodness!) the medical school student body, and when economic resources finally have been stretched to their limits in the United States, thus forcing us to set some priorities in what soon will be known as the nation's second-largest enterprise, the health business.

Especially in times such as these, we are all in need of common goals and principles, a set of common denominators from which we can work, a firm platform of common purpose to which we can return for guidance, a reference standard against which we can compare our activities. If such a document is not possible, would it not be of great value to get a clearer understanding of the motivations, goals, and satisfactions of some of the world's outstanding physicians? From such a collection of personal statements the interested reader could distill aspects that have meaning for him. This book represents such an effort. One can hope that this collection of personal statements is a step toward a serious forum on values, ethics, and moral considerations in the medical profession.

Medicine has become enormously complex. Physicians these days not only carry on general patient care, but they may become highly trained specialists, research scientists, full-time teachers, or administrators concerning themselves with medical education, delivering health care services, or organizing our vast biomedical research efforts. A book such as this that proposes to speak of motivation must also speak to students, medical and premedical, in an effort to give them a glimpse of what it is that prompts these men and women to pursue a medical career. If this book is to have any significance, the statements must be able to cross the so-called ''generation gap'' and carry an immediacy and a meaning that is, I suspect, highly personal, much the same as the Hippocratic Oath is really a very personal statement, one which affords some insight into the man Hippocrates was.

To me, the meaning of the Hippocratic Oath and the reason for its enduring value is this highly personal quality which reflects the basic concepts of devotion to people and a desire to serve them. I believe that these two concepts should be the common denominator which was mentioned earlier. In his statement, Hippocrates makes everything else emanate therefrom: the physician's relation with his patient is sacrosanct; what follows is a great respect for teaching and, by implication, for research and the acquisition of new knowledge. The humanistic basis for Hippocrates' actions is still tenable for most modern physicians and I believe for most modern medical and university students. Is it not likely that this particular interest in people is crucial not only to the makeup of the practitioner of medicine (like Hippocrates), but is also an important ingredient in the medical specialist, researcher, and administrator? If so, then it is clear that school admission committees and medical educators generally should be concerning themselves more with the nature and quality of motivation in prospective medical students, once a necessary basic intelligence and training level has been established. The tendency in the past 50 or 60 years has been to test motivation through the establishment of a kind of academic obstacle-survival course and to make final selections from among the survivors on the basis of academic standing.

This policy has shifted somewhat in recent years, and it is hoped that the present volume will add perspectives which will enhance our consideration of this problem.

MEDICAL SCHOOLS

Since the early twentieth century and the Flexner Report, there has been a major emphasis in medical schools on scientific and technical competence, accomplished by setting rigorous standards, forcing students to master a certain voluminous body of knowledge. This particular characteristic of medical school, which most graduate students in the arts and sciences would find abhorrent, has not prevented an ample number of intelligent students from clamoring for entrance. At the same time, there has been an increasing amount of criticism on the part of some people regarding the dehumanization and depersonalization of medical practice. Although our whole society has undergone this same process of depersonalization, there is no simple answer to the questions raised by medical critics. Suffice it to say that the medical profession, including medical educators and our society as a whole, recognizes the great need for many more physicians trained and motivated to deliver medical care. Too many of our practicing physicians have been trained in foreign, often underdeveloped, countries which can ill afford to lose their precious manpower; too large a proportion of our graduates forego the practice of medicine for other careers within the biomedical health complex.

There are massive efforts at reorientation. Medical schools are rewriting their curricula to build free, unprogrammed, elective time with flexibility to allow for student individuality. Some are providing a multiplicity of pathways from which the student may choose; thus he may select a pathway aimed at training family or "primary contact" physicians, or he may choose specialty medicine, biomedical research, or "administrative medicine." At the postgraduate level, the prestigious Millis Commission's recent report strongly recommended a residency program to train primary physicians; the report suggested that the humanities and behavorial sciences be included in the residency period, and went on to imply that if this did not succeed in producing the necessary humanism in the end product, there should be a reexamination of medical school admission policies.

I believe that medical care of the type delivered by family physicians, primary physicians, general practitioners, obstetricians, pediatricians, internists, and most surgeons must be based primarily on the desire to serve.

I believe that medical care of the type delivered by family physicians, primary physicians, general practitioners, obstetricians, pediatricians, internists, and most surgeons must be based primarily on the desire to serve. In order to produce a growing number of people who will spend their lives in these activities, it is not enough to encourage them to read Tolstoy, Freud, and Riesman during their residency; rather, it would be ideal if they could be chosen primarily on the basis of estimating the nature of their motivation, a motivation that may have led them to concentrate in the humanities and social sciences before entering medical school.

The quality of our motivation is surely not the sole factor responsible for the dehumanizing tendencies of the twentieth century. In addition to the motivational issue, other sociologic and economic factors have played a significant role—among them, the emphasis on professionalization, which occurs through long and intensely arduous training years, the excess of patient demands and expectations, and the overload in requests for help. Of interest in the latter regard is the Good Samaritan study conducted with graduating theology students at Princeton. A test situation was established for each student (unaware that he was participating in a test) so that he passed a supposed suffering fellow man under the same conditions as did his colleagues, except for a number of variables: some were rushing to an appointment and some had time to spare; some thought they were on their way to give a television talk on the parable of the Good Samaritan, and others thought they were going to an interview for a first-rate position. Reportedly, the only variable that showed a positive correlation with stopping to help the man in trouble was not being in a hurry. If this sort of thing holds true for medical practice, then it suggests that changes in the organization of health care can, in fact, be instrumental in aiding the reemergence of humanitarianism.

Similar kinds of considerations regarding these and other issues could be made about medical specialists, researchers, and administrators. These points and conflicting ones will be made and developed by some of the other contributors to this volume.

The term "motivation" may be too restrictive. The aim here is to get the various contributors to talk about medicine and their own careers in terms of meaning and satisfaction, challenge and responsibility, creativity and opportunity. The people on both sides of the "generation gap" are all involved in a great search for meaning, or so we are told. It seems to me that "the search for meaning" is a phrase that applies to all of us everywhere.

A technocratic society such as ours, which deifies data and the hard sciences and fears platitudes, may also be a little afraid of and somewhat embarrassed by the philosophic quest for meaning.

A technocratic society such as ours, which deifies data and the hard sciences and fears platitudes, may also be a little afraid of and

somewhat embarrassed by the philosophic quest for meaning. On the other hand, even our politicians recognize the nature of the problem. Listen to what Nelson Rockefeller says in *Foreign Affairs*:

> The deepest problem before America, then, is moral or psychological. Since much of the current uneasiness reflects a search less for solutions than for meaning, remedies depend for their effectiveness on the philosophy or values which inspire them. The student unrest is impressive, not because some of it is fomented by agitators, but because it includes some of the most idealistic elements of our youth. In fact, much that disquiets us today gives us cause for hope, for it reflects not cynicism but disappointed idealism.
>
> Nelson A. Rockefeller: *Policy and the People*[1]

Governor Rockefeller went on to make other observations relevant to our purposes in this book:

> Decades of "debunking" and materialism have left the young generation without moral support in face of the challenges of a revolutionary age. Leaders at all levels are seen to have been asking not too much of our people but too little. The contemporary discontent proves, among other things, that man cannot live by economics alone; he needs quality and purpose in addition to material well-being; he needs significance and meaning beyond physical comfort. The quality and success of the Peace Corps can be explained on no other ground. The spirit of idealism which it has fostered should —and can—animate our actions in meeting a wide variety of challenges.
>
> For a people grown great in the experience of the frontier, the twin challenges of a technocratic bureaucracy and

helping the world find a modern structure offer an adventurous opportunity. This is an exciting age. The current uneasiness exists because people care—and yet do not see the way to make their aspirations come true. The task is to prove that their aspirations are relevant and attainable. This cannot be the responsibility of the President alone; it is the responsibility of all public officials, of leaders in all walks of life—indeed, of all of us.

> Nelson A. Rockefeller: *Policy and the People*[2]

It is not difficult to list other leaders who are capable of speaking articulately about our society's goals and directions, its meaning, challenges, and opportunities. Few modern men have spoken more poignantly about the nature and meaning of their own lives than did Dag Hammarskjöld in his autobiographical book *Markings*.[3] Although many people may not share his religiosity, the crux of his ideas can, I believe, have significance for all of us with a major interest in medicine. Some examples, which are particularly pertinent, follow:

Conscious of the reality of evil and the tragedy of the individual life, and conscious, too, of the demand that life be conducted with decency. . . .

"To fail"—Are you satisfied because you have curbed and canalized the worst in you? In any human situation, it is cheating not to be, at every moment, one's best. How much more so in a position where others have faith in you. . . .

For someone whose job so obviously mirrors man's extraordinary possibilities and responsibilities, there is no excuse if he loses his sense of "having been called." So long as he keeps that, everything he can do has a meaning, nothing a price. Therefore: if he complains, he is accusing—himself.

Finally, Mr. Hammarskjöld aims a question at his own attempts to pass wisdom on to others, which he might well have aimed at all those who have written in this book:

The scientist only records what he has been able to establish as indisputable fact. In the same way, only what is unique in a person's experience is worth writing down as a guide and a warning to others. In the same way, too, an explorer leaves it to others to pass their time taking notes on the quaint customs of the natives, or making devastating remarks about the foibles of their traveling companions.

True—and which do you?

> Dag Hammarskjöld: *Markings*.[3] Translated by W. H. Auden and Leif Sjöberg. Copyright © 1964 by Alfred A. Knopf, Inc. Reprinted by permission of the publisher.

ON BEING A PHYSICIAN

But excellence implies more than competence. It implies a striving for the highest standards in every phase of life. We need individual excellence in all its forms, in every kind of creative endeavor, in political life, in education, in industry, in short, universally.

> John Gardner: *Excellence: Can We Be Equal and Excellent Too?*[4]

The striving for excellence, the quest for meaning through service, a sense of satisfaction, and a kind of sacramental attitude concerning work are aspects of human character and personality that are not peculiar to the medical profession. One would expect, in fact, that these attributes would characterize productive workers in many fields. What then, if anything, is peculiar and special about medicine?

DIFFERENT FROM OTHER PROFESSIONS It has always seemed to me that medicine as a profession offers three particular qualities to its practitioners, qualities which, indeed, do provide distinctive benefits to our profession. The first is the constant contact with suffering and death which is afforded physicians; it is terribly difficult for a sensitive physician to ignore the realities of life, to fail to question and requestion the deeper meanings and purposes and quests of human existence, and to misappropriate one's own priorities so that false values and ultimately meaningless goals become paramount. It must be admitted that there is a danger in having to face daily the human suffering and death of one's patients and friends, and that danger is a kind of attitude of fatalistic cynicism which some doctors and nurses seem particularly prone to develop.

The second special attribute the medical profession offers its practitioners has something to do with age—the later years of the physician's career and life. The physician has the great opportunity of continually developing his trade. The degree to which he develops this art will, in many instances, determine his effectiveness; its development, in turn, will depend upon his continued growth as a sensitive, cognitive, participating member of the human race. Thus, the physician who can maintain his scientific and technical knowledge base is offered the almost unique opportunity of becoming increasingly more valuable to and effective in society as he grows older. He seldom needs to be concerned that, as he approaches 50, his job will be better done by the younger men. Surely, he may begin to see fewer patients, but those he sees can be cared for very well. A career which offers continued, lifelong utility, with the potential for increasing value as the years go by, is a career which should be highly desirable to people seeking to live a life of high quality and excellence which is somehow related in their minds to hard work and service.

A third characteristic of medicine which makes it a distinctive profession is a characteristic which is seen in other areas of human endeavor, though not to so great a degree. This characteristic is at the source of the observation frequently made by outsiders when they comment on how boring it is to be with a group of doctors: "All they ever talk about is medicine!" Aside from an intrinsic interest in human biology, the ideal physician usually shares with other physicians an almost morbid concern for medical knowledge. Some newly learned fact may save an unknown patient's life; some recently published paper may indicate a way to aid in diagnosing or treating other patients whose maladies are poorly understood by the physician or whose treatment is currently unsuccessful. Sometimes physicians allow this quest for new information to become such a passion or even compulsion that they cease to develop effectively other aspects of their intellectual and aesthetic lives. Such physicians may be said to be enhancing their technical side at the expense of their "artful" side. Occasionally, of course, some physicians may develop a skill in handling various personalities far in excess of their ability to carry out the technical aspects of treating disease. At this point they may be "successful" and popular, but perhaps inadequate.

Medicine offers maximum opportunity for self-fulfillment, particularly for those who can either intuitively or rationally relate such fulfillment with giving of self. With every opportunity comes both a responsibility and a challenge. For the good physician, the responsibility is to deliver the best possible care to his patients, and the challenge is to develop and maintain the necessary scientific, technical know-how and personal attributes which will allow him to carry out his responsibility.

These high-sounding sentiments may have meaning for some people, but others will raise many different questions which demand answers. These days, people seem to question the physician's honesty and competence more often. Does this seriously detract from practice? What would happen if the worst fears of some people were realized and doctors became salaried? Francis Peabody said that the first rule of good patient care is to care for the patient. This implies responsibility. Is the essence of the personal physician the fact that an individual physician accepts personal responsibility for the health and welfare of his patient? Is that really important in practice to physicians? Must that go down the drain in the future world of supermarket medicine, where services are supplied in quantity by superb physician-technician specialists? Is there to be a role in the future for a family or personal physician—and, if so, what will be his best characteristics and the nature of his work satisfactions?

What about physician-technician specialists? An objectionable term, perhaps, but more and more an appropriate one! Do we need them? Obviously! Are they an entirely different breed from the personal physician? Must they have different skills and aptitudes? Doesn't the cardiovascular surgeon also have more than just technical responsibilities? Does he gain anything by his daily confrontation with death and long-term suffering? How can he best deal with these things—or better, how can he show the rest of us how to best deal with them? Are there any rewards from caring for terminally ill patients (the threat of severe illness is, after all, usually the threat of death), and if, according to the latest style, death is only molecular disintegration, how can anyone consider it a constructive occupation to deal with such patients? Does such an occupation force a special wisdom and acceptance of death on aware physicians? Are these thoughts mere platitudes?

What about medical scientists? Are they the same type of people as family physicians and physician-specialists? Do we actually divide our entering classes to medical school according to these three categories? Or should we? What are the rewards for the medical scientist or clinical investigator? Are they purely intellectual, or do action and experimentation emanate from the bedside experience? Is there a humanism here too? Or are clinical investigators biologists with a primary intellectual interest in the human species?

What about the clinical teacher? He used to be the practitioner who freely donated his time to pass on the art. Of late, there has been a trend toward having full-time faculty members carry out most of this function. Often these people have to carry out productive research programs and seldom actually care for patients by themselves, as a personal physician must do. Does this matter? Is it good or bad? Should it be modified? What should teachers be, basically? What are their satisfactions and what is it they want to pass on to their students? Should we be teaching a method, a set of facts, a logical approach? Or should we be an example since all the preceding things are in books—and, if an example, what sort of an example?

What about medicine and society? What are the medical administrator's goals, ambitions, and motivating forces; how does he get his satisfactions?

THE HEALTH MANPOWER CRISIS

Hippocrates once said to one of his students: "Let your best means of treating people be your love for them, your interest in their affairs, your knowledge of their condition, and your recognized attentiveness to them."
Muslim tradition

Studies show that medical students' attitudes are different than one might expect; something may happen to them in current medical schools—the human aspect of medicine may be emphasized less. Still others say this isn't so, that the current situation is the best that could be expected. At the personal level, some say our medical schools are failing to turn out service-oriented doctors. Some members of society say that we have failed to set up an excellent system for delivering health care; diminished federal funding suggests a future decrease in the rapid rate of growth of national investment in research, and research will become somewhat less accessible than it once was to bright, young, aspiring physicians. There is a great and urgent need to develop manpower at many levels. Twenty-five percent of physicians in this country are foreign trained, a fact which is appalling in what it says about our own inadequate training programs, not to mention the implication that we are draining valuable resources from disadvantaged nations. Thus, our society demands and will continue to demand in increasing fashion sweeping changes in the anachronistic, expensive, and fragmented type of health care delivery system now prevalent in the United States.

Such changes will mean organization, priorities, allocation of resources, economic limitations, systems analysis—in other words, the coming of age of a national health enterprise.

There is abroad an undercurrent suggesting that the solution of health manpower problems will follow hard upon the definition of the problems. Certainly our medical schools cannot produce the required number of physicians unless that number can be accurately predetermined. Perhaps by having economists defining the needs in terms of the number of physicians required and by having educators and sociologists combine to make medical school more palatable and to offer sufficient incentives to entice people into medicine, we will be able to produce bodies in sufficient quantity to solve the numbers problem.

I believe, however, that even if such analyses are possible, they would not be a true or complete solution. Once again, I would like to suggest that part of the solution lies in an understanding of motivation. If we can define what motivates a happy and satisfied physician, one who does his job well and competently and is happy with doing it for a lifetime, one who is capable of communicating his knowledge, advice, and concern to his patients—if we can do this, then we will be able to pick out college students with these motivations and encourage them to go to medical school. By selecting our students more on the basis of their motivations, goals, and satis-

By selecting our students more on the basis of their motivations, goals, and satisfactions, we will be able to produce more physicians truly concerned and vitally interested in their profession.

factions, we will be able to produce more physicians truly concerned and vitally interested in their profession. More than the numbers will have been met; an appropriate and important step will have been taken toward resolving the problem of depersonalization.

It is my contention that there is a great untapped source of future family physicians. They are to be found among the many young men and women who never get to medical school, but who have the proper motivation and basic ability to communicate with patients, and who would thrive on the kinds of demands made on the practicing physician. A significant number of these students possess the necessary scientific aptitude to acquire medical skills and to attain excellence in the physician's trade, but too often are discouraged from medical school for invalid reasons. One of the greatest obstacles that keeps many of these people from clinical medicine could be overcome by developing a basic science aptitude test which could accurately establish at the 16-, 17-, or 18-year-old level whether or not the student has enough ability to succeed in medical school. The results of such a test should be made known to the students, who should then be encouraged to pursue whatever intellectual interests they wish in college, secure in the knowledge that a collegiate emphasis outside of the natural sciences will not preclude their becoming physicians, and may, in fact, be helpful.

WHY THIS BOOK?

No one in my own medical student experience ever said very much that I recognized, at any rate, as dealing with some of these important matters in a meaningful way, until a physician named Herrman Blumgart talked long into the night with a group of fourth-year students about caring for dying patients. Later in that same year, Chester Jones, another venerable and kind physician, in a matter of a few short minutes on two separate occasions made me feel that he was welcoming me into a very important and special profession, and left me with a lasting impression of his concept of and concern for all that is involved with being a physician. It is pertinent, if somewhat distressing, to note that in my eight years' experience teaching medical students, I have too seldom talked with them about this sort of thing.

Perhaps wisdom exists only in the mind of the listener or reader, but perhaps also every life incorporates or uncovers a little insight and wisdom from which others may profit. Those people who are sufficiently articulate may communicate these things. In my own life, such episodes of illumination from others occurred all too infrequently and often the lasting lessons and impressions were not fully understood by me until long afterward.

In college, I took an introductory course in the natural sciences given by Professor Leonard Nash. Professor Nash's lectures were intriguing partly because they were so unique. He almost never told us anything; that is, he almost never lectured. Rather he would conduct an experiment on the stage of the lecture hall, which was just as likely not to work as it was to be successful. Only in retrospect did I realize fully that Professor Nash was setting an example for us all in his own behavior and reactions, demonstrating curiosity, honesty, imagination, and persistence.

He showed us what science was by his daily interaction with it, and we learned from a master things we never forgot and could never get from a book. I am now convinced that those pedagogical lessons are the most important and significant things I know about my own profession of teaching medical students and house officers.

After college and before medical school, I spent a year at Cambridge University in England, and during this period had an opportunity to make the acquaintance of T. S. Eliot. I had read all his works during my college years and one day spent a wonderful half hour discussing the difficulties of reconciling involvement in the affairs of people with the capacity to maintain a degree of indifference to their sufferings sufficient that one would not disintegrate in the face of others' misfortunes. During the course of this animated conversation, he found out that I was a Roman Catholic and later, after I had expressed some ambivalence about going to medical school, he said in a way I have never forgotten, "The world needs good Catholic doctors." Many times since I have recalled those words, which still seem to thunder down at me from some mountaintop oracle. He could just as easily have said, "The world needs good agnostic doctors" or "good atheist doctors" or "good Buddhist doctors," because what he was telling me was that the world needed good doctors and he thought I had the stuff to be one. That thought was particularly important at a later time when I felt that Mr. Eliot's confidence in me apparently was not shared to the same degree by some of the medical school faculty. I chose to rely on Mr. Eliot and, for better or worse, I am glad I did.

The kind of thing we are asking our authors to express here was exemplified by the practicing physician who told me, when discussing his job, that some of the most rewarding experience of his professional life came from helping and observing some of his patients as they came to terms with their own death. As he talked, I was impressed with the significance being a physician held for this man. His words and reactions evoked a response from me at a time when I was considering a medical career and his comments were, in fact, important in encouraging me to give it a try.

During my last year of medical school, a highly respected and successful practicing physician told us about the most important rule in his daily life as a physician. His rule, which he said required frequent repeating to himself, was always to sit down when visiting a patient on rounds, even if his visit was to be only 30 seconds long. He pointed out that the patient frequently relaxed, more easily communicating what was on his or her mind, or at least felt that the physician was willing to spend some time and had a personal interest in his patient. His obvious success in accomplishing these goals, which he demonstrated to us each day on rounds, planted seeds which are still bearing fruit.

The following statement made in 1895 by William Osler, the father of modern American medicine, has been helpful to me again and again since the time I first came across it. It is important not only because he said it, but because so many of us can recognize the tendency to slip away from what might be considered an underlying assumption in any physician's basic philosophy.

In these days of aggressive self assertion, when the stress of competition is so keen, and the desire to make the most of oneself so universal, it may seem a little old fashioned to preach the necessity of humility; but I insist for its own sake and for the sake of what it brings, that due humility should take the place of honour in the list. For its own sake, since with it comes not only a reverence for truth, but also a proper estimation of the difficulties encountered in our search for it. More perhaps than any other professional man, the doctor has a curious, shall I say morbid? sensitiveness to (what he regards) personal error. In a way this is right; but it is too often accompanied by a cocksureness of opinion, which, if encouraged, leads him to so lively a conceit that the mere suggestion of a mistake under any circumstances is regarded as a reflection of his honour, a reflection equally resented, whether of lay or professional origin. Start out with the conviction that absolute truth is hard to reach in matters relating to our fellow creatures, healthy

or diseased, that slips in observation are inevitable, even with the best trained faculties, that errors in judgment must occur in the practice of an art which consists largely in balancing possibilities— start, I say, with this in mind, and mistakes will be acknowledged and regretted; but instead of a slow process of self deception, with ever increasing inability to recognize truth, you will draw from your errors the very lessons which will enable you to avoid their repetition.

William Osler: *Aequanimitas.*[5] Copyright © 1932 by Blakiston, Inc. Used with permission of McGraw-Hill Book Company.

We will know someday how to measure motivation—how to direct individuals with different goals and satisfactions. Right now, however, we need help from some of the more articulate and thoughtful members of our profession. We are asking our authors for wisdom; we are asking them to unlock a little of what is inside them and expose it for public view.

Admittedly, we are posing very difficult questions to them, questions which really can be answered only by the most integrated or perfected of men. This is one reason why the people who have been asked these questions were chosen.

The people who have contributed to this book are men who, directly or indirectly, have had some effect on my own thinking about medicine. Many of them are people with whom I have had close personal contact; others I have known either through their writings or through their influence on others. This explains why many well-known and highly respected physicians are not included and also why several men are included who are not national figures. Furthermore, among the many superb physicians I know who could easily have contributed excellently to an endeavor such as this one, some are not included because of the desire to get a variety of points of view concerning the various activities open to the modern physician. The fact that I am a specialist in internal medicine, with subspecialty interest in infectious diseases, serves to explain why so many of the contributors are related to these areas. It should in no way be construed that there is a dearth of intelligent and sensitive people in the many specialties of medicine not represented here.

REFERENCES

1 Rockefeller NA: Policy and the people. *Foreign Affairs* 46:231 (1968).
2 *Ibid.*, p. 234.
3 Hammarskjöld D: *Markings.* L Sjöberg and WH Auden (trans), New York, Alfred A Knopf, 1965, pp 111, 154, 156, 173.
4 Gardner J: *Excellence: Can We Be Equal and Excellent Too?* New York, Harper & Row Publishers Inc, 1961, p 160.
5 Osler W: Teacher and student. *Aequanimitas.* Philadelphia, P Blakiston's Son & Co Inc, 1932, p 38.

Chapter 2
Hippocrates and History:
The Arrogance of Humanism
Dickinson W. Richards, MD

*If man is to keep the world in balance, he needs more than knowledge;
he must have responsibility, humility, magnanimity, self-denial: in
science, government, industry, and education.*

What a pleasing title this book has, and what an open invitation to anyone interested in the Father of Medicine. In this essay, what I shall try to do is this: first, to describe Hippocrates as a living person, what he looked like, how he thought and expressed himself, how he was regarded by his contemporaries of the fifth and fourth centuries BC; next, to describe Hippocrates as a physician and surgeon, his powers of observation, and the range of his clinical experience. After this, I shall consider Hippocrates' broader philosophy, his ideas about medicine and the natural order, man and nature. So much for Hippocrates himself: then I shall review the Hippocratic Corpus, the whole 400-year collection of writings gathered under his name; then, briefly, how his views and teachings fared down the ages; and, finally, how his ideas relate to some of the urgent problems of the present day.

Editor's Note: Dr. Richards is a well-known physician, teacher, and medical scientist. In 1956 he was awarded the Nobel Prize in Medicine for his part in the development and utilization of cardiac catheterization in the study of human disease and physiology. A student of Hippocrates, Dr. Richards has published several articles about him and his times.

Hippocrates lived in the great age of Greece. His long life (460–370 BC) spanned approximately those of Socrates and Plato combined; he died when Aristotle was a young man, and a decade or so before the birth of Alexander the Great.

There are two clear references by Plato, Hippocrates' contemporary. In the *Protagoras*,[1] Socrates postulates that a young colleague, also named Hippocrates, might go to Hippocrates of Cos, the Asklepiad, to be instructed in medicine. (Asklepiad was a term apparently used to describe a member of the general guild of physicians.) In the *Phaedrus*[2] of Plato it is recorded that Hippocrates the Asklepiad teaches that an understanding of natural events is the necessary approach to a knowledge of medicine (literally "the body").

In his *Politics*,[3] Aristotle has an interesting comment: "When one says 'the Great Hippocrates'," he writes, "one means not the man, but the physician." From this brief but authoritative statement we can deduce that Hippocrates was a man, that he was well known to Aristotle, and that then, a generation after his death, he was already a commanding figure. Some have even thought that there is here an implication that Hippocrates was a man of small stature, and this may well be so.

PHYSICAL FEATURES   The pertinent question is raised, however, of what Hippocrates did indeed look like. This question has occupied archeologists for more than three centuries.[4]

The first evidence that was found, early in the seventeenth century, was a Roman coin of Cos, of the first century AD, on which were depicted a head in profile, "hip" in Greek letters, and a serpent staff. The head was rounded, bald, with a short beard; the nose large with broad nares. The design is, of course, crude but gives a definite idea of the kind of head and countenance the man had. There was much interest through the latter eighteenth and the nineteenth centuries in finding an antique sculptured head or other portrait that would resemble the head on the coin sufficiently to enable scholars to call the head Hippocrates. There was a head in the Capitoline Museum in Rome, another of the same man in the British Museum, and still others familiar to all and for many years accepted as that of Hippocrates. The fit was not good, the face being much narrower than that on the coin. Half a century ago, with much additional evidence, this head was clearly identified as that of the Stoic philosopher, Chrysippus. There was then, at that point, no accepted representation of Hippocrates, except the coin.

In 1940, in the excavation of a burying ground near Ostia Antica, the ancient seaport of imperial Rome, there was found within the family tomb of a distinguished Greco-Roman physician of the first century AD a pedestal, on which was an inscription beginning, "Life is short." Near the pedestal, on the ground, was the sculptured head, or herm, of an elderly man, the right side of the face much damaged. The contour of the head and details of the face were found to correspond closely with those on the Roman coin of Cos. The

remainder of the inscription on the pedestal did not complete the Hippocratic First Aphorism, but was an appropriate funerary sentiment: "Short is the life, but long the aeons that we mortals spend beneath the earth. To all is given part in the divine fate, whatever it be." Further examination of existing sculpture has revealed four additional heads that correspond quite closely to that at Ostia: one is in the Museo Chiaramonti, the Vatican; one in the Uffizi, Florence; one in the National Museum, Naples; and one in the Ny Carlesberg Glyptothek, Copenhagen. A fifth head, quite like that in Copenhagen, was found two years ago lying in a field near Rome. All these indicate that this was a personage of note, recognized in the Greco-Roman world.

The sum total of evidence, granting that it is circumstantial, has led most archeologists to believe, with some confidence, that the head represents what antiquity accepted as Hippocrates' likeness. This Ostia head is a fine Roman copy of an earlier Greek original (Figs 1-3). It is seen to be a head and countenance of great power, expressing strength and sorrow in almost equal measure, the face of a man who has seen all human experience. The Hellenistic style places the Greek original at about 280 to 300 BC, or somewhat less than 100 years after Hippocrates' death.

WHAT ENDURED?   What were the enduring creations that came out of the life of this remarkable man? As in all history, there are not many certainties, and we must deal with records of greatly varying authenticity.

One certainty is the Hippocratic *Corpus*, the whole mass of medical treatises (over 70 of them still surviving) that were gathered over a period probably of some 400 years, and that have survived over a period of 24 centuries. This in itself is an astonishing product. We have, of course, writings on religion, collected over much longer periods, and still with us; but where else, in either ancient or modern times, have we a collection of objective and interpretative writings, in a scientific field, assembled in one man's name,

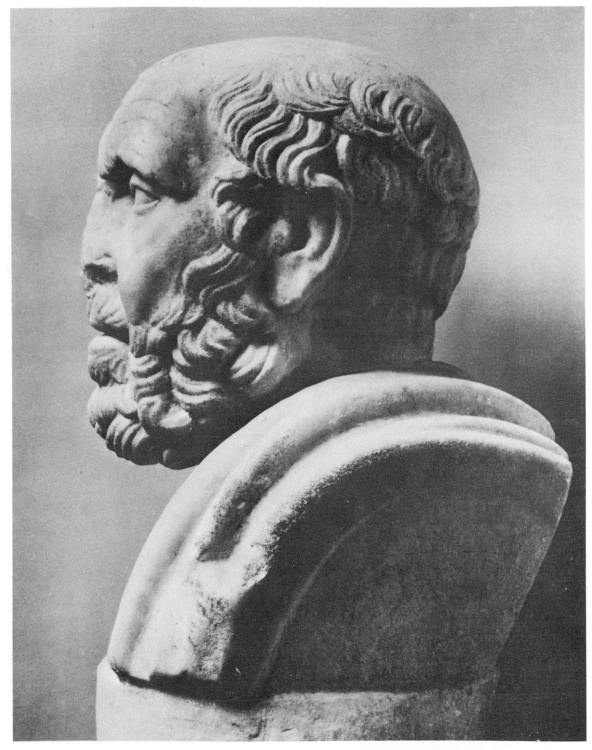

Figure 1. Hippocrates of Ostia, side view. (From DW Richards: Hippocrates of Ostia. *JAMA* **204**, June 24, 1968, pp 1049–1056. Copyright 1968, American Medical Association.)

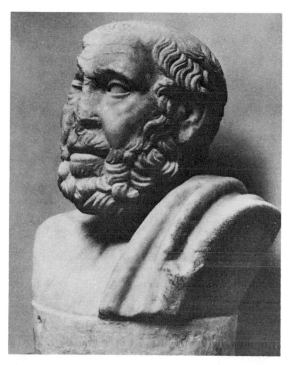

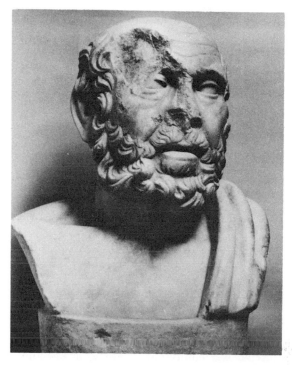

Figure 2. Hippocrates of Ostia, seen from the left side. (From DW Richards: Hippocrates of Ostia. *JAMA* **204**, June 24, 1968, pp 1049–1056. Copyright 1968, American Medical Association.)

Figure 3. Hippocrates of Ostia, seen from the right side. (From DW Richards: Hippocrates of Ostia. *JAMA* **204**, June 24, 1968, pp 1049 1056. Copyright 1968, American Medical Association.)

over so long a period, so sedulously protected and so earnestly studied and used, over so great a span of time? Plato and Aristotle, to be sure, and of course Galen wrote more extensively, but within one or two generations they and their schools had completed their work. The Stoics continued teaching and writing for centuries, but their works were scattered, never held together by one dominating personality, and in great part lost.

It is fairly certain that there existed a school of medicine at Cos even before Hippocrates the Great.[5] His biographer, Soranus (not a reliable authority, to be sure), mentions his grandfather, Hippocrates the First, and at least two of the writings in the *Corpus* have been dated, with some assurance, before Hippocrates.

What were the truly fundamental contributions to medicine of Hippocrates himself? The evidence is largely internal, and authorities naturally vary as to which treatises are

"genuine," meaning by this either written by himself or his immediate students or associates. I believe that by reference to a few of these one can reach the primary features of his teaching.

One of the more severe critics, Deichgräber,[6] admits only one, the *Epidemics*, Books I and III, as surely by Hippocrates himself. These are in simple form. They consist, first, of a discourse on "Constitution," that is, the meteorological conditions, and the kinds of disease occurring in a particular season; and second, three series of most detailed and exact descriptions of individual clinical cases. These are, moreover, complete. These are no single visits to a prestigious patient by a prestigious consultant. The physician here sees every kind of patient, from the wealthy aristocrat to the artisan, the domestic, even the slave; and he follows the patient from the beginning of his disease to its end, whether recovery or death, and whether the disease lasts two days or four months. He is concerned about the patient's mental and emotional state, as well as the physical strains or excesses that led up to the illness; and he is not in the least concerned about himself or enhancing his own reputation. Just as one example, here is a case of fulminating diphtheria:[5]

The woman suffering from angina (sore throat) who lay sick in the house of Aristion began her complaint with indistinctness of speech. Tongue red, and grew parched.

On the first day, shivered, and grew hot.

On the third day, rigor, acute fever; a reddish hard swelling in the neck, extending to the breast on either side; extremities cold and livid, breathing elevated; drink returned through the nostrils, she could not swallow, stools and urine ceased.

On the fourth day, all symptoms worse.

On the fifth day, she died.

Hippocrates:
Epidemics III, Case VII

In the annals of medicine, it would be difficult to find a more concise, exact, or vivid description of this dread disease.

This kind of exact description was new. Here is an accurate observer of natural events; not a philosopher proving a system or priest demonstrating his magic or justifying his gods. As Hippocrates himself insists over and over again, he is a practitioner of his craft; and a craft is perhaps as good a name for Hippocratic medicine as the traditional word "art," although the Greek word actually has an even larger meaning than either or both of these terms.[7]

OTHER WORKS What else does he think and do in the broad field of medicine? There are a number of other works which are considered by most authorities to have been written by Hippocrates or one of his colleagues asso-

ciated in contemporary practice and teaching. The treatise *Regimen in Acute Diseases* indicates the broad principles of therapy, using the means then available: diets, purges, emetics, bleeding, and general daily regimen. The *Prognostic*[8] gives the evaluation of symptoms and signs, favorable and unfavorable. The surgical treatises on fractures, dislocations, and wounds of the head are an extraordinary group, detailing most accurately the anatomy and signs of these various injuries, when to use the knife, how to reduce the fracture or dislocation, precisely how to dress or bandage the injury, what will happen on succeeding days, and how to deal with these events, right on to the long-drawn-out problems of gangrene and amputation.

Hippocrates' primary interest is in the patient and his care. "It is especially necessary, in my opinion," he writes, "for one who discusses this art to discuss things familiar to ordinary folk. For the subject of our inquiry is simply and solely the sufferings of these ordinary folk when they are sick or in pain."[5] His more general observations on medicine and its practice are apt to be added as terse comments in the midst of some case report or clinical discussion, like so many of our great clinicians, whose finest truths are often offered, almost casually, at the bedside. "State the past, diagnose the present, foretell the future," Hippocrates writes in the *Epidemics*. "Practise all this. As to diseases, make a habit of two things: to help, or at least not to harm. The art is of three parts: the disease, the sick man, the physician. The physician is a laborer for the art."

Here is another, from the treatise on *Joints* (Dislocations): "What you should put first in all the practice of our art is how to make the patient well; and if he can be made well in many ways, one should choose the least troublesome. This is more honorable, and more in accord with the art; that is, for anyone who is not covetous of the false coin of popular advertisement."

This discussion is most frank and outspoken. While severely criticizing unskillful practitioners, the author admits that there is much that he does not know, that he is "at a loss" about how to treat some conditions, that others will be fatal in spite of all treatment. Even more unusual, especially for that generally dogmatic philosophic age, Hippocrates is perfectly willing to describe a treatment that he has tried and that has failed. "I write this on purpose," he states, "for those things also give instruction, which after trial show themselves failures, and show why they failed."[9] Where else, in ancient times, can one find a natural philosopher as disarmingly honest as this? His contemporary, Socrates, no doubt, was equally honest but hardly elsewhere in ancient times does one encounter this attitude.

This is not so much humility as it is respect, respect for man's fallibility, represented here in the physician, recognition that man cannot know all, that the best of his endeavors are limited, full of error. This is important, and I shall come back to it.

In the chapter on *Airs, Waters, and Places*[5] Hippocrates reaches out further, and endeavors to place man in relation to his environment—man and nature—as it were, together: what kind of human beings develop in such and such a climate or ecological state, as well as what diseases they will have. While he describes accurately malarial climates, and the chronic malarial state in man, other sections are wide of the mark as we would interpret them now; but the point here is the breadth of Hippocrates' conception of medicine, and the identification of man, both in health and disease, as a part of nature.

HIPPOCRATES' PHILOSOPHY Hippocrates' attitude, his philosophy, at the foundation of his medical "art" or "craft," is perhaps best set forth in a very early chapter called *Ancient Medicine*.[5] In this he begins by stating that medicine has no need of hypotheses. Here one must distinguish, as Jones[5] notes, the ancient from the modern notion of "hypothesis." In the modern, a hypothesis is a postulate which, once stated, can be investigated. Not so in

ancient times. Then, a hypothesis was a thesis, a declaration of underlying truth, to be accepted and thereafter used to explain phenomena, but never questioned. To such hypotheses Hippocrates was opposed. He does not accept, for example, Empedocles' proposition that, in order to know nature, one must first know the origin of man, how he came into being, and out of what elements.

He admits certain general processes and forces, which can be derived from the study and observation of man himself. As one would expect, these are not especially original, but relate to a number of philosophic generalities current in the fifth century BC. The state of health is one of harmony, or balance of forces.[5] An acute disease, for example, with sharp acrid discharges, is caused by an imbalance of forces, to be restored by "coction," into thicker, more purulent secretions that lead to healing, and this through mixture or "blending." The so-called "humors," in this early era, were recognized; they were numerous and of various kinds. The fixed doctrine came later.

THE BASIS OF MEDICAL CARE

In all cases, the basis of medical care is to understand "physis," that is, nature or the natural order. The function of medicine and the physician is to assist nature to restore the balance of forces in the body, which is the state of health.

It is necessary now to define our terms even more precisely, if we are to know what Hippocrates is talking about. The word "physis," nature, originates from a more fundamental one, meaning to grow, spring forth, or come into being. As Hippocrates uses "physis," it means both the natural order in the large sense, and also the nature, or constitution, of man himself. As Galdston notes,[10] man "is in effect considered part of the natural order under whose sway he has his being."

The other word of importance is "iatriké," medicine or the art of healing, and this too is very broad. In Hippocrates' conception, it signifies the guidance of man by the physician, in health and disease, and in all man's relations with nature. It does not include the idea of experimentation as a planned action to demonstrate a process; but Hippocrates was very much aware of the experimental or exploratory aspects of medicine. The Greek word for trial, which he uses for "treatment" in the *First Aphorism*,[11] shows that for him every therapeutic effort in medicine is an experiment, as indeed it is.

In this same treatise, *Ancient Medicine*, Hippocrates makes the boldest and most inclusive statement of all. "I hold," he writes, "that clear knowledge about nature can be obtained from medicine and from no other source." This is presumptuous indeed. It may be no more than a naive statement by a craftsman trying to advance the prestige of his own trade. Perhaps; but I believe that it is more than this. Since man and nature are one, we must seek this knowledge through the study of man, and man in nature. This is medicine in its broadest sense. I believe that Hippocrates had this large concept in mind, though the language was not then available to give it more precise expression. There may be also the thought that at that (pre-Aristotelian) time, only in medicine were wholly objective observations being made.

I should mention the Hippocratic *Aphorisms*. These terse statements, some four hundred of them, are of variable quality and origin; many are brilliant clinical observations, many obscure and hard to interpret, many of post-Hippocratic and some of pre-Hippocratic origin. They were revered and memorized in later ages by scores of generations of Greek, Roman, Hebrew, Arabic, and medieval physicians. The *First Aphorism* by itself is almost a sufficient moral precept for the practice of medicine:[11] "The life short, the art long, the right time but an instant, the trial (of therapy) precarious, the crisis grievous. It is necessary for the physician to provide not only the needed treatment, but to provide for the patient himself, and those beside him, and for his outside affairs."

SACRED DISEASE   We must examine one more Hippocratic or early post-Hippocratic treatise, that on epilepsy—*On the Sacred Disease*—in which he contrasts medicine with religion and magic.

The name "sacred disease" for epilepsy came out of the tradition of some past age. But why this, asks Hippocrates, more than any other? All diseases are divine, he insists, and all are human. Each has a nature, and proceeds according to its natural order.

Hippocrates is opposed to nonrational magic, but not at all opposed to religion in and for itself. Bring the sick man to the sanctuary, he says, "at least it is godhead that purifies and cleanses us from the greatest of our sins."

While thus not denying religion, he holds as absolutely to the mechanical order in his description of nature as Democritus himself. Incidentally, while there is multiple evidence that Hippocrates and Democritus of Abdera were friends over many years,[12] Hippocrates did not use, or appear to need, atomistic theory in all its detail. He might have been interested in Aristotle's biology, but not his cosmogeny. Plato's idealism was the antithesis of Hippocrates' primary concern with objective living events. Man belongs to nature, according to Hippocrates, but nature does not belong to man. This is not a direct quotation, but is, I believe, the essence of Hippocrates' attitude toward man and nature. Hippocrates' attitude is thus one of intense and continued inquiry into the processes of health and disease, combined with an underlying humility which recognizes his own limitations in the understanding of nature, and his own fallibility in the alleviation of man's suffering.

THE HEBREW CULTURE   In another Mediterranean culture at about this time, the Hebrew, there were writings which proclaimed another doctrine which was to carry down through history with profound effect on future times: the doctrine that man, under a beneficent Deity, is Lord of Creation.

This would appear to be the very opposite

of Hippocrates' belief, of man as a part of nature, as nature's servant, with nature—all knowing, all containing, and all powerful—the master. This contrast is basic to our longer story of Hippocrates and history, and we should therefore examine these Judaic writings, both in their relation to Hebrew attitudes of the time, and in their later development and influence.

The particular idea of man, under God, as Lord of Creation, is expressed most eloquently in the Old Testament:

When I consider thy heavens, the work of thy fingers, the moon and the stars, which thou has ordained, What is man, that thou art mindful of him? and the son of man, that thou visitest him? For thou has made him a little lower than the angels, and has crowned him with glory and honour. Thou madest him to have dominion over the works of thy hands; thou has put all things under his feet; all sheep and oxen, yea, and the beasts of the field; The fowl of the air, and the fish of the sea, and whatsoever passeth through the paths of the seas.

Psalm 8

This seems at first sight like a broad dominion indeed, but looked at more closely, one sees that the Lord has delivered to man a very limited part of nature, chiefly the living creatures with which man came in contact. All the other vast works of God are beyond man's control or understanding. In this great realm the Lord reigns, and man bows down. Even within his small "dominion," man holds only a stewardship under the ever watchful eye of his Creator.

This attitude is set in its place by a consideration of the Book of Psalms as a whole. These are a collection of hymns and poems, of many ages and origins, believed now to have been assembled about the time of the building of the second temple (516 BC) just after the death of Cyrus the Great, or about a century before Hippocrates.

There is expressed here every kind of attitude of man toward God, and God toward man:

Confidence and assurance, as in the Eighth Psalm just quoted.

Praise and adoration: "The heavens declare the glory of God; and the firmament sheweth his handiwork."
    Psalm 19

Thanksgiving and mercy: "O give thanks unto the Lord; for he is good; for his mercy endureth forever."
    Psalm 136

Trust: "I will say of the Lord, He is my refuge and my fortress: my God; in him will I trust."
    Psalm 91

Humility and fear: "For we are consumed by thine anger, and by thy wrath are we troubled. Thou hast set our iniquities before thee, our secret sins in the light of thy countenance. For all our days are passed away in thy wrath: we spend our years as a tale that is told."
    Psalm 90

Supplication: "Out of the depths have I cried unto thee, O Lord."
    Psalm 130

Despair: "My God, my God, why hast thou forsaken me?"
    Psalm 22

More profound than any of these, the Book of Job declares the all pervading power of God, and the complete and abject submission of man:

Then the Lord answered Job out of the whirlwind, and said, Who is this that darkeneth counsel by words without knowledge?" ". . . Where wast thou when I laid the foundations of the earth?" (Chapter 38) And he proceeds then to declare His wondrous works, across the range of the earth, the sea, the air, and the heavens. Man cannot comprehend the Almighty, and dares not question Him. The Lord answers Job as He answered Moses a thousand years before: "I am that I am." [13]

With this deeper relationship between man and God (or man and nature) one can believe that Hippocrates would concur. The important later course of the simplistic, cheerful, and confident doctrine of man, under a kindly Deity, as Lord of Creation, we shall come back to. White[14] has also discussed this simplistic aspect of Judaic doctrine and its consequences.

HIPPOCRATES THROUGH HISTORY

So much for Hippocrates, the man and the physician, and his teaching. Now we must pursue the adventures, misadventures, and distortions of himself and his doctrines through the course of history. We must keep separate at all times the two main features of this teaching—one is the actual clinical instruction, in practical medicine; the other is the larger philosophical scheme of man in nature—because these two have very different histories.

THE SCHOOL OF HIPPOCRATES   Let us examine first the course of Hippocratic medicine within his school itself, as more and more medical writings came to be added to the collection. These were from many sources, and with many different philosophic backgrounds, Pythagorean, Aristotelian, Stoic, Epicurean, and so forth. The whole, as we have it now, was probably a part of the library of this school.

As is so often the case with a leader of thought, the wide-ranging philosophy of Hippocrates became increasingly restricted and dogmatized as time went on, to end eventually, and unhappily, in that rigid rubric which continued down the ages as the Hippocratic doctrine of the four humors, combining these with the four forces or powers. This, as we have noted, Hippocrates himself had been at much pains to denounce, as the wrong way to approach the art and science of medicine. Figure 4 gives the pattern. Like so many the-

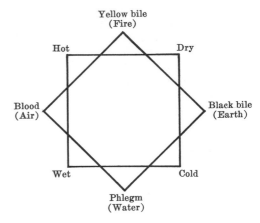

Figure 4. The Galenic and medieval doctrine of "elements" (fire, earth, air and water); "humors" (yellow bile, black bile, blood and phlegm); and "qualities" (hot, cold, moist and dry). (From DW Richards: Hippocrates of Ostia. *JAMA* **204**, June 24, 1968, pp 1049–1056. Copyright 1968, American Medical Association.)

ories, it is so neat that it ought to be true even if it is not, and therefore was thought worthy of being perpetuated.

THE OATH   Even more, perhaps, than his scientific attitude, Hippocrates as a man was stripped of his human qualities and made into a figurehead, if not a semideity. He was solemnly pronounced nineteenth in lineal descent from Asklepios, and twentieth in lineal descent from Hercules; he was set up as an actual disciple of Asklepios. Nowhere is this more apparent than in the so-called Hippocratic Oath, and one of the most refreshing examples of recent historical criticism has been that of the late Professor Edelstein. Edelstein demon-

Edelstein demonstrated that the Oath was not Hippocratic at all, but a sort of manifesto by a Pythagorean cult, written a generation or so after Hippocrates' death.

strated[15] that the Oath was not Hippocratic at all, but a sort of manifesto by a Pythagorean cult, written a generation or so after Hippocrates' death. The removal of Hippocrates from his so-called Oath restores him to us as a living and responsive human being.

This is worth just a word or two of further comment. Take the Oath's sententious beginning: "I swear by Apollo, physician, by Asklepios, by Hygeia, by Panacea, by all the gods and goddesses," and so forth and so forth. In the true Hippocratic writings, Hippocrates does not swear, either by Apollo or anyone else. Least of all would he have sworn by Asklepios, and the latter's suppositious daughters, Hygeia and Panacea. Hippocrates' doctrine of rational medicine was the opposite of the Asklepian rites of magic and dream-ritual, for which he had nothing but contempt. In the genuine Hippocratic writings, the name of Asklepios is never even mentioned. There is, in fact, a legend cited by Pliny that Hippocrates himself burned to the ground an earlier temple of Asklepios on the Island of Cos.[16] Though probably apocryphal, this legend may still represent Hippocrates' opinion.

Similarly, all the strong provisions in the Oath against surgery, therapeutic abortion, and so forth are wholly in accord with Pythagorean doctrine, and wholly at a variance with the Hippocratic doctrine.

Thus, the so-called Hippocratic Oath is not Hippocratic, but a document written a generation after Hippocrates died by another later cult of philosophers and physicians.

Upon reflection, is it not odd that for thousands of years, hundreds of thousands of eager young physicians should have employed the first moment of their medical careers in swearing a mighty Oath, whereas the Father of Medicine himself never saw the Oath, never swore this Oath, and indeed, so far as the record goes, never swore at all? There are, of course, many excellent ethical precepts in the Oath; these also can be found, stated in brief and reasonable words, in the true writings of Hippocrates.

In the later works of the *Corpus*, if one leaves aside the medical philosophy and looks only at the medical and surgical observation, one finds that there still is much of value, and of the widest range. This solid foundation of practical clinical medicine is what continued to be valued by successive generations of physicians, and what therefore held the *Corpus* together as a sort of textbook on a grand scale. The long list of commentators provides abundant proof of this. Aristotle comments on the treatise, "The Nature of Man"; his student, Menon, lists a number of the writings.[5] Herophilus, the anatomist of the Alexandrian school, around 300 BC, was a commentator, and more extensively, his student Bacchius. Eoritan, in the time of Nero, listed the works known to him. To complete our study, the great Renaissance compiler and editor, Anutius Foesius,[17] assembled some 200 commentators on the works of Hippocrates, Greek, Roman, Hebrew, and Arabic, as well as medieval and Rennaissance.

But it was, of course, Galen at the end of the second century AD who truly and authoritatively brought to life again the major writings of the Hippocratic School. It is extraordinary how absolute the devotion which this arrogant and overweening man paid to the Father of Medicine. To be sure, if Galen did not agree with the Hippocratic writing, he sometimes reinterpreted it in the direction of his own ideas. He wrote commentaries on, or mentioned over 30 chapters,[18] including all but one of those that we now accept as "genuinely" Hippocratic. It is interesting that Galen does not mention the Oath. But Galen also accepted, and made his own, that same rigid humoral philosophy worked out in the post Hippocratic period; and he successfully passed this on to later Roman and medieval times.

We can skip now over vast centuries. With medical theory and philosophy fixed, and with experimental inquiry as yet unborn, practical medical knowledge was derived largely from the ancients, and even this in fragmentary form. Some of Galen's medicine and physiology survived, much of his *materia medica*. Greek medicine was delivered largely through Arabic sources, though Hippocrates' *Aphorisms*, *Prognostic*, and *Dietetics* were available in Latin translation.

These sources formed the textbooks in the better schools for a thousand years. Surgery declined to the level of barber-surgeon practitioners. Medicine as a practical healing art was reduced to bleeding, purging, and using empirical formulae, mixed with astrology, superstition, and magic. Its total impotence during the ravages of the Black Death, from the mid-fourteenth century on, diminished its standing still further.

MEDICINE DURING THE RENAISSANCE Medicine was late in joining the Revival of Learning, slumbering on in Galenic tradition for nearly two centuries after the first flowering of art and literature in Italy. This was only partly because of the stubborn adherence of medical leaders to Galenic doctrine; partly because other science was late in starting, and partly also because the full texts of the medical knowledge of the ancients arrived from the East only toward the end of the fifteenth and early sixteenth centuries. The Hippocratic *Corpus* was a part of this new or newly restored learning. The first editions of the *Corpus,* with Latin translations, were published in 1525 and 1526.

This was a time of great events, in which, as it turned out, Hippocrates and his doctrines played a diminishing role. Let us consider again the two aspects of this doctrine: on one hand, the clinical descriptions and teaching, and on the other, the broader ideas of medicine and philosophy. In the former, as one would expect, it was the clinicians who seized avidly upon the newly discovered writings, whereas the anatomists and physiologists, such as Vesalius and William Harvey, stayed with Galen and Aristotle, at least as long as they could.

Outstanding among these clinicians were Ambroise Paré of France in the sixteenth century, Thomas Sydenham of England in the seventeenth, and Hermann Boerhaave of Holland in the early eighteenth century.

Paré, the surgeon, contemporary of Vesalius, was a man of humble origin and no learn-ing. He has been thought to have hired some assistant to put into his writings Hippocratic quotations, but Paré did more than this. In his great textbook of surgery, the section on fractures and dislocations is modelled exactly after the Hippocratic treatises; in fact it reads like an extension of these.[19] Paré was a true disciple of the Father of Medicine.

Thomas Sydenham went further: not only did he follow, in his textbook *Processus Integri,* the Hippocratic method of exact clinical description, but he accepted also his broader ideas of health and disease in the natural order, and made explorations in the field of epidemiology. These, however, were not taken up by his successors, and were soon forgotten.

AGE OF DISCOVERY

But these more or less isolated events in clinical medicine, over a two-century span, are small indeed when compared to the momentous discoveries and revolutions in the whole realm of science. I realize that these are familiar to everyone, but I must look at them briefly in their relation to medicine, both looking backward to the ancients, and also forward as they transformed all science, philosophy, and society in the generations ahead. The dominant force, of course, was the discovery and elaboration of the methods of experiment, which had been absent from the work of almost all in ancient times.

There was a resurrection also of the old Judaic, now Judeo-Christian, doctrine of man, under a beneficent Deity, as Lord of Creation. This belief, which we left with the Hebrews two thousand years back, had had a variable course down the centuries. There had been a reappearance with the "good news" of earlier Christianity, and from then on it was strengthened in good times when God was merciful and man prospered, blotted out in times of poverty, defeat, pestilence, and despair, or when some priest or prophet thundered God's wrath and damnation, and even Christ was preached more as judge than as Savior.

But in the later sixteenth and throughout the seventeenth century, the "Century of Genius," the exhilaration of discovery pervaded all Western Europe, especially as freedom of thought finally emerged from the repression of the Church. Yet most of the great scientists of the age—one thinks especially of the British school, Robert Boyle, Isaac Newton, Stephen Hales—where devout and pious men who recognized in all humility the limitations of their work and set forth their discoveries as demonstrations of the wondrous works of God.[20] Just as with the early Hebrews, theirs was not only an inquiry but a stewardship under the surveillance of an all-wise Creator, and in no sense a conquest.

In the eighteenth century, the scene changed again. This was the Age of Enlightenment, in philosophy, literature, science, and politics. Disregarding Voltaire's satire, the general view was that indeed "all was for the best, in the best of all possible worlds."

In the physical sciences, in this brave new world, man was all but overwhelmed by his own success. Whitehead has said that "the Middle Ages were the Age of Faith based on Reason, the eighteenth century the Age of Reason based on Faith."[21] It was faith in science and its limitless possibilities. It was also faith in man and his limitless capability. The Deity was referred to as Divine Providence, and appeared to be benign, and in accord with man as prospective Lord of Creation. The earlier doctrine of Francis Bacon, that knowledge is power, gave philosophic blessing to the advances of technology. Man was the master; nature in its limitless profusion was his servant. There was something also of the Crusader added to the conception, man conquering the infidels of a baleful nature, or at least of the baleful and antihuman features of man's environment. In any event, the prospect was pleasing. By taking thought and exerting himself, man would soon learn to live forever in prosperity and peace. The immense achievements of science and technology through the eighteenth and nineteenth cen-

turies could not but serve as proofs of the validity of this conception. By the end of the nineteenth century Providence disappeared, man was on his own, and the Age of Humanism had arrived.

In the new scheme of things it is apparent that Hippocrates' ideas had long faded into the background. As emphasized recently by Galdston,[10] whatever was left of the Hippocratic idea of medicine assisting nature in the restoration of health gave way to the experimental approach and its consequences. Diseases became specific entities, with etiologic agents, cures, and preventions, and in the ever-strengthening anthropocentric philosophy of our age, they came to be looked upon as enemies to be put down and stamped out under the foot of the Lord of Creation. Each discovery was another battle won, in man's total conquest of nature. One by one, infections, surgical conditions, deficiency states, metabolic defects, have been brought under control by surgery, miracle drugs, or other agents; even persisting chronic diseases have been alleviated. In our environment, pests unfavorable to our food products, animal or vegetable, have been destroyed by powerful poisons; predatory animals wiped out. Heredity in plants and animals has been rearranged to man's benefit, and even in man, heredity is about to be placed under favorable control, at least in the minds of some. Man has, in fact, all but reached his goal as Lord of Creation. Even two world wars, with their insane and ghastly devastation, did not disturb the dream, still resting in the confident scientific philosophy of the eighteenth century.

Then, at first slowly, later with increasing momentum, something happened. God disappeared from his heaven, and all was not right with the world. Man's power became ever greater, but this, curiously, made matters worse and not better, because his power became too great for his own understanding, and moved even further beyond his awareness of consequences. It began to be apparent that on this earth there is no longer a physical frontier: the limitless horizons of the eighteenth century have been closed in. One physical event, man-induced, can reach around the world. There is now no place to hide, as many have said on numerous occasions.

One is reminded of that moment in the life of Niels Bohr,[22] that great and good man, when he awoke to the somber realization that the true and the good are not the same, that the true, in fact, can be appallingly evil. I refer, obviously, to the explosion of the first atomic bomb. There is no need to continue this story: everyone is aware of the subsequent destruction, the radioactivity that has been loosed upon the world, and the present threat of annihilation. It was the same event that brought Robert Oppenheimer to remark, drily, that for the first time, science has discovered the meaning of sin.

But already man, in his rash expenditure of power, has pushed nature beyond its capacity. Nature is no longer indefinitely extensive and extending; it is returning upon itself, and upon us. Man's unbridled use of his technological armament throws whole segments of the natural order out of balance, with the full meaning of this obscure, the outcome unknown.

In a word, the world has moved from an open to a closed system. This is something new for the world, or at least newly apprehended, and it must be reckoned with, because it is irrevocable. Examples of this are everywhere, and beyond enumeration, but a few may be identified.

Having reached this point, this crisis or turning point in the world's history, we must (as my further argument) consider how it relates to our prime dilemma: the established and still believed eighteenth century philosophy, versus that of our now forgotten friend Hippocrates. Is man still master of his fate, still Lord of Creation, and if not, what are his prospects?

NATURE AND MAN   There are two worlds: the world of nature and the world of man; or if you prefer, the ecological world and the politico-socio-military-economic world, each acting on the other. I appreciate that everyone these days is talking, writing, meeting, protesting, and organizing on all these problems; any repetition would seem unnecessary. But perhaps I can identify a very few, and from this suggest—which, after all, is the topic I began with—how Hippocrates might respond to the situation before us.

However much we don't like to talk or even think about it these days, the nuclear sword of Damocles hangs over us all the same, the sword heavier with each succeeding year, and the thread more tenuous. We do not even know what our existing excess radiation will have done a century from now. And the politico-military industrialists go on building up, and building, the supplies above and beneath the earth, and placing them in trigger-releasable form, at least in Russia and the USA. Small bits of information about these materials filter through the politicomilitary curtain, from time to time.

There is that curious Pentagonian euphemism called Broken Arrow,[23] "accidental damage to a nuclear weapon, resulting in actual or potential hazard to life and property." There have been several of these, from crash of bombers and breakage of hydrogen bombs, releasing plutonium dust. I know very little about these things, but read that this radioactive substance has a half-life of 24,000 years, and two billionths of a gram is lethal to a human being. One such event occurred in northern Spain in 1966, turning the area into a radioactive wasteland; another in northern Greenland in 1968, causing the military to spend millions frantically digging and dredging up tons of radioactive snow and ice.

Then there is the Hanford Atom Products Operation in south central Washington State, where in the years just before and after the end of World War II the Hanford reactors produced, in the words of Sheldon Novick,[24] "enough plutonium to end the world in one incandescent flash." Now there are stored there, in addition, in steel and concrete tanks, 75 million gallons of intensely active radioactive wastes, "about as much radioactivity as would be produced by the explosion of all the plutonium war heads in our nuclear stockpile." It was not realized at the time these were built that this is a fairly active earthquake area; and the tanks were not built to withstand such shocks. Dr. Glenn T. Seaborg, of the Atomic Energy Commission, commenting at the end of Novick's paper, while not denying the inadequacy of early geologic surveys, states that all this has been checked, and that the Atomic Energy Commission is watching the situation, and working to solidify the wastes. We hope so. The main point here, however, is the magnitude of even the secondary possibilities of our nuclear threat. We applaud the peaceful uses of nuclear power, but what are the consequences of the heat and other effluents into nearby waters, and of possible diffusion of radioactive tritium into the air? [25]

To turn to another problem that we do talk about: DDT was hailed as a great discovery, and indeed it was. Who would have thought it would persist and find its way into fish and bird life, to the extinction by sterilization of countless millions? It also is in us. What will it do to us? We don't exactly know. There are, of course, strong and probably eventually effective measures to eliminate DDT. But are other pesticides any better?

The Canadian Government,[26] more forthright than some others in such matters, distributes information on the present state of affairs; for example, how, in the fruit-growing regions, milder pesticides which soon lose their effectiveness are being succeeded by stronger chemicals. What do we know about the late or ultimate effects of these chemicals? The farm hands, formerly spraying in blue denims, now have to wear insulating suits and masks. But they are in a bind: the pestiferous insects are still becoming immune and increase, while the favorable predatory insects have all been killed off and the birds and insect-eating animals killed or driven away.[27] Yet if the farmers do not spray they lose 30% of their crop sales. And who can stand up against the power of money?

Take oil, and the other fossilized fuels that have so fabulously enriched so many, brought prosperity to so many more, and so many material benefits to untold thousands across the world. The primary product of combustion, carbon dioxide, while colossal, seems now likely to be controllable, at least for a while, by reason of the vast absorbing capacity of our oceans, so that the "hothouse effect" will not be death-dealing.[28] Of course, there is prodigious pollution by other gases within populated places, but these are small compared with the world's surface, and are receiving much attention anyway.

What about the never-ending spillage and outpouring of oil and its various products of combustion, down our streams into coastal waters, and out on the open ocean, destroying uncountable quantities of aquatic and marine life, of all varieties and in all stages of their life cycles? [29] When Thor Heyerdahl reports the same fouling of surface water all across the Atlantic,[30] we can wonder what other poisons, such as DDT, are doing to the surface and life below. We know, incidentally, that it is marine plant life which is largely responsible for the replenishment of atmospheric oxygen[28] (though the cycle is a slow one). Is this not cause for some concern? Politicians make high-sounding speeches about how all this will be brought under strict control; but the dire demand now, in economic terms, is simply that almost everything moves by oil and the larger part of all our applied energy is supplied by this substance. Knowing this, we are forced to ask: will there ever be control, or can there be?

Other local ravages of waters, forests, and minerals by many industries and many governments are being more seriously dealt with, because man with his myopic vision can discern them. But still the wastage goes on.

Population, of course, presents another vast

problem. Solutions are technically feasible, but socially generations away. It has not reached a point of disaster in this country but it has in India, and other crowded nations are not far from it, where people not only have no place to hide, but no place to live, and nowhere to go.

And then there is war, ever more costly and dehumanizing at home, as power increases; devastating, ghastly, and genocidal abroad. But war on this scale seems now to be strictly an American specialty, and I should apologize to Hippocrates for being so parochial. However, he would understand. He was said to have been an honorary citizen of Athens, saw both the greatness, the defeat, and the downfall of Athens, and lived for a score of years after. (This reputed honor was probably apocryphal, but then, so is my fancy.) In the prosperous days of Athens one imagines how he might have called on one of his comfortable Athenian patients sitting in his olive grove with his friends, and hearing them say of their enemies, By Zeus, after all, why do we bother, why not just go over and kill them all?

To come back, finally, to our primary question once more: how about man as Lord of Creation? If one is to be Lord of Creation, one must foresee all, anticipate all consequences, not wait for disaster to occur, unknown or even unimagined; then frantically spend half of one's time and energy correcting past blunders. But man does not anticipate, and he does not or has not the knowledge to count the cost. If one is to be Lord of Creation, one must act for the good of all, not for a favored few. Man acts for the favored few, the strong against the weak.

The plain fact is, man is not Lord of Creation and never will be. Once an eager explorer, then a confident builder, he has become, by a curious turn of fate, the destroyer, at the moment destroying his habitation and not far from destroying himself. "They have sown to the wind," said the prophet, three centuries before Hippocrates, "and they shall reap the whirlwind." [31]

And nature, on her side, can indeed be de-ranged, but if sufficiently deranged, may she not simply dispose of her one-time little conqueror?

Man, proud man,
Drest in a little brief authority,
Most ignorant of what he's most assured,
His glassy essence, like an angry ape,
Plays such fantastic tricks before high
*   heaven*
As make the angels weep.
        Shakespeare:
        "Measure for Measure"

Or, if you find Shakespeare bitter, try Euripides:

Oh, vain is man,
Who glorieth in his joy, and hath no fears,
While to and fro the chances of the years
Dance like an idiot in the wind.
        Euripedes: *Daughters of Troy*

It is not hard to judge how Hippocrates would react to all this; how he would accept, in our present circumstances, the somber verdict of the two tremendous visionaries whom I have just quoted,[32, 33] one of them an immediate contemporary, the other flourishing two thousand years later. Hippocrates would stress that man must be the servant of nature and can never be its master; man must be nature's protector, and not its despoiler; nature is now seen to be finite and limited, yet man is more finite and infinitely more limited. Man must have respect, as Hippocrates himself did, for his own errors and frailties. With the "chances of the years," by reason of man's immense and ill-expended power, the world has reached a turning point: it is now a closed system. Man has himself now passed his day of freedom on this planet; he cannot have all he wants, but he must learn what things are too big for him: too big for his conquest, too big for his consciousness.[34] In the larger humanism, man must learn to conform, not imperiously strive to impose his will on things infinitely greater and more complex than he is.

All this is easy to say, hard to do. There must be a program, no doubt. What I am arguing for is not a program—I have none—but a state of mind. The Lord and nature know, and are in ultimate command; man does not know, and is not in command. He needs vast extension of his knowledge—everyone is aware of this. His search into the unknown will always be incomplete and inadequate. Everyone is not aware of this. If the Lord and nature are ruthless at times, they keep the world *in balance*. If man is even to approach this, he needs more than knowledge; he must have responsibility, humility, magnanimity, self-denial: in science, government, industry, education, by all those in power everywhere.

Can man measure up, and is there still time? Who can tell?

These are some of the considerations that emerge from a contemplation of Hippocrates and history.

REFERENCES

1 Plato: *Protagoras*, 311, B.
2 Plato: *Phaedrus*, 270, C-E.
3 Aristotle: *Politics*, VII 4, 1326a.
4 Richter GMA: *Portraits of the Greeks*. London, Phaidon Press Ltd, 1965.
5 Jones WHS: *Hippocrates 1*. Loeb Classical Library. London, William Heinemann Ltd, 1923.
6 Deichgräber K: Die Epidemien und das corpus hippokraticum. *Abhandlungen der preussischen akad der wissenschaften; phil-hist klasse nr 3*, 1933.
7 Richards DW: Medical Priesthoods, Past and Present. *Trans Ass Amer Physicians*, Baltimore, 1962.
8 Jones WHS: *Hippocrates 11*. Loeb Classical Library. London, William Heinemann Ltd, 1923.
9 Withington ET: *Hippocrates III*. Loeb Classical Library. London, William Heinemann Ltd, 1928.
10 Galdston I: The Decline and Resurgence of Hippocratic Medicine. *Bull NY Acad Med* 44:1237, 1968.
11 Richards DW: The First Aphorism of Hippocrates. *Perspect Biol Med* 5:61, 1961.
12 Diogenes Laertius: *Lives of the Philosophers*. Bohn's Classical Library, London, 1853.
13 Chamberlin RB, Feldman H: *The Dartmouth Bible*. Houghton Mifflin, 1965.
14 White L Jr: The historical roots of our ecological crisis. *Science* 155:203–207, 1967.
15 Edelstein L: The Hippocratic Oath: Text, translation, and interpretation. *Bull Hist Med*, suppl 1, 1943.
16 Herzog A: *Kos Asklepieion*, vol I. Ergebnissen der Deutshen Ausgrabungen und Forschungen. Berlin, Heinrich Keller, 1932.
17 Foesius A: *Magni Hippocratis Medicorum Om-nium Facile Princeps, Opera Omnia quae Extant*. Geneva, Samuel Chouet, 1657.
18 Garrison FH: *An Introduction to the History of Medicine*. Philadelphia, WB Saunders Co, 1924.
19 Richards DW: Shock and collapse in internal medicine. VII International Congress of Internal Medicine. Stuttgart, Georg Thieme, 1963.
20 Hales S: *Vegetable Staticks*. 1727.
21 Whitehead AN: *Science and the Modern World*. New York, MacMillan Co, 1925.
22 Moore R: *Niels Bohr, His Science, and the World They Changed*. New York, AA Knopf, 1966.
23 Larus J: Nuclear accidents and the ABM. *Saturday Review*, May 31, 1969.
24 Novick O: Earthquake at Casa. *Environment* 12, Jan 1970.
25 Radford EP, et al. Nuclear power plants of the Chesapeake Bay: a statement of concern. *Environment* 11, Sept 1969.
26 Canadian Government Department of Agriculture. Documentary film, 1969.
27 Dickinson JC III: Hydra-headed pesticides. *Science* 171:16, 1971.
28 Restoring the quality of our environment. Report of the Environmental Panel, President's Science Advisory Committee. Office of Science and Technology. The White House, November 1965.
29 Abelson PH: Marine pollution. *Science* 171:21, 1971.
30 Heyerdahl T: *National Geographic Magazine*, January 1971, p 55.
31 Hosea 8:7.
32 Shakespeare W: *Measure for Measure*.
33 Euripides: *Daughters of Troy*.
34 Galdston I: Prometheus and the Gods. An essay on ecology. *Bull NY Acad Med* 40:560, 1964.

Part II
On Caring for the Patient

Chapter 3
Medicine:
The Art and the Science
Herrman L. Blumgart, MD

*The science of medicine and the art of medicine are not mutually an-
tagonistic. On the contrary, they complement each other; together they
constitute a continuum in the service of mankind.*

The science of medicine consists of the entire
stockpile of knowledge accumulated about man
as a biologic entity. The art of medicine consists in the skillful application of scientific
knowledge to a particular person for the
maintenance of health or the amelioration of
disease. For the individual physician, the
meeting place of the science of medicine and
the art of medicine is the patient.

The skillful application of available knowledge is not confined to the doctor-patient relationship. Government, for instance, also has a
major responsibility in delivering medical care
by applying skillfully all available knowledge
for the benefit of society. This entails even
more intricate problems that traverse not only
government as such, but also economics, sociology, politics, and cultural anthropology. Momentous problems are being debated. How
much of the tax dollar should be appropriated
for health? And what are the priorities? Will

Editor's Note: Dr. Blumgart has had a long and
illustrious career in teaching and practicing internal
medicine and in clinical investigation at the Harvard
Medical School.

an additional health dollar purchase more
health by spending it for housing, for pure
water and air, for nutrition? Or should it be
spent for medical and paramedical education?
Or for research?

Whatever the form of medical care, the one-
to-one doctor-patient relationship is the essential unit or building block which, in the aggregate, must form the edifice of medical care
whatever its ultimate architecture. Regardless
of the machinery or the method of delivering
medical care, I believe that this vital personal
interaction between doctor and patient can be
preserved, provided the physician wills it so.
This, at least, has been my experience, having
observed salaried physicians in hospital services, physicians in army camps under hardship
conditions, and physicians caring for patients
on a fee for service in civilian life.

The quality, the intimacy, and the understanding displayed in the doctor-patient relationship were not influenced by the method of
delivering medical care nor by the method of
payment; they were determined by the motivation of the doctor, and of course to some extent by the characteristics of the patient.

THE SCIENCE AND THE ART OF MEDICINE

In recent years, one has heard repeated outcries that science of medicine has so engulfed physicians that they are no longer interested in the patient as a person. The patient, it is said, knows how he feels, but does not know what he has, while the doctor knows what the patient has, but does not know how he feels. It is contended that fascination with the disease has excluded compassionate regard for the patient who is suffering. A robot generation of milliequivalent doctors is being produced.

In defense of molecular biology and, indeed, of the broad scientific approach to medicine, certain brief comments are in order. The great advances in science have revolutionized the American way of life. The average life expectancy has increased from 63 to 72 in the past 20 years due to scientific progress, not to the dawn of greater compassion. More than three million Americans are alive today who would be dead except for these advances of the past 20 years.

To acknowledge the scientific triumphs of medicine is not to denigrate the ministry of medicine. The science of medicine and the art of medicine are not mutually antagonistic. On the contrary, they complement each other; together they constitute a continuum in the service of mankind. It is of more than historic interest in this connection that many great scientific contributions have been achieved by practitioners who apparently conceived mankind as a whole to be their patient: Harvey, Withering, Koch, Jenner, Morgagni, Auenbrugger, Laennec, Bright, Laveran, MacKenzie, Banting, and Minot, to name but a few.

Without scientific knowledge, a compassionate wish to serve mankind's health is meaningless.

Without scientific knowledge, a compassionate wish to serve mankind's health is meaningless. But scientific knowledge is more readily taught, whereas the application of knowledge at the bedside is largely a function of sagacity inherent in or personally developed by the individual physician. That the science and the art of medicine may be combined was felicitously expressed by the Harveian Orator of the Royal Society of Physicians in 1686, 284 years ago, when he said of William Harvey, "He practiced medicine with such grace that he seemed to have been born with the skill rather than to have learned it."

To combine the science and the art of medicine at the bedside, to weigh the evidence, and to decide wisely are ever more difficult. As science progresses, the interests of the investigators become narrower and narrower, whereas the scope of the clinicians must become broader and broader. The necessity of gradually knowing more and more about less and less is an inevitable consequence of expanding frontiers and a fixed cerebral capacity—all of which confirms Ralph Barton Perry's remark that, "It is comparatively easy to get educated; it is hard to stay educated." But this ingredient of the art of medicine—that is, the wise, discriminating selection of the knowledge applicable to the scientific problem—is of basic importance.

As specialization becomes increasingly necessary, the perplexed patient searches the more avidly for the broad-visioned physician who is learned in one circumscribed segment of medicine, but who can nevertheless analyze the clinical problem, identify the area of knowledge applicable to the patient's disability, and refer him to the appropriate consultant when that is indicated. Never before has it been so crucial that each physician be equally clear about both what he knows and what he does not know.

The great scientific advances of the first seven decades of this century in controlling the external environment also have brought into increased prominence the fact that man's own behavior now determines many of the causes of his own illness and death. As I look back in my own lifetime, I see in kaleidoscopic succession triumph after triumph in the control of tuberculosis, pernicious anemia, the infectious diseases, malaria, diabetes, and hyperthyroidism—to mention but a few. It is difficult for me to realize that the medical student of today may see none or only one to two cases of many classical infectious diseases such as typhoid, amebiasis, polio, bone tuberculosis, or meningococcal meningitis. As pointed out by our colleagues in public health, especially Lester Breslow, man's own behavior to an ever-increasing degree now tends to undermine his health and determines the pattern of disease.

In the social environment, particularly in the more highly developed Western countries, the increasing physical and chemical pollutions of air, water and soil are only now beginning to be more fully appreciated. To paraphrase Lawrence J. Henderson, we are demonstrating the "unfitness of our environment." In waging war, we sorrowfully point to the 50,000 American deaths and hundreds of thousands wounded in Vietnam and the expenditure of vast resources for munitions and billions for materials that, devoted to peaceful pursuits, might have resulted in better housing, education, and nutrition. Lung cancer still is on the increase and will account for one fourth of all cancer deaths. The annual 50,000 deaths and hundreds of thousands of severe injuries resulting from automobile accidents continue without any significant counter moves. The influence of alcohol and the widespread use of psychopharmacologic drugs, not to speak of the relation of smoking to emphysema, the relation of obesity and overeating to diabetes and heart disease, are other areas of increasing concern. This is not to mention food additives, insecticides, fumigants, herbicides, repellents, powerful detergents, preservatives, contraceptive pills, inhalants, and smog.

The physician, more than anyone, can exert great influence not only as an informed citizen, but also in the direct guidance of his patient during illness or at the time of periodic health checkups.

DRUGS AND POISONS

The selection of drugs is an important component of the art of medicine. By virtue of our scientific advances, one possesses a power, heretofore unknown in medicine, to manipulate the chemical composition of the intracellular and extracellular environment of the body. Never has the responsibility in using drugs been so great. Despite their vigilance, physicians are inevitably ignorant of all the potentialities of drugs for good or evil, often because knowledge regarding these agents is incomplete. The recent past illustrates how illness and even death may be inflicted inadvertently. The grim tragedy of thalidomide and phocemelia, chloromycetin and aplastic anemia, and yellow fever vaccine with its thousands of cases of hepatitis (although this misfortune in turn opened up new vistas in our understanding of the latter disease) are but a few examples. With approximately 500 new drugs entering the market each year, the problems confronting physician and patient grow rapidly.

The problem is unfortunately even more complex. The testing of new drugs is inadequate and fraught with unnecessary error. The recent exposé by the New York Times of fraudulent reports regarding the testing of as much as a third of all new drugs is shocking. The Food and Drug Administration of the United States Department of Health, Education, and Welfare has had superb leadership and dedicated staff. But the appropriations by Congress have been inadequate and efforts to facilitate the wise prescription of drugs have been defeated by the powerful drug interests when profits have been endangered. Efforts to eliminate the crazy-quilt confusion of as many as 20 or 30 names for the same drug, to produce uniformity by generic designation, and to aid the physician by a compendium of drugs similar to the Physician's Desk Reference but utilizing generic or equivalent terminology have to date been blocked by the commercial drug lobby, despite valiant efforts by Dr. Goddard, Dr. Herbert Ley, and others. The design of the initial studies and of subsequent therapeutic trials of new drugs is excellent. The fault lies in the inadequate financial means of the FDA to carry them out on a sufficiently extensive basis. (Sixty thousand companies sell approximately $130 billion of drugs, cosmetics, and food a year.)

Even the most commonly used agents such as quinidine, digitalis, the thiazides, and hormonal agents such as thyroid, insulin, steroids, and progestins carry considerable risk. Drugs can be standardized, but patients cannot. The art of medicine demands adjusting the drug to the unique characteristics of the individual patient.

The art of medicine demands adjusting the drug to the unique characteristics of the individual patient.

In some instances, independent beneficial effects of widely used drugs have been discovered by astute clinicians. The discovery of digitalis by Withering, vaccination by Jenner, quinine for arrhythmias by Wenckebach and, more recently, diazepam (Valium®) for musculospastic disorders (night leg cramps) and L-dopa for Parkinsonism are but a few brilliant examples.

In the use of many drugs, the upper therapeutic range is perilously close to the level that causes toxic and other untoward effects. The prevalence of this toxicity in everyday practice has been vividly portrayed by several studies. In one of the leading teaching hospitals, a record was kept of unfortunate sequellae and accidents attributable to accepted and well-intentioned diagnostic and therapeutic measures. Major toxic reactions and accidents were encountered in 5% of the hos-

pitalized patients. Approximately 3% of all hospital admissions are due to similar causes. A particularly well-documented study is the excellent treatise aptly entitled *Diseases of Medical Progress* by Robert H. Moser.

HUMAN EXPERIMENTATION AND THE DOCTOR–PATIENT RELATIONSHIP

Every time a physician administers a drug to a patient, he is, in a certain sense, performing an experiment. It is done, however, with therapeutic intent and within the doctor–patient relationship. The doctor–patient relationship has the welfare of the patient as its prime objective and may be characterized as a therapeutic alliance. In contrast, the experimenter-subject relationship has the discovery of new knowledge as its primary objective and may be termed a scientific alliance.

When so much can be accomplished medically for those who are ill, it would be tragic if the patient could not be completely confident that his welfare, and not scientific progress, were the physician's main concern. In a world frequently indifferent and sometimes hostile, the patient often cherishes his relationship with the physician as his main refuge and comfort. This relationship must remain inviolate. Everyone recognizes the importance of acquiring new knowledge regarding disease and its treatment. This must never violate the patient's traditional trust in his physician. Furthermore, a similar concern must govern the scientific investigator in his relation to the experimental subject.

In all instances the physician must be certain that the expected benefit of a particular drug or procedure outweighs the estimated risk. When the uninfluenced course of the disease entails a grave prognosis, one may rightfully consider drugs or surgery with high risk. But fully informed consent is mandatory. Within the recent past, there seem to have been an increasing number of investigations that conferred little or no conceivable benefit to the subject undergoing hazardous examination. Specifically, I refer to such studies as the catheterization of the urinary tract of healthy female babies in a foundling home to establish the identity of normal bacterial flora, and the cardiac catheterization and coronary angiography of patients without heart disease with inadvertent production of myocardial infarction.

Such studies are to be considered a violation of the doctor-patient relationship; fortunately they are in the minority. More debatable and more widespread is coronary arteriography in certain patients in whom the morbidity and mortality of the procedure are accepted even though no information affecting therapeutics or patient welfare is anticipated.

The tendency of medical science to consider its mission solely the increase of knowledge, regardless of the use to which it is put, has been implicit in a certain few scientific articles. Science, pursued for its own sake, has yielded rich rewards, but these must be viewed in the context of humanistic criteria. The thesis that science itself contains within its domain social values and social responsibilities requires reaffirmation.

The governing ethical principles relating to various clinical and research efforts entail an infinite variety of concrete problems and conflicting values. When do kidney transplantation, cardiac transplantation, and hypophyseal ablation for carcinoma of the breast or diabetic retinitis cease to be sheer experimentation and achieve the status of therapeutic procedures? And, in the latter instance, in which patients is the admittedly great risk justified? These problems preclude the formulation of an exact generalization that can be neatly applied to a specific instance. As Justice Holmes cautioned, "General propositions do not decide concrete cases." The increasing complexity and scope of medical science will undoubtedly only add to the present difficulties. In the future, as in the present, the ultimate guardian is the wise, responsible, and humane physician, acting singly or in concert with others.

In the past several years, certain constructive steps have been taken both to protect the rights of the subject and to ensure human experimentation for the welfare of society. Widespread open discussions have encouraged development of an informed public opinion. Reports of investigations on human subjects increasingly contain validations by investigators regarding the propriety of the study and observance of the rights, privacy, and welfare of the subjects. Public granting agencies, such as the National Institutes of Health, and private agencies such as the American Heart Association, insist on detailed descriptions of all protocols of any investigation involving human subjects, with approval and continuing supervision by appropriate review boards. Review committees of hospital and medical schools are assuming active participation. Publishers and editors in the medical field, as witness the *New England Journal of Medicine*, are insisting that authors include statements regarding informed consent and safeguards relating to the safety of human subjects.

COMMUNICATION—THE DOCTOR AND PATIENT

In all the aforementioned matters relating to the patient, the physician must recognize the individual's right to participate in decisions affecting his physical welfare. Most patients are comforted when the nature of their illness and its expected course are explained in kindly and considerate terms. No condition is so complex that it can not be explained in simple, intelligible language. To clothe the illness in unintelligible terminology only increases the patient's anxiety. The physician must adapt his conduct to the specific needs of the particular person; firmness, deliberateness, and encouragement are supports frequently of greater importance than the choice of sedatives. With other patients, particularly those who have been accustomed to authoritative, autocratic parents, a more severe and positive attitude is necessary. Such patients may be disquieted by explanation, misinterpreting this as an indication of weakness and uncertainty on the physician's part.

SYMPATHY AND EMPATHY

It is commonly believed that a physician, in caring for his patient, should exercise sympathy. One cannot fully appreciate the problems of others, it is said, unless one can put oneself in another's place. The act or capacity of entering into or sharing the feelings of another is known as sympathy.

I should like to submit, however, as so ably stated by Charles D. Aring, that "entering into the feelings of another and becoming similarly affected may not be the constructive method that has been supposed." To do so involves loss of objectivity and perspective and leads to "feedback" mechanisms that may serve to aggravate the fears, the sorrows, and the perplexities of the patient. "The physician able to determine his emotional boundaries, that is, where he leaves off and where someone else begins, and who does not indulge completely in the other's emotional problems, functions more usefully, happily, and gracefully." This attitude has been aptly denoted by the term "neutral empathy." "Compassionate detachment" is, perhaps, more precisely descriptive. One enters into the feelings of one's patient without losing an awareness of one's own separateness. *Appreciation* of another's feelings and his problems is quite

---

Appreciation *of another's feelings and his problems is quite different from* joining *in them.*

---

different from *joining* in them. Once having achieved "neutral empathy" a physician will have attained maximum freedom to act for the patient's greater benefit. To function independently in this manner demands, above all, inner security, full knowledge of one's self and self-acceptance. These, in turn, require a way of life epitomized by one of our great

physicians as follows, "I have had three ideals; first, to do the day's work well and not to worry about tomorrow; second, to act the golden rule, as far as in me lay, towards my professional brethren and towards the patients committed to my care; and third, to cultivate such a measure of equanimity as would enable me to bear success with humility, the affection of my friends without pride, and to be ready when the day of sorrows and grief came to meet it with the courage befitting a man." Such goals are not easy objectives, but in lesser or greater measure each physician in his lifetime can strive toward them.

THE HISTORY AND PHYSICAL EXAMINATION IN THE DOCTOR-PATIENT RELATIONSHIP

Each illness constitutes an emotional crisis for every patient, and his eventual health will depend not only on his physical but also on his emotional recovery. When one sits with a patient to write down his present illness, one is engaged in one of the most intensely personal experiences in clinical medicine; one is learning his habits, his fears, his hopes. There are two technics in taking a history; they have two different objectives. The first of these may be called the "cross-examination technic." This technic has as its object the accurate identification of the hallmarks of organic disease.

The other is the "listening technic," during which the physician should be mostly silent. This enables the patient to relate his experiences in terms of his own values and concerns. Permitting the patient to relate freely what is uppermost in his mind encourages him to verbalize the experiences that are of the greatest emotional significance to him. In describing his symptoms in detail, the patient transfers to the physician the material that has become the focus of his anxiety; in a very real sense his anxieties become the doctor's problem rather than his own.

These two technics are not wholly separate; frequently, they overlap and merge. They always supplement each other in an understanding of the disease and the person. Each symptom has a beginning or onset. It also has its course, which is called the clinical course. It has a life history of its own. But the physician will not know the person or the disease unless he knows both and thereby understands the intimate interrelation that exists between the life history of the individual and the life history of the signs and symptoms of disease.

The quality of the history reflects the competence of the physician and, when excellent, is a revealing portrait of the patient as a person as well as of the disease.

HISTORY TAKING AS HISTORY

It is of interest to reflect on the essential nature of history taking and some of the qualities that determine its excellence. It has much in common with the discipline of historical science. As Walshe stated in the Linacre Lecture in 1950, "We are in fact seeking to collect a record of past events that for us are not sense data, but things that have happened not under our eyes; things that, more often than not, we cannot submit to any process of scientific verification." Out of the myriad of episodes often subjectively colored and interpreted by the patient, the physician selects, discards, analyzes, and assembles data in the light of his appraisal of the patient. Similarly, the professional historian is not concerned with simple events as such, but attempts to discern beneath their external sequence their innermost meaning in terms of the social, economic, and cultural forces operating at the time. So it is with clinical history taking and particularly with the formulation of the present illness.

Parenthetically, it is of more than passing interest in this connection to note that much of the debate over whether psychiatry should be regarded as science may have been due to the fact that many have tried to force it erroneously into the mold of the natural sciences rather than the field of historical science.

One frequently hears the comment, "Well, there is the problem of time. We are too busy determining the fundamental organic status of the patient to probe into his personality to ascertain the kind of person who has the disease." My reply is clear. In the first place, unless one knows the person, the diagnosis will frequently be incomplete or inaccurate. In the second place, if the physician tries to learn about the person with the disease from the very first moment they meet, it will take very little more time, and in some cases no more time than the usual trite, narrow approach to the patient. In the third place, unless one knows the patient, the treatment may be inappropriate. And, finally, the physician will be missing one of the most fascinating and rewarding aspects of our profession.

Many illnesses demand immediate remedial measures. Thus, a Colles fracture, a sore throat, bleeding peptic ulcer, or life-threatening acute myocardial infarction requires instant specific treatment. This is the foremost concern of the patient and the physician. A patient enveloped by the pain or shock of an acute heart attack is like a survivor of a shipwreck swimming in the Atlantic Ocean; his world is limited to the few feet immediately surrounding him. But, especially under such circumstances, alleviation of anxiety by the feeling of security engendered by confidence in the physician is of utmost importance to patient and family and may be the deciding factor in determining a successful outcome.

Beneath the immediate requirements of an illness, the physician must perceive the secondary, tertiary, or more remote factors requiring support or remedial action. These may be physical or psychological. For example, paroxysmal atrial fibrillation may be based on predisposing thyrotoxicosis that in turn is related to emotional problems. The degree to which these factors are operative, when, if, and how they should be treated are matters that will tax the subtle resources of the most gifted physician. Among other considerations he must decide as a psychologist at what levels he will explain the physical and emotional problems to the patient and family. In Osler's phrase, "He must have triocular vision."

PSYCHOSOMATIC MEDICINE

The modern emphasis of "psychosomatic medicine" is encouraging in intent. But so far as it denotes something new and apart from medicine, it is a retrogressive concept, for all medicine is psychosomatic. Just as there can be no disease without a patient, there can be no organic disease without emotional reverberations. Nor can there be emotional upheavals without bodily representation. Knowledge of the extent to which each of these two factors is operative and an estimate of their relative importance in each patient are essential to accurate diagnosis and successful therapy.

Approximately half the patients who consult a physician have no organic disease or only minor disorders. The other half may have an engulfing catastrophe such as acute myocardial infarction, cancer, or serious metabolic disorders such as diabetes mellitus that may pose equally devastating emotional problems. And there is the middle group that requires professional judgment to determine in which half the patient belongs—that is, whether the elevated blood pressure is due to renal disease or to frequent encounters with someone who raises his blood pressure; whether the nausea and heartburn are due to gastrointestinal cancer or cholecystitis, or perhaps merely due to a person who makes him "sick in the stomach." Or, in this middle group, one may find the young woman of 20 who experiences lassitude, chronic fatigue, and loss of weight, having assumed within several years the responsibilities of wife, household, and two children —plainly, the syndrome of "mother insufficiency." The experience of one of the leading rehabilitation centers is instructive. All 631 patients who were undergoing rehabilitation because of disabling heart disease were re-examined by a team of outstanding cardiologists to ascertain the degree of effort that these patients could undertake without harm. Some 175 or 28% of the patients were found to be completely normal. They were disabled not by heart disease but by the fear of heart disease, instilled in them by a false diagnosis of heart disease.

One of the many lessons of this experience is that every diagnosis of a psychologic, psychiatric, or organic disorder should be founded on positive data. There is nothing more dangerous than the diagnosis based on exclusion. In all these categories one can rehabilitate patients and abolish their disabling symptoms most successfully only so far as one understands their fears and anxieties.

Every physician encounters patients who have continuing multiple subjective complaints as a necessary ingredient of their lives. They require lifelong repeated reassurance. They usually are not suitable candidates for psychoanalysis, lobotomy, or electric shock. It is essential that the physician recognize that the production of symptoms is part of the sustenance of life for such patients and that the continued production of symptoms is not a reflection of his incompetence or inadequacy. Recognizing this, a physician can often be the support that enables such a patient to walk successfully through life. The patient is released from some of his anxiety, feels secure despite his continued inner turbulence, and is confident that any organic disturbance requiring specific treatment will be identified.

In all this, while we are observing and trying to understand the patient, we must remember that he is observing and evaluating us. As John Donne remarked in his *Devotions* in 1623, some 367 years ago, "I observe the physician with the same diligence as he the disease." Unknowing and unskilled in medical matters, the patient can judge only by the familiar hallmarks of his own experience. He notes whether his physician is like the surgeons of medieval times who washed their hands only once—after the operation was over. The patient observes whether the physician places the stethoscope over the mitral area, seems to lose himself in reflection, and then reapplies and reapplies this instrument. After several such reapplications the patient surely ponders the meaning of this stammering performance by the physician with a wandering stethoscope.

EXPLANATION AS A THERAPEUTIC TOOL

Virtually all patients should be told the nature of their ailment. The physician should bear in mind that the actual situation must be imparted as a painter paints a picture: Different colors must be used in terms of the subjective impression to be conveyed, as a snow scene may be painted various shades of gray or white or, on a bright, sunlit day, as predominantly blue.

THE CARE OF THE DYING PATIENT

Of all the questions regarding what to say—and what not to say—to one's patient, none are more difficult than what to inform the dying patient or the patient with incurable cancer. I do not believe there is an easy single or uniform reply, but certain considerations afford valuable guidance. The underlying guiding principle is that we conduct ourselves to support the specific needs and strengthen the particular defenses of the particular patient for whom we have accepted responsibility. Some patients

> *Fear death as children fear to go in the dark. And as that natural fear in children is increased with tales, so is the other.*
> Francis Bacon: *Essays of Death*

Such men protect themselves by denial of reality. Not infrequently, they have previously said to other members of the family or to their physician, "If I ever have such a condition, I do not want to know it." They may express satisfaction in their fancied improvement even as they waste away. Every physician has observed many such patients who peacefully and calmly pass into eternity, successfully protected from their fear by barriers that they themselves have constructed.

In treating fatal illnesses such as malignancy, it is the physician's responsibility to maintain the comfort of his patient. Obviously, neither the law nor the tenets of any religious faith require postponement of death or continued suffering by adherence to the usual time schedule of the usual doses of sedatives and narcotics. There is no need for the dying to envy the dead.

How one deals with patients is influenced by their cultural and religious background. A poignant example was Pope John XXIII, who said to his confessor as he received the Sacrament of the Sick, "I have been able to follow the course of my death step by step. Now I am going sweetly to my end. I am on the point of leaving. We are going to the House of the Lord." Indeed, all Catholics look upon death as a brief interlude. Similarly, all devout Christians, Jews, Hindus, and Moslems, as well as members of other faiths, believe in life after death. For such people, as well as others, the plain unvarnished truth is for them:

> *One short sleep past, we wake eternally. And death shall be no more; death thou shalt die.*
> John Donne: *Holy Sonnets X*

I recall a poignant example in a fine old Negro who was at the Thorndike Memorial Laboratory. He was approximately 69 years of age. Progressive congestive heart failure had developed. He could see, and the physician saw, the inexorable increase in the edema of the legs, swelling of the abdomen, and finally swelling of the arms. At that time the young assistant resident responsible for his care jauntily and very optimistically reported that all was going well; he was definitely better and everything would be fine. The patient became more and more terrified because in his isolation his sole contact with reality was through his physician, who from the best of motives was telling him that the illness was disappearing when he knew he was getting worse. I shall never forget him asking one of us, "Will you tell me, Doctor, just what my condition is?" We said to him, "You are a very sick man." He said, "I am going to die, am I not?" We replied, "The chances are against you because we can see you are getting worse. However, we have seen patients as sick as you who, while taking the medicine we are giving, finally recover and have years still to live. We shall do what we can to have you recover, but we must admit that the chances are against you."

I shall never forget his relief in finding one or two doctors he could trust to give him accurate and truthful information. He said, "I am relieved to know just how things stand. Actually, I have had a full and good life and have seen my four children established honorably and successfully." Two days later he quietly entered his dreamless sleep; contented, with equanimity and without fear.

It is sometimes said that people come into the world alone and that they die alone.

Surely, no greater solace can be afforded to some patients than to stand vigil with them as they pass into eternity.

Illness brings many other moments of vast loneliness, none more difficult than the long journey on a flat, hard, uncomfortable stretcher from the ward or room to the operating theater. Never have I known patients more appreciative of a familiar figure than during that anxious trek and during those moments as they lose consciousness.

Increasing our skill and our ability to treat patients is a lifelong fascinating journey. Understanding the interrelationship between the patient and his disease and the effects of the social, economic, and physical environment is a never-ending quest and gratification. No physician can ask more of his destiny. Nor should he be satisfied with less. Finally, all these reflections are, I believe, but a reaffirmation of the ancient aphorism of Hippocrates, uttered 2400 years ago, "Where there is love of humanity, there is love of the art of medicine."

BIBLIOGRAPHY

Aring CD: Sympathy and empathy. *JAMA* **167**:448, 1958.

Barr DP: Hazards of modern diagnosis and therapy: price we pay. *JAMA* **159**:1452–1456, 1955.

Blumgart HL: Caring for the patient. *New Eng J Med* **270**:449–56, 1964.

Langer E: Human experimentation: New York verdict affirms patients' rights. *Science* **151**:663–666, 1966.

Moser RH: *Diseases of Medical Progress: A Contemporary Analysis of Illness Produced by Drugs and Other Therapeutic Procedures*, ed 2. Springfield, Ill, Charles C Thomas, 1964.

Pappworth MH: *Human Guinea Pigs: Experimentation on Man*. Boston, Beacon Press, 1968.

Walshe FMR: Humanism, history and natural science in medicine. *Brit Med J* **2**:379–384, 1950.

Chapter 4
Science and Humanism:
Medicine and Existential Anguish[1]
Richard M. Magraw, MD

The doctor's fundamental work is inextricably interwoven with what philosophers call the "existential anguish" of his patients.

SCIENCE AND HUMANISM

The mention of *science* and *humanism* in medicine brings to mind a way of thinking about the doctor's work that involves the integration of two contrasting philosophies, two kinds of problem solving, and two distinct value systems—each pair understood to be opposite poles. According to this view of things, all physicians might be expected to have an awareness (as undoubtedly many do) that their practical day-to-day work with patients involves a successful continuing reconciliation of certain antipodal and basically contradictory responsibilities and modes of operation. While the continuing pressures of daily medical work are largely felt by doctors in terms

Editor's Note: Dr. Magraw is both an internist and psychiatrist who for many years served on the full-time faculty at the University of Minnesota Medical School. In 1969 he left a postion in the Department of Health, Education, and Welfare to participate in the development of four new medical schools in the University of Illinois system. Portions of this article previously appeared in Magraw RM: An interpretation of medical humanism. *The Pharos of Alpha Omega Alpha* 32 (1):10, 11, 17, 1969.

of how busy they are and the demands on their time, the strains of practice are also understood as resulting from the conflicting (and subliminal) tugs of unresolved antitheses.

If we take this view of things in medicine, we are likely to assume that the paired polarities involved (that is, the contrasting values, philosophies, and views of professional work) have their origin in the shifting needs of patients during their illnesses, in the physician's own emotional needs and capacities (that is, his personal character structure), and not least in the physician's training.

In recent years, since the publication of C. P. Snow's essay on two cultures, it has been usual to describe the assumed antithetical poles in medicine as those of medical science and medical humanism. However, these ideas have a history long antedating Snow. They have, for instance, been considered earlier in terms of the mind and body dualism of Descartes.

The device of presenting contrasting elements in medicine is a way of simplifying medical education and is promoted or made necessary by the complexity of learning to be a doctor. The process involved is a kind of reductionism. Instead of attempting simultaneously to master sciences like microbiology, pharmacology, pathology, and to learn processes like interviewing, physical diagnosis, bedside care, along with acquiring wisdom such as that concerning man as a social being and the way families and individuals live, and then finally to fuse the entire lot into the "applied anthropology" which is medical care, the student is assigned a reduced and more manageable task. He is permitted a reductionistic approach in that he takes up his study piecemeal. It is assumed that ultimately a synthesis of the pieces will occur.

The student then studies biological science and clinical phenomena as "medical science"; the rest of the necessary clinical wisdom and skill is to be acquired through human (or humanitarian) practice with patients, and this might be called "medical humanism."

However, as has been pointed out many times, what often happens is that the two-cultures idea tends to become strengthened and fixed in all the young doctor's subsequent medical work by what is essentially an arrangement for presenting a simplistic model of the professional task for the sake of the beginner—the student.

Thus, following the conditioning of his medical training, the doctor may continue to perceive molecular biology, pathology, and so forth as the science of medical practice instead of understanding them as subsets of a larger medical science which we would here define as "medical humanism." By that we mean the knowledge (the *scientific* knowledge) about man and his diseases which the doctor needs to do his professional work.

Issues of pervasive importance and considerable subtlety are thus presented as a kind of medical Yang and Yin with emphasis on the contrasting, opposing, or irreconcilable elements of the two, rather than on their consonance or convergence. Hence, as noted above, medical practice is seen as involving one principle (science) with another principle (humanitarianism) which must be brought together to achieve a balanced and productive whole. It is assumed that this Yang and Yin do not belong together, but must be brought together with effort (and hence, only at times).

One point of this essay is to emphasize that, useful as this approach is for the early professional development of these students, it may later hamper professional effectiveness. The ideas to be emphasized in this essay can be simply stated as follows.

First, the concept wherein medical science and medical humanism are seen as antithetical or antipodal elements in medicine is primarily useful to the learner in medicine although it also may be useful in certain highly technical (and reductionistic) aspects of clinical medicine whereby the patient's well-being is further advanced if he is considered an object rather than a person, that is, if he is considered in the "I-it" frame of reference rather than the "I-thou" frame of reference of Martin Buber.

Second, a useful perspective as to the roles which medical education and the process of professionalization play in determining the attitudes of medical practitioners toward these concepts can be obtained by tracing the series of patient models from which students learn during their training.

Third, with maturation of professional skills and attitudes, doctors, and particularly those doctors who provide primary care or care to patients in the context of their daily lives, come to see medical science and medical humanism as identical or congruent elements rather than as antithetical and contrasting poles.

To consider whether medical science and medical humanism are more usefully conceived of as polar opposites or as regions along a spectrum, as contrasting and counterbalancing concepts on the one hand or essentially congruent concepts on the other, we must come to definitions.

DEFINING TERMS The definitions I wish to focus on first are those concerning humanism, since those are likely to be misunderstood. In particular, there are several terms pertinent to the phrase medical humanism which are oftentimes considered to have similar, if not identical, meanings, but which are not at all synonymous. These are: humanism, humanistic, humanitarian, and humane. Their connotations may be about as helpful to us as their denotations. Their use as synonyms is likely to obscure ideas which are important to all physicians and particularly to medical students.

Humane is the first term to consider. It denotes benevolence. It connotes a quiet, tolerant concern for others, and also connotes a degree of good will which stops short of any radical or unseemly solutions. It suggests a wish to spare suffering or relieve pain, most particularly physical pain, and also carries overtones of at least a mild commitment to reform.

Humanitarian indicates an active philanthropy. It connotes a giver with more than the usual commitment to the well-being of others, particularly those less fortunate than himself. The difference in meaning between humane and humanitarian is suggested if we state that a missionary may be humane but he is certainly a humanitarian. In a sense the presence of the unfortunate, that is, those who need help, is required for the humanitarian "to do his thing." Thus, there is an implication that humanitarianism shines most brightly in an hierarchical world; that is, one where there is a significant difference between the state of the high and the low.

Humanism or *humanistic* are terms that have a variety of meanings, often quite technical, although they are apt to be used quite loosely. Correspondingly, there are numerous individual interpretations of what humanism is in the medical context. Once again it will be useful to analyze the various meanings of the term humanism as a point of departure.

HUMANISM OR HUMANISTIC SCHOLARSHIP One meaning of humanism derives from the study of the humanities. As will be noted subsequently, the flowering of this study toward the end of the Middle Ages, and with the Renaissance, was associated with at least a partial reconciliation between the concepts and cultures of the classical civilizations and those of Christianity. As time went on the idea of humanistic scholarship per se was refined to mean the production, through study of the humanities and especially the classics, of a broadly cultured, civilized, and presumably wise man. This is what some of our senior clinicians have in mind when, noting the phenomena of specialization in medical education and the narrowing fields of expertness and interest observed in clinical work, they make a nostalgic plea for a return to a Renaissance ideal of scholarship. Elder statesmen of medicine, particularly those who are themselves essayists or editorialists, are prone to ask for an infusion of humanism in medicine by reviving the study of the humanities. Such a course of study, it is hoped, would offset the narrow technical education regarded as characteristic of the specialist scientist. Although this humanism is very useful to the doctor and his patients, it is not in my opinion the most important one in the medical context.

PHILOSOPHY AND ETHICS In philosophy and ethics, humanism has had a succession of meanings. In general, it described a view of life which emphasizes the dignity and freedom of man. As noted above, it signified an attempted synthesis of the values of Greek and Roman civilizations with Christianity. For some, it came to mean a human-centered, self-sufficient view of life, and for others it has meant essentially an atheistic view—one that holds that man must rely on himself (only) in coping with life. The optimists assume (and humanism is optimistic) that man can perfect his character by his own efforts.

Since physicians often, if not usually, come to such a humanistic view in their personal lives, this philosophy or "theology" might be thought of as "medical" humanism. Furthermore, although medical care in every culture inevitably involves situations which border on the domain of religion, religious considerations (in part because of the doctrinal issues) may be awkward and embarrassing in clinical discussions. By contrast, humanism, in the sense of a moral commitment to act out of regard for one's fellow man, carries the common denominator of Western religious thought without such embarrassment and without the encumbrance of denomination or doctrine. This is then one kind of "humanism" observed among physicians and it has a place in medicine, but it is not what I have in mind as medical humanism.

HUMAN LIFE   I believe the most fruitful use of the term medical humanism is to indicate a pervasive awareness that the proper study of medicine is the human being and human life. The real conceptual field of medicine is not biology, pathology, or diseases per se, but dis–eases of men or man and his dis–eases. According to this view, the daily work of the doctor is better understood as applied anthropology rather than in the frame of reference of reductionistic biology. If the scientist's first loyalty is to his material, then the first loyalty of the physician is to man in the context of his life.

The philosophical polarities of academic medicine (or "biomedicine" as it is fashionable to term it in some circles) between reductionistic biology and the care of the human being have not confused or dismayed the medical humanist, since one of his fundamental premises is that biology and medicine are not the same. No matter how closely related and mutually dependent, they are not congruent. He understands also that a mechanistically based study of component elements of the individual patients with necessary subdivisive analysis and specialization is inevitably studded with artefacts and that it results in care which is often incomplete. Finally, he understands that the individual patient cannot be reassembled into a whole by some simple process of addition or recombination any more than Humpty Dumpty could; for

while the term "individual" is often used to express the idea of single or separate, its more generic meaning is "undividable." Thus, nothing human can retain its human quality if it is subdivided or reduced below the unit of an individual any more than the substance of an atom of iron can remain iron when the atom is fragmented into subatomic particles and becomes muons, pions, and so forth.

All interest in disease and death is only another expression of interest in life, as is proven by the humanistic faculty of medicine that addresses life and its ails always so politely in Latin; it is only a division of the great and pressing concern which, in all sympathy, is now named by its name: the human being, the delicate child of life, man.
      Thomas Mann: *The Magic Mountain*
      Copyright © 1927 by Alfred A. Knopf, Inc.

Humane, humanitarian, humanist: each adjective describes an important characteristic in those who care for the sick. In today's medicine, and particularly in today's medical education, perhaps the most important of these attributes is the last. This current importance derives from the tensions within society at large but also from the principal philosophical struggles now going on in medical schools. These are the struggles between an emphasis on reductionistic biology and an emphasis on the entire human being (both of these are scientific, both are "medical science" —one, reductionistic biology, is a subset of the other); the self-replicating, specialized professional training with its partially irrelevant virtuosity, as opposed to an education oriented directly to service needs and geared to changing patterns of work and professional roles.

There is yet another reason why the attribute of humanism is more necessary in the physician at present than those of humanitarianism or humaneness, important as these latter are. This relates to the changes in our society at present and can be understood in the light of the eighth stage of charity in

Maimonides' famous progression of eight stages of charity cited below. It relates also to the fact that humanism has both an egalitarian implication (in contrast to humanitarianism) and an implied expectation of change in human institutions.

Recognizing that all acts of giving were not equally effective, Maimonides once made a formal ranking of eight stages of charity:

Giving grudgingly.

Giving ungrudgingly but inadequately.

Giving on solicitation (that is, after having been asked).

Giving before being asked but with the gift and giving known to both giver and receiver.

Giving in which the giver is known to the recipient but the donor does not know to whom it goes.

Giving in which the recipient is known to the donor but the giver is not known to the recipient. (Indeed, the fact of the gift may be unknown.)

Giving without knowing to whom the gift is going and in such a way that the recipient does not know who has given.

Conducting one's own life in a way that takes away the occasion for charity and influencing society toward that end.

The attributes of the humane and the humanitarian are those of benevolence, charity, and relieving suffering. These will surely always remain among those most important qualities of the physician. However, it is as the medical humanist that the physician studies man in the contexts of his life and society as a first order of business rather than incidentally. It is out of this study that understandings and approaches evolve which mature to an egalitarian approach to others in work and life and the adaptability to social change; these are implicitly required by the eighth stage of charity described by Maimonides and are also required by medical tradition and the usages of new social arrangements.

As traditions of charity medicine give way to a new set of arrangements, human and charitable attitudes of the physician toward the sick will never be outmoded. However, a new, more penetrating understanding of man is required when the doctor, in his confrontation with the individual patient, is not bolstered by an imprinting with the hierarchical usages of charity medicine during his formative professional experiences.

Similarly, a new and more penetrating understanding of society and of man as a social being is required of the physician as medicine moves from an individual enterprise to a cooperative venture or a social venture. The understanding or, if you will, the "medical science" required is that of humanism.

Having defined "medical humanism" as "the scientific understanding of man required to provide optimal medical care to human beings, in the context of their lives," some comment concerning the nature of medical care is required.

THE NATURE OF MEDICAL CARE

One way of conceiving of medical care and personal health service is to state that regardless of what technique a physician may use to accomplish any particular task, basically his role is to assist the patient with disease, the pains of life, injury and illness, and death. Except in terms of techniques used, it doesn't matter whether the illness is heart disease, cancer, stroke, or alcoholism or whether the injury is a fracture, the discouragement of being fired from the job, or the bilateral bruising of parents and their offspring during the maturation of adolescence. I think we will not be much off the mark if we say that the best generalization we can make about personal health service is that the doctor's fundamental task is to help the people who come to him in any way he can. He is to alleviate the pains of living or lighten in any way he can the anguish of existence. I believe I can say this more provocatively using the language of philosophers to state that the doctor's fundamental work is inextricably interwoven with what philosophers call the "existential anguish" of his patients.

Nonetheless, having made the point that the doctor's fundamental work and goal is tied to the human realities of his patients' lives, it must still be emphasized that in some ways

---

The best generalization we can make about personal health service is that the doctor's fundamental task is to help the people who come to him in any way he can.

---

and sometimes the patient can be better helped and his well-being further advanced if he is dealt with as a thing or object; at other times the patient is better helped if the physician focuses on the whole person. In order to "see" the problem and to help, the doctor's role requires him to be a virtuoso of focus. His function is more that of a zoom lens with an infinite number of stops along the spectrum of focus, rather than being limited to a restricted number of lens stops.

Perhaps all of us should pay more attention than we do to the fact that a physician's training consists not only in progressively acquiring an enlarged data base and set of skills, but also in encountering a graded series of "patient models" and in getting perspectives about the dimensions of responsibility to his patients. In other words, we may say that as a student in medicine moves through his professional training he is introduced to a series of "different" patients at different levels of complexity.

It is this succession of patient models that the medical student is exposed to in his professional development that makes up his repertoire in later professional work.

The first "patient" the student is introduced to is the cadaver. The cadaver is obviously a highly complex model for the beginning student, yet understanding the cadaver is often easier than trying to understand the

living, responding, feeling persons whom the student will ultimately meet and work with when he becomes a practitioner.

Subsequently, the student in training meets other segments or perspectives of the "patient." He meets these other segments in such forms as tissue specimens from normal and diseased organs (what physiologists euphemistically term "heart-lung preparations") and specimens of blood and urine. Specimens from that surrounding universe of animal and vegetable life which make up each individual human being's symbiotic microcosm are also encountered by the medical student.

As the student moves into other phases of his training, he is introduced to other "patient" segments representing larger or smaller elements of the whole. These may be in the form of simulated heart sounds, synthetic pelves and the like, or patient models in forms like motion pictures or video tapes of patients. These obviously incomplete models are all understood as something less than the whole patient. Those of us in medical education, however, are less discriminating about what makes up the complete or whole patient when the student begins to deal with real or live patients. Thus, the first human patients the student examines in his physical diagnosis course and later talks to are in a sense functioning as manikins for him. His interaction with them is quite perfunctory. He plays little or no professional role with them and undertakes no professional responsibility.

Progressively, however, the student is introduced to increasingly "human" human beings. They begin to talk back, to interact, and to negotiate with him. The heart-lung preparation is superseded by successively more complicated models of the patient. This evolves through the display of physiology and pathophysiology of organs to a synthesis of the entire human organism. Having developed an understanding of the symbiotic universe of microbiology, the student must progressively understand the social symbiosis of the patient's real life as well as of the hospital or clinic.

In clinical work the student moves progressively from perceiving or diagnosing his patient as a case of pneumonia (no small feat in itself) to understanding him in human terms—first as a feeling human being and then as a part in a complex fabric or network of family, marital, social, and occupational contexts.

Before he can regularly perceive and deal with the whole patient and the anguish of the patient's existence, the student must achieve some excellence in the techniques required in handling all of the simpler patient models, and this takes time and experience. Until he has acquired sureness in his professional functioning at a simpler level of defining the patient, the student or physician is limited in his capacity to move to the next level of complexity. He is inclined to define the patient at no higher level of complexity than he can comfortably handle, even though such a level may be less than optimal for the patient and even though the patient model or prototype the doctor chooses to address himself to may be less than fully human.

It is just here that the idea of "medical science" as synonymous with reductionistic biology rather than with medical humanism is likely to be used as a psychological defense by the physician. It is a device for increasing the "social distance" between physician and patient and controlling the demand which the patient may make on the physician. Such a defense is appropriate for the student (and indeed for all physicians at times of psychological and emotional depletion), but is inappropriate as a philosophy on which to base a lifetime of professional practice.

FOOTNOTE

1 Taken in part, by permission of the publisher, from Dr. Magraw's article, An Interpretation of Medical Humanism, *The Pharos of Alpha Omega Alpha,* vol. 32, no. 1, Jan 1969, pp 10, 11, 17.

Chapter 5
The Care of the Patient
Francis Weld Peabody, MD

One of the essential qualities of the clinician is interest in humanity,
for the secret of the care of the patient is in caring for the patient.

It is probably fortunate that most systems of education are constantly under the fire of general criticism, for if education were left solely in the hands of teachers the chances are good that it would soon deteriorate. Medical education, however, is less likely to suffer from stagnation, for whenever the lay public stops criticizing the type of modern doctor, the medical profession itself may be counted on to stir up the stagnant pool and cleanse it of its sedimentary deposit. The most common criticism made at present by older practitioners is that young graduates have been taught a great deal about the mechanisms of disease, but very little about the practice of medicine —or, to put it more bluntly, they are too "scientific" and do not know how to take care of patients.

Editor's Note: Originally delivered as a lecture to Harvard Medical School students, Dr. Peabody's essay was first published in Peabody FW: The care of the patient. *JAMA* 88:877, 1927, and later in the same year as a booklet by the Harvard University Press. Although written 45 years ago, today's physicians and academicians can still attest to the unerring accuracy and insight of this great teacher and doctor.

One is, of course, somewhat tempted to question how completely fitted for his life work the practitioner of the older generation was when he first entered it, and how much the haze of time has led him to confuse what he learned in the school of medicine with what he acquired in the harder school of experience. The indictment is a serious one, agreed upon by numerous recent graduates, who find that in the actual practice of medicine they encounter many situations which they had not been led to anticipate and which they are not prepared to meet effectively. Where there is so much smoke, there is undoubtedly a good deal of fire, and the problem for teachers and for students is to consider what they can do to extinguish whatever is left of this smoldering distrust.

THE ART AND SCIENCE OF MEDICINE

To begin with, the fact must be accepted that one cannot expect to become a skillful practitioner of medicine in the four or five years allotted to the medical curriculum. Medicine is not a trade to be learned but a profession to be entered. It is an ever-widening field that requires continued study and prolonged experience in close contact with the sick. All that the medical school can hope to do is to supply the foundations on which to build. When one considers the amazing progress of science in its relation to medicine during the last 30 years, and the enormous mass of scientific material which must be made available to the modern physician, it is not surprising that the schools have tended to concern themselves more and more with this phase of the educational problem. And while they have been absorbed in the difficult task of digesting and correlating new knowledge, it has been easy to overlook the fact that the application of the principles of science to the diagnosis and treatment of disease is only one limited aspect of medical practice. The practice of medicine in its broadest sense includes the whole relationship of the physician with his patient. It is an art, based to an increasing extent on the medical sciences, but comprising much that still remains outside the realm of any science. The art of medicine and the science of medicine are not antagonistic but supplementary to each other. There is no more contradiction between the science of medicine and the art of medicine than between the science of aeronautics and the art of flying. Good practice presupposes an understanding of the sciences which contribute to the structure of modern medicine, but it is obvious that sound professional training should include a much broader equipment.

The problem that I wish to consider, therefore, is whether this larger view of the profession cannot be approached even under the conditions imposed by the present curriculum of the medical school. Can the practitioner's art be grafted on the main trunk of the fundamental sciences in such a way that there may arise a symmetrical growth, like an expanding tree, the leaves of which shall be for the "healing of the nations"?

The physician who speaks of patient care is naturally thinking about circumstances as they exist in the practice of medicine; but the teacher who is attempting to train medical students is immediately confronted by the fact that, even if he would, he cannot make the conditions under which he has to teach clinical medicine exactly similar to those of actual practice.

The primary difficulty is that instruction has to be carried out largely in the wards and dispensaries of hospitals rather than in the patient's home and the physician's office. Now, the essence of practicing medicine is that it is an intensely personal matter, and one of the chief differences between private practice and hospital practice is that the latter always tends to become impersonal. At first sight this may not appear to be a very vital point, but it is, as a matter of fact, the crux of the whole situation. The treatment of a disease may be entirely impersonal; the care of a patient must be completely personal. The significance of the intimate personal relationship between physician and patient cannot be too strongly emphasized, for in an extraordinarily large number of cases both diagnosis and treatment are directly dependent on it, and the failure of the young physician to establish this relationship accounts for much of his ineffectiveness in the care of patients.

HOSPITALS Hospitals—like other institutions founded with the highest human ideals—are apt to deteriorate into dehumanized machines, and even the physician who has the patient's welfare most at heart finds that the pressure of work forces him to give most of his attention to the critically sick and to those whose diseases are a menace to the public health. In such cases he must first treat the specific disease, and then there remains little time in which to cultivate more than a superficial personal contact with the patients. Moreover, the circumstances under which the physician sees the patient are not wholly favorable to establishing the intimate personal relationship that exists in private practice, for one of the outstanding features of hospitalization is that it completely removes the patient from his ac-

> *Hospitals—like other institutions founded with the highest human ideals—are apt to deteriorate into dehumanized machines, and even the physician who has the patient's welfare most at heart finds that the pressure of work forces him to give most of his attention to the critically sick and to those whose diseases are a menace to the public health.*

customed environment. This may, of course, be entirely desirable, and one of the main reasons for sending a person into the hospital is to get him away from home surroundings, which, be he rich or poor, are often unfavorable for recovery; but at the same time it is equally important for the physician to know the exact character of those surroundings.

Everybody, sick or well, is affected in one way or another, consciously or subconsciously, by the material and spiritual forces that bear on his life, and especially to the sick such forces may act as powerful stimulants or depressants. When the general practitioner goes into the home of a patient, he may know the whole background of the family life from past experience; but even when he comes as a stranger he has every opportunity to find out what manner of man his patient is, and what kind of circumstances make his life. He gets a hint of financial anxiety or of domestic incompatibility; he may find himself confronted by a querulous, exacting, self-centered patient, or by a gentle invalid overawed by a dominating family; as he appreciates how these circumstances are affecting the patient he dispenses sympathy, encouragement, or discipline. What is spoken of as a "clinical picture" is not just a photograph of a man sick in bed; it is an impressionistic painting of the patient surrounded by his home, his work, his relations, his friends, his joys, sorrows, hopes, and fears. Now, all of this background of sickness which bears so strongly on

the symptomatology is liable to be lost sight of in the hospital. (I say "liable to" because it is not by any means always lost sight of and because I believe that by making a constant and conscious effort one can almost always bring it out into its proper perspective.) The difficulty is that in the hospital one gets into the habit of using the oil immersion lens instead of the low power, and focuses too intently on the center of the field.

> *When a patient enters a hospital, the first thing that commonly happens to him is that he loses his personal identity.*

When a patient enters a hospital, the first thing that commonly happens to him is that he loses his personal identity. He is generally referred to not as Henry Jones, but as "that case of mitral stenosis in the second bed on the left." There are plenty of reasons why this is so, and the point is, in itself, relatively unimportant; but the trouble is that it leads more or less directly to the patient being treated as a case of mitral stenosis, and not as a sick man. The disease is treated, but Henry Jones, lying awake nights while he worries about his wife and children, represents a problem that is much more complex than the pathologic physiology of mitral stenosis, and he is apt to improve very slowly unless a discerning intern discovers why it is that even large doses of digitalis fail to slow his heart rate. Henry happens to have heart disease, but he is not disturbed so much by dyspnea as he is by anxiety for the future. A talk with an understanding physician who tries to make the situation clear to him, and then gets the social service worker to find a suitable occupation, does more to straighten him out than a book full of drugs and diets. Henry has an excellent example of a certain type of heart disease, and he is glad that all the staff find him interesting, for it makes him feel that they will do the best they can to cure him; but just because he is an interesting case he does not cease to be a human being with very human hopes and fears. Sickness produces an abnormally sensitive emotional state in almost everyone, and in many cases the emotional state repercusses, as it were, on the organic disease. The pneumonia would probably run its course in a week, regardless of treatment, but the experienced physician knows that by quieting the cough, getting the patient to sleep, and giving a bit of encouragement, he can save his patient's strength and lift him through many distressing hours. The institutional eye tends to become focused on the lung, and it forgets that the lung is only one part of the body.

SYMPTOMS WITHOUT ORGANIC CAUSES But if teachers and students are inclined to take a limited point of view even toward interesting cases of organic disease, they fall into much more serious error in their attitude toward a large group of patients who do not show objective, organic pathologic conditions, and who are generally spoken of as having "nothing the matter with them." Up to a certain point these patients will command attention as long as the physicians think there is a diagnostic problem, but as soon as the physician has assured himself that they do not have an organic disease, he passes over them lightly.

Take the case of a young woman, for instance, who entered the hospital with a history of nausea and discomfort in the upper part of the abdomen after eating. Mrs. Brown had "suffered many things of many physicians." Each of them gave her a tonic and limited her diet. She stopped eating everything that any of her physicians advised her to omit, and is now living on a little milk with a few crackers, but her symptoms persist. The history suggests a possible gastric ulcer or gallstones, and with a proper desire to study the case thoroughly, she is given a test meal, gastric analysis, and duodenal intubation; roentgen-ray examinations are made of the gastrointestinal tract and gallbladder. All of these diagnostic methods give negative results; that is, they do not show evidence of

any structural change. The case immediately becomes much less interesting than if it had turned out to be a gastric ulcer with atypical symptoms. The visiting physician walks by and says, "Well, there's nothing the matter with her." The clinical clerk says, "I did an awful lot of work on that case and it turned out to be nothing at all." The intern, who wants to clear out the ward so as to make room for some interesting cases, says, "Mrs. Brown, you can send for your clothes and go home tomorrow. There really is nothing the matter with you, and fortunately you have not got any of the serious trouble we suspected. We have used all the most modern and scientific methods and we find that there is no reason why you should not eat anything you want to. I will give you a tonic to take when you go home." Same story, same colored medicine! Mrs. Brown goes home, somewhat better for her rest in new surroundings, thinking that nurses are kind and physicians are pleasant, but that they do not seem to know much about the sort of medicine that will touch her trouble. She takes up her life and the symptoms return and then she tries chiropractic, or perhaps Christian Science.

It is rather fashionable to say that the modern physician has become "too scientific." Now, was it too scientific, with all the stomach tubes and blood counts and roentgen-ray examinations? Not at all. Mrs. Brown's symptoms might have been due to a gastric ulcer or to gallstones, and after such a long course it was only proper to use every method that might help to clear the diagnosis. Was it, perhaps, not scientific enough? The popular conception of a scientist as a man who works in a laboratory and who uses instruments of precision is as inaccurate as it is superficial, for a scientist is known, not by his technical processes, but by his intellectual processes; and the essence of the scientific method of thought is that it proceeds in an orderly manner toward establishing a truth. The chief criticism to be made of the way Mrs. Brown's case was handled is that the staff was contented with a half-truth. The investigation of the patient was decidedly unscientific in that it stopped short of even an attempt to determine the real cause of the symptoms. As soon as organic disease could be excluded the whole problem was given up, but the symptoms persisted. Speaking candidly, the case was a medical failure in spite of the fact that the patient went home with the assurance that there was "nothing the matter" with her.

A good many "Mrs. Browns," male and female, come to hospitals, and a great many more go to private physicians. They are all characterized by the presence of symptoms that cannot be accounted for by organic disease, and they are all liable to be told that they have "nothing the matter" with them. Now, my own experience as a hospital physician has been rather long and varied, and I have always found that, from my point of view, hospitals are particularly interesting and cheerful places; but I am fairly certain that, except for a few people who want to get in out of the cold, there are not many people who become hospital patients unless there is something the matter with them. And, by the same token, I doubt whether there are many people, except for those who would rather go to the physician than go to the theater, who spend their money on visiting private physicians unless there is something the matter with them. In the hospital and in private practice, however, one finds this same type of

Many physicians whom I have questioned agree that, excluding cases of acute infection, approximately half of their patients complained of symptoms for which an adequate organic cause could not be discovered. . . . Medically speaking, cases where there are symptoms without organic causes are not serious as regards prospective death, but they are often extremely serious as regards prospective life.

patient, and many physicians whom I have questioned agree that, excluding cases of acute infection, approximately half of their patients complained of symptoms for which an adequate organic cause could not be discovered. Numerically, then, these patients constitute a large group, and their fees go a long way toward spreading butter on the doctor's bread. Medically speaking, they are not serious cases as regards prospective death, but they are often extremely serious as regards prospective life. Their symptoms will rarely prove fatal, but their lives will be long and miserable, and they may end by nearly exhausting their families and friends. Death is not the worst thing in the world, and to help a man have a happy and useful career may be more of a service than saving life.

What is the matter with all these patients? Technically, most of them come under the broad heading of the "psychoneurotics"; but for practical purposes many of them may be regarded as patients whose subjective symptoms are due to disturbances of the physiologic activity of one or more organs or systems. These symptoms may depend on an increase or a decrease of a normal function, on an abnormality of function, or merely on the subjects becoming conscious of wholly normal function that normally goes on unnoticed; and this last conception indicates that there is a close relation between the appearance of the symptoms and the threshold of the patient's nervous reactions. The ultimate causes of these disturbances are to be found not in any gross structural changes of the organs involved, but rather in nervous influences emanating from the emotional or intellectual life which, directly or indirectly, affect in one way or another organs that are under either voluntary or involuntary control.

All of you have had experiences that have brought home the way in which emotional reactions affect organic functions. Some of you have been nauseated while anxiously waiting for an important examination to begin, and a few may even have vomited; others have been seized by an attack of diarrhea under the same circumstances. Some of you have had polyuria before making a speech, and others have felt thumping extrasystoles or a pounding tachycardia before a football game. Some have noticed rapid shallow breathing when listening to a piece of bad news, and others know the type of occipital headache, with pain down the muscles of the back of the neck, that comes from nervous anxiety and fatigue.

These are all simple examples of the way that emotional reactions may upset the normal functioning of an organ. Vomiting and diarrhea are due to abnormalities of the motor function of the gastrointestinal tract—one to the production of an active reversed peristalsis of the stomach and a relaxation of the cardia sphincter, the other to hyperperistalsis of the large intestine. The polyuria is caused by vasomotor changes that take place in the peripheral vessels in blushing and blanching of the skin, and in addition there are quite possibly associated changes in the rate of blood flow and in blood pressure. Tachycardia and extrasystoles indicate that not only the rate but also the rhythm of the heart is under a nervous control that can be demonstrated in the intact human being as well as in the laboratory animal. The ventilatory function of the respiration is extraordinarily subject to nervous influences; so much so, in fact, that the study of respiration in man is associated with peculiar difficulties. Rate, depth, and rhythm of breathing are easily upset by even minor stimuli, and in extreme cases the disturbance in total ventilation is sometimes so great that gaseous exchange becomes affected. Thus, I remember an emotional young woman who developed a respiratory neurosis with deep and rapid breathing and expired so much carbon dioxide that the symptoms of tetany ensued.

The explanation of the occipital headaches and of so many pains in the muscles of the back is not entirely clear, but they appear to be associated with changes in muscular tone or with prolonged states of contraction. There is certainly a very intimate correlation between mental tenseness and muscular tense-

ness, and whatever methods are used to produce mental relaxation will usually cause muscular relaxation, together with relief of this type of pain. A similar condition is found in so-called writers' cramp, in which the painful muscles of the hand result not from manual work but from mental work.

One might go much further, but these few illustrations will suffice to recall the infinite number of ways in which physiologic functions may be upset by emotional stimuli, and the manner in which the resulting disturbances of function manifest themselves as symptoms. These symptoms, although obviously not due to anatomic changes, may nevertheless be very disturbing and distressing, and there is nothing imaginary about them. Emotional vomiting is just as real as the vomiting due to pyloric obstruction, and so-called nervous headaches may be as painful as headaches resulting from a brain tumor. Moreover, it must be remembered that symptoms based on functional disturbances may be present in a patient who has, at the same time, organic disease, and in such cases the determination of the causes of the different symptoms may be an extremely difficult matter. Everyone accepts the relationship between the common function symptoms and nervous reactions, for convincing evidence is to be found in the fact that under ordinary circumstances the symptoms disappear just as soon as the emotional cause has passed. But what happens if the cause does not pass away? What if, instead of having to face a single three-hour examination, one has to face a life of being constantly ill? The emotional stimulus persists and continues to produce the disturbances of function. As with all nervous reactions, the longer the process goes on, or the more frequently it goes on, the easier it is for it to continue. The unusual nervous track becomes an established path. After a time, the symptom and the subjective discomfort that it produces come to occupy the center of the picture, and the causative factors recede into a hazy background. The patient no longer thinks, "I cannot stand this life," but he says aloud, "I cannot stand this nausea and vomiting. I must go to see a stomach specialist.''

Quite possibly your comment on this will be that the symptoms of such "neurotic" patients are well known, and they ought to go to a neurologist or a psychiatrist and not to an internist or a general practitioner. In an era of internal medicine, however, which takes pride in the fact that it concerns itself with the functional capacity of organs rather than with mere structural changes, and which has developed so many "functional tests" for kidneys, heart, and liver, is it not rather narrow-minded to limit one's interest to those disturbances of function which are based on anatomic abnormalities?

There are other reasons, too, why most of these "functional" cases belong to the field of general medicine. In the first place, the differential diagnosis between organic disease and pure functional disturbance is often extremely difficult, and it needs the broad training in the use of general clinical and laboratory methods which forms the equipment of the internist. Diagnosis is the first step in treatment. In the second place, the patients themselves frequently prefer to go to a medical practitioner rather than to a psychiatrist, and in the long run it is probably better for them to get straightened out without having what they often consider the stigma of having been "nervous" cases. A limited number, it is true, are so refractory or so complex that the aid of the psychiatrist must be sought, but the majority can be helped by the internist without highly specialized psychologic technic, if he will appreciate the significance of functional disturbances and interest himself in their treatment. The physician who does take these cases seriously—one might say scientifically—has the great satisfaction of seeing some of his patients get well, not as the result of drugs or as the result of the disease having run its course, but as the result of his own individual efforts.

Here, then, is a great group of patients in which it is not the disease but the man or the woman who needs to be treated. In general, hospital practice physicians are so busy with the critically sick, and in clinical teaching they are so concerned with training students in physical diagnosis and attempting to show them all types of organic disease, that they do not pay as much attention as they should to the functional disorders. Many a student enters upon his career having hardly heard of them except in his course in psychiatry, and without the faintest conception of how large a part they will play in his future practice. At best, his method of treatment is apt to be a cheerful reassurance combined with a placebo. The successful diagnosis and treatment of these patients, however, depend almost entirely upon establishing that intimate personal contact between physician and patient which forms the basis of private practice. Without this, it is virtually impossible for the physician to get an idea of the problems and troubles that lie behind so many functional disorders. If students are to obtain any insight into this field of medicine, they must also be given opportunities to build up the same type of personal relationship with their patients.

TEACHING CONDITIONS Is there, then, anything inherent in the conditions of clinical teaching in a general hospital that makes this impossible? Can you form a personal relationship in an impersonal institution? Can you accept the fact that your patient is entirely removed from his natural environment and then reconstruct the background of environment from the history, the family, a visit to the home or workshop, and from the information obtained by the social service worker? And while you are building up this environmental background, can you enter into the same personal relationship that you ought to have in private practice? If you can do all this, and I know from experience that you can, then the study of medicine in the hospital actually becomes the practice of medicine, and the treatment of disease immediately takes its proper place in the larger problem of caring for the patient.

When a patient goes to a physician he usually has confidence that the physician is the best, or at least the best available, person to help him with his trouble. He relies on the physician as a sympathetic adviser and a wise professional counselor. When a patient goes to a hospital he has confidence in the reputation of the institution, but it is hardly necessary to add that he also hopes to come into contact with some individual who personifies the institution and will also take a human interest in him. It is obvious that the first physician to see the patient is in the strategic position and in hospitals all students can have the satisfaction of being regarded as physicians.

For example, consider the poor man who has just been jolted to the hospital in an ambulance. A string of questions about himself and his family has been fired at him, his valuables and even his clothes have been taken away from him, and he is wheeled into the ward on a truck, miserable, scared, defenseless, and, in his nakedness, unable to run away. He is lifted into a bed, becomes conscious of the fact that he is the center of interest in the ward, wishes that he had stayed at home among friends, and, just as he is beginning to take stock of his surroundings, finds that a thermometer is being stuck under his tongue. It is all strange and new, and he wonders what is going to happen next. The next thing that does happen is that a man in a long white coat sits down by his bedside, and starts to talk to him.

Now, it happens that according to our system of clinical instruction that man is usually a medical student. Do you see what an opportunity you have? The foundation of your whole relation with that patient is laid in those first few minutes of contact, just as happens in private practice. Here is a worried, lonely, suffering man, and if you begin by approaching him with sympathy, tact, and consideration, you get his confidence and he becomes *your* patient. Interns and visiting physicians may come and go, and the hierarchy gives them a precedence; but if you make the most of your opportunities he will regard you as his personal physician, and all the rest as mere consultants. Of course, you must not drop him after you have taken the history and made your physical examination. Once your relationship with him has been established, you must foster it by every means. Watch his condition closely and he will see that you are alert professionally. Make time to have little talks with him—and these talks need not always be about his symptoms. Remember that you want to know him as a man, and this means you must know about his family and friends, his work and his play. What kind of person is he—cheerful, depressed, introspective, careless, conscientious, mentally keen or dull? Look out for all the little incidental things that you can do for his comfort. These, too, are a part of "caring for the patient." Some of them will fall technically into the field of "nursing," but you will always be profoundly grateful for any nursing technic that you have acquired. It is worth your while to get the nurse to teach you the right way to feed a patient, change the bed, or give a bed pan. Do you know the practical tricks that make a dyspneic patient comfortable? Assume some responsibility for these apparently minor points and you will find that it is when you are doing some such friendly service, rather than when you are a formal questioner, that the patient suddenly starts to unburden himself, and a flood of light is thrown on the situation.

Meantime, of course, you will have been active along strictly medical lines, and by the time your clinical and laboratory examinations are completed you will be surprised to see how intimately you know your patient, not only as an interesting case but also as a sick human being. Everything you have picked up about him will be of value in handling the situation later. Suppose, for instance, you find conclusive evidence that his symptoms are due to organic disease: say, to a gastric ulcer. As soon as you face the problem of laying out his

---

You find that it is one thing to write an examination paper on treating gastric ulcer and quite another thing to treat John Smith, who happens to have a gastric ulcer.

---

regimen you find that it is one thing to write an examination paper on treating gastric ulcer and quite another thing to treat John Smith, who happens to have a gastric ulcer. You want to begin by giving him rest in bed and a special diet for eight weeks. Rest means both nervous and physical rest. Can he get it best at home or in the hospital? What are the conditions at home? If you keep him in the hospital, it is probably good for him to see certain people, and bad for him to see others. He has business problems that must be considered. What kind of compromise can you make on them? How about the financial implications of eight weeks in bed followed by a period of convalescence? Is it, on the whole, wiser to try a strict regimen for a shorter period, and, if he does not improve, take up the question of operation sooner than is in general advisable? These and many similar problems arise in the course of treating almost every patient, and they have to be considered, not from the abstract point of view of treating the disease, but from the concrete point of view of caring for the individual.

Suppose, on the other hand, that all your clinical and laboratory examinations turn out entirely negative as far as revealing any evidence of organic disease is concerned. Then you are in the difficult position of not having discovered the explanation of the patient's symptoms. You have merely assured yourself that certain conditions are not present. Of course, the first thing you have to consider is whether these symptoms are the result of or-

ganic disease in such an early stage that you cannot definitely recognize it. This problem is often extremely perplexing, requiring great clinical experience for its solution, and often you will be forced to fall back on time in which to watch developments. If, however, you finally exclude recognizable organic disease, and the probability of early or very slight organic disease, it becomes necessary to consider whether the symptomatology may be due to a functional disorder which is caused by nervous or emotional influences. You know a good deal about the personal life of your patient by this time, but perhaps there is nothing that stands out as an obvious etiologic factor, and it becomes necessary to sit down for a long intimate talk with him to discover what has remained hidden.

EMOTIONAL CONDITIONS Sometimes it is well to explain to the patient, by obvious examples, how it is that emotional states may bring about symptoms similar to his own, so that he will understand what you are driving at and will cooperate with you. Often the best way is to go back to the very beginning and try to find out the circumstances of the patient's life at the time the symptoms first began. The association between symptoms and cause may have been simpler and more direct at the onset, at least in the patient's mind, for as time goes on, and the symptoms become more pronounced and distressing, there is a natural tendency for the symptoms to occupy so much of the foreground of the picture that the background is completely obliterated. Sorrow, disappointment, anxiety, self-distrust, thwarted ideals or ambitions in social, business, or personal life, and particularly what are called maladaptations to these conditions—these are among the most common and simplest factors that initiate and perpetuate the functional disturbances.

Perhaps you will find that the digestive disturbances began at the time the patient was in serious financial difficulties, and that they have recurred whenever he is worried about money matters. Or you may find that ten years ago a physician told the patient he had heart disease, cautioning him "not to worry about it." For ten years the patient has never mentioned the subject, but he has avoided every exertion, and has lived with the idea that sudden death was in store for him. You will find that physicians, by wrong diagnoses

---

You will find that physicians, by wrong diagnoses and ill-considered statements, are responsible for many wrecked lives, and you will discover that it is much easier to make a wrong diagnosis than it is to "unmake" it.

---

and ill-considered statements, are responsible for many wrecked lives, and you will discover that it is much easier to make a wrong diagnosis than it is to "unmake" it. Or, again, you may find that the pain in this woman's back made its appearance when she first felt her domestic unhappiness, and that this man's headaches have been associated, not with long hours of work, but with a constant depression due to unfulfilled ambitions. The causes are manifold and the manifestations protean. Sometimes the mechanism of cause and effect is obvious; sometimes it becomes apparent only after a very tangled skein has been unraveled.

If the establishment of an intimate personal relationship is necessary in diagnosing functional disturbances, it becomes doubly necessary in their treatment. Unless there is complete confidence in the sympathetic understanding of the physician as well as in his professional skill, very little can be accomplished; assuming that you have been able to get close enough to the patient to discover the cause of the trouble, you will find that a general hospital is not at all an impossible place for treating functional disturbances. The hospital has, indeed, the advantage that the entire reputation of the institution, and all that it represents in the way of facilities for diagnosis and treatment, help to enhance the confidence which the patient has in the individual physician who represents it. This gives the very young physician a hold on his patients that he could scarcely hope to have without its support. Another advantage is that hospital patients are removed from their usual environment, for treating functional disturbances is often easier when patients are away from friends, relatives, home, work, and, indeed, everything that is associated with their daily life. It is true that in a public ward one cannot obtain complete isolation in the sense that this is a part of the Weir Mitchell treatment, but the main object is accomplished if one has obtained the psychologic effect of isolation which comes with an entirely new and unaccustomed atmosphere. The conditions, therefore, under which you as students come into contact with patients with functional disturbances are not wholly unfavorable, and with very little effort they can be made to simulate closely the conditions in private practice.

It is not my purpose, however, to go into a discussion of the methods of treating functional disturbances, and I have dwelled on the subject only because these cases illustrate so clearly the vital importance of the personal relationship between physician and patient in the practice of medicine. In all your patients whose symptoms are of functional origin, the whole problem of diagnosis and treatment depends on your insight into the patient's character and personal life, and in every case of organic disease there are complex interactions between the pathologic processes and the intellectual processes which you must appreciate and consider if you would be a wise clinician. There are moments, of course, in cases of serious illness when you will think solely of the disease and its treatment; but when the corner is turned and the immediate crisis is passed, you must give your attention to the patient. Disease in man is never exactly the same as disease in an experimental animal, for in man the disease at once affects and is affected by what we call the emotional life. Thus, the physician who attempts to take care of a patient while he neglects this factor is as unscientific as the investigator who neglects to control all the conditions that may affect his experiment. The good physician knows his patients through and through, and his knowledge is bought dearly. Time, sympathy, and understanding must be lavishly dispensed, but the reward is to be found in that personal bond which forms the greatest satisfaction of the practice of medicine. One of the essential qualities of the clinician is interest in humanity, for the secret of the care of the patient is in caring *for* the patient.

Chapter 6
What Is a Clinician and What Does He Do?
Philip A. Tumulty, MD

*A first-rate clinician trains himself to do two things exceedingly well:
to talk to his patients, and to listen to them.*

What is a clinician and what does he do? Sometimes it is easier to describe what something is not than to define what it is, and since a succinct definition of the term "clinician" is not easily conceived, it might be helpful to start with this approach. Thus, a clinician is not someone whose prime function is to diagnose or to cure illness, for in many cases he is not able to accomplish either of these.

A clinician is more accurately defined as one whose prime function is to manage a sick person with the purpose of alleviating most effectively the total impact of the illness upon that person. Several terms used in this definition require development.

MANAGEMENT OF A SICK PERSON

Managing a sick person is entirely different from diagnosing an illness and prescribing

Editor's Note: Dr. Tumulty's essay is reprinted from Tumulty PA: What is a clinician and what does he do? *New Eng J Med* 283:20–24, 1970, and was presented to third-year students at Johns Hopkins University School of Medicine as the opening lecture in a course entitled, "Introduction to Clinical Medicine."

therapy for it. For example, consider a mother who has three young and perpetually active children and a husband who is preoccupied by his work. She doesn't see much of him, and when she does they are both tired and the children are boisterous. She visits her physician with complaints of headaches, stiffness, and soreness in the back of her neck, persistent fatigability, frequent loose stools with mucus, and a 10-pound weight loss. Her symptoms have reached an intensity that makes it difficult for her to care for her family. After appropriate examination and studies, the final diagnosis is as follows: "anxiety state with tension headaches and a spastic colon." The physician prescribes diazepam (Valium®), propantheline (Pro-Banthīne®), psyllium mucilloide (Metamucil®), and propoxyphene (Darvon®). She is told to return in six weeks for follow-up examination.

Thus, the physician has correctly diagnosed her condition, and has prescribed appropriate medications—but has he managed this sick person? Emphatically not!

Managing this patient would require these additional ingredients:

An explanation, in terms highly meaningful to her, of the relationship between her symptoms and factors in her personality and home situation.

A review of all the elements in her circumstances that might be creating stress.

Some constructive advice about children's behavior and discipline, and about being a young wife.

Insistence on an hour's rest period every day after lunch, free of the children.

Writing down a well-organized weekly work schedule to bring some order out of household chaos and insisting upon adherence to it.

Suggesting that she employ a day worker every week or two to help with the heavy house cleaning.

A conference with the husband to ensure that he understands how to support his wife's position (inquiries about sex adjustment would be apropos at this juncture).

An admonition to go light on relaxing cocktails and nightcaps during this stressful period, lest dependencies develop.

Clearly, managing a sick person entails much more than diagnosis and prescribing medicines.

Clearly, managing a sick person entails much more than diagnosis and prescribing medicines, and it demands much more of the physician. Also, it gives back much more to the patient.

Management means that the physician comprehends the total problem and is sensitive to the total effects of an illness on the person, the spiritual effects as well as the physical, the social as well as the economic. With the wisdom born of education and experience, the clinician attempts to prevent, diminish, or heal this sum total of effects. Specific forms of therapy are brought to bear directly upon a pathologic process. Management is concerned

with the sickened person, the family, and the community.

Today, even highly sophisticated treatment schedules can be put on tapes, to be printed out at the push of the proper button. Computers are being successfully employed in diagnosis. But the ways of wise management of a sick person can only come out of an understanding spirit, and a sensitive as well as perceptive and educated mind.

A patient given specific therapy has something done to him to aid his recovery. A patient who is well managed is capable of helping himself to recover, for he has been provided with insight and knowledge, hope and security, and the motivation to do whatever may be required.

In incurable illness, treating the disease may become a hopeless, vain gesture, and anguished suffering and ultimate death are stark admissions of its failure. However, if the sick person is thoughtfully managed, the effects of incurable illness can be made immeasurably less devastating for both the patient and the family, and possibly some of the most mortal effects of fatal illness can be overcome which are often far more psychologic than physical.

TOTAL IMPACT OF ILLNESS

In defining "clinician," I employed the expression, "alleviating most effectively the total impact of the illness upon that person." Two concepts here require further development.

The impact of sickness upon a person is always multifocal, the effects highly complex. They involve the whole person, with his spiritual, intellectual, emotional, social, and economic components.

A pair of kidneys will never come to the physician for diagnosis and treatment. They will be contained within an anxious, fearful, wondering person, asking puzzled questions about an obscure future, weighed down by the responsibilities of a loved family, a job to be held, and bills to be paid. A biochemist or a physiologist ignores all these secondary factors; he can confine his attention to the kidneys. But the clinician must learn the facts about it all, comprehend it all, and develop a plan of management for all of it. Otherwise, his approach is superficial.

Finally, sickness rarely affects only the patient. If he is the member of a family, the entire family is inevitably affected, to greater or lesser degrees. Hence, in a peculiar and special sense, all clinicians have family practices—even the most erudite and "hard to get to see" consultants. This magnifies the clinician's responsibility greatly, for his success or failure in managing a patient's problem will be reflected in the welfare of the

---

Few, indeed, shoulder a burden of personal responsibility heavier than the clinician's.

---

patient's family members. Few, indeed, shoulder a burden of personal responsibility heavier than the clinician's.

A CLINICIAN'S FUNCTION

So much for what a clinician is. How does he function?

He listens thoughtfully to the patient's complaint.

He proceeds to gather together all the available clinical evidence pertinent to it, beginning with the history and physical examination.

Through logical analysis of this clinical evidence, he formulates a reasoned explanation for the cause of the patient's complaint, in the light of his knowledge and past experience.

He develops a program of management for the patient, in the terms already discussed.

CLINICAL EVIDENCE Clinical evidence is the basic material with which the clinician works. He gathers it from several sources: the history; the physical examination; laboratory studies and special technics (such as x-ray study); and consulting opinions.

The source of the clinical evidence is not the essential point, although experience daily points out the primacy of the history and physical examination. The essential point is that the evidence be both complete and valid, that its total implications be understood, and that it be critically reviewed in relation to other evidence already at hand.

It is foolish to argue that the history is a more important source of clinical evidence than the physical examination, or that the latter is a more valuable source than laboratory or x-ray study. The key evidence in understanding a particular patient's complaint may be disclosed by any of these evidence-gathering techniques. A clinician must be equally adept in employing all of them. Facts are his concern, no matter how they are harvested, and he must seek them by every means available.

Clinicians must regard themselves as indomitable gatherers of clinical evidence. They must hunt for evidence anywhere that it might be hidden, in the history or physical examination, in some special test, in conversation with a family member, or tucked away in some previous medical report.

Today, in contrast to the past, a diagnosis must often be specifically correct if the patient is to get well, for so many modern forms of therapy have highly specific actions. This scientific advancement compels the clinician to sharpen his clinical skills to the very keenest edge, so that he can extract from a meticulous history and physical examination every particle of pertinent clinical evidence, which he can then coordinate with evidence gathered by other means. Never before has such a premium been placed upon expertise in the performance of the history and physical examination as the prime steps in the diagnostic process from which all other investigative steps logically proceed.

Once analysis of the clinical evidence has led to a diagnosis and a plan of management for the patient's problem has been constructed, the physician comes to a highly critical point in his relationship with his patient: he must explain to him the nature of his illness and formulate for him the program of management.

Once analysis of the clinical evidence has led to a diagnosis and a plan of management for the patient's problem has been constructed, the physician comes to a highly critical point in his relationship with his patient: he must explain to him the nature of his illness and formulate for him the program of management. Unless these matters are handled with clarity and sensitivity, so the patient can understand fully what is wrong and also has the will to marshal his personal resources to cooperate fully, the correct diagnosis and therapy may have no practical meaning whatever for the patient. Ignorance, misconceptions, fears, insecurities, resentments, hopelessness, and unanswered queries may block his response.

COMMUNICATING
WITH THE PATIENT

This brings us to one of the last but surely one of the most essential considerations of what it is a clinician does. A clinician spends a great amount of his working hours communicating with his patients. What the scalpel is to the surgeon, words are to the clinician. When he uses them effectively, his patients do well. If not, the results may well be disastrous.

You are surely aware that physicians are not as highly esteemed now by the general public as they were in the past. It seems unlikely that the public, so easily impressed by what appears to be scientific, resents the fact that physicians nowadays have become more scientific in their education and methods. Actually, what many patients miss and resent today is their inability to communicate with their physician in a meaningful way. Patients have questions that they want answered, their fears require dissipating, their misunderstandings need clarifying, and abysmal ignorance about themselves demands enlightenment. Today, many patients with serious health problems leave their physicians' offices with less comprehension of what is wrong and what they must do to get well than the average customer understands about his car when he drives it out of the repair shop. "Pay your bill and drive off." "Get these prescriptions filled and come back in two months." And, if the patient feels deprived of adequate communication with his physician, family members often are totally devoid of it.

We clinicians are better educated and more scientific than ever before, but we have a great failing: we sometimes do not communicate effectively with our patients or with their families.

No wonder the resentments. We clinicians are better educated and more scientific than ever before, but we have a great failing: we sometimes do not communicate effectively with our patients or with their families. Some of us do not provide the time or make the effort. Others simply do not know how to talk to sick persons. If this seems exaggerated, it might be recalled that in the entire Marburg Building at Johns Hopkins, there is but one small room suitable for serious family conferences. The general daily practice, therefore, is to discuss critical and frequently shocking issues with relatives while standing in noisy halls, dodging food trucks and litters. Critical information and advice are given to sick persons and their families buffet style—standing up!

An effective clinician must have a number of skills, and these the clinician must endeavor to make his own. He must be a scientist. He must be knowledgeable about the natural course of common and uncommon diseases. He must be able to harvest clinical evidence from all available sources. He must be a keen analyst of these gathered facts, and through logic proceed to a reasonable conclusion concerning their significance. But, in addition, if these capabilities are to have a practical effect upon the patient, the clinician must have the facility to communicate with him and his family members.

The wisdom of Thomas Aquinas, the logic of Newman, and the clinical genius of Osler will not be effective in making well a patient who does not fully understand why he is sick, or what he must do to get well. A first-rate clinician trains himself to do two things exceedingly well: to talk to his patients, and to listen to them. And he acts similarly with responsible family members.

Through well-conceived conversations, the physician hopes to accomplish a number of indispensable purposes, the first being the extraction of all the clinical evidence about the historical development of the patient's illness, followed by quieting the patient's anxieties. Here it is essential to realize that all illness in all persons is inevitably productive of varying degrees of fear and anxiety, though they are often well submerged under seeming indifference, bravado, or sophistication. These emotions may spring from many causes and assume many forms but they are always there. If the doctor is powerless to do anything else to aid a patient, he has accomplished a great deal and has justified his being that patient's physician if, through his conversation, he strips from an illness ugly, eroding, and undermining fears. The fear of cancer is widespread. No less prevalent is the cancer of fear in people who are ill. Its only

cure is therapeutic conversation with the physician.

In addition, the clinician must constantly ask patients to undergo diagnostic and therapeutic maneuvers that are costly, unpleasant, or very hard for the patient to accomplish. Recovery from illness often depends on the ability of the patient to exert stern self-discipline over himself. Only full understanding of the problem by the patient can lead to adequate motivation. Only the clinician can bring this about, and only to the degree that he is able and willing to converse with his patient.

The clinician has to learn to talk to his patients and even more important he has to like talking to his patients.

Therefore, he has to learn to talk to his patients and even more important he has to like talking to his patients. It is his greatest asset as a clinician. The most rewarding study of man is man. No one has the privilege of knowing man so intimately, at times of such great personal moment, and under such highly sensitive circumstances, as the physician. He becomes intimately familiar with man as he is born, as he sickens, and as he dies. Like no one else, he has the opportunity to listen to the laughter and to the cries. Like no other man, he has the opportunity to speak to man, and through his words he can guide and correct him, heal him, and give him solace to the very edge of eternity.

When the clinician is exceedingly busy, as most clinicians are, there is a widespread tendency to substitute tests for talk, and various therapeutic maneuvers take the place of enlightenment and motivation. One must remember that talk is indeed cheap, but it can also be healing.

SOME GUIDELINES Here are some practical guidelines in talking to patients.

Almost all patients, regardless of intel

lectual capacity, are naive and simplistic when dealing with their own health problems. One should assume nothing, start from basic facts, and build upward. A brilliant person is often a dull patient. A less endowed patient is often like a child.

Patients quickly forget what they are told, and are easily confused if told too much at once. Therapeutic conversation should be administered in small but continued dosages, in a preplanned fashion.

Very often, patients will retain only the part of the conversation which agrees with their own ideas, or is pleasant to them. Gentle, firm, persistent reiteration is essential if important concepts are to be acted upon. One must emphasize, again and again.

Because of anxiety and tension, patients are easily confused and poorly retentive. Therefore, dissipating anxiety and tension is always the first order of business. Frequently, one accomplishes more with subsequent conversations than with the initial conversation, as rapport develops and first fears fall away. First conferences often merely set the stage for subsequent effective ones. One proceeds in a stepwise manner. If the first are not well handled, not much can be expected later.

Effective conversation with patients must be planned ahead, and cannot be just off the cuff. Careless or ill-planned conversations can be disastrous to the patient, and may have a profound effect upon him.

Needless details and technicalities should be avoided. They will not be understood, and may prompt a host of new anxieties.

Above all else, the clinician should be protective of the patient's position, and not of his own. He must be a wise censor, filtering out matters that will either cause needless worries or fail to achieve positive motivation. The physician who is impelled to tell the patient or the family (or both) all the facts is frequently protecting his own insecurity.

It must be remembered that conversation is therapeutic only to the degree that the patient has confidence in what the clinician says. This, in turn, is directly related to the pa-

tient's respect and trust. Most laymen will take clinical abilities for granted, and will not judge the physician in terms of his basic medical skills, which they assume he possesses merely because he is a physician. He will be judged, and then trusted accordingly, solely in terms of the following:

The genuineness of his interest.

The thoroughness of his approach to the problem.

His personal warmth, understanding, and compassion.

The degree of clarity with which he gives the patient insight into what is wrong, and what must be done.

CONCLUSION

This brings us back once again to the primacy of the history and physical examination. They set the tone and create the background for future therapeutic relations between the patient and his physician. The patient has the opportunity to see his physician functioning at his best, and he judges him, assaying the qualities of the man and the abilities of the physician.

He becomes willing to entrust himself to this person who gathers so meticulously each relevant fact from the history and who misses no clue during his searching physical examination—each fact, each clue being scientifically scrutinized, and eventually so understandingly interpreted for the patient, whose confidence grows. He begins to feel better. He knows he has found a superb clinician.

AN IMAGE In conclusion, today's young people seek models. Here is an image of a clinician:

He is meticulous in accumulating the historical and physical data from the patient. His questioning of the patient is searching and incisive, like that of a wise barrister. He interprets the clues derived from the physical changes with the precision of an experienced detective. His analysis of the clinical evidence is methodical and disciplined, so that no diagnostic or therapeutic possibility can be over-looked. The reasonableness of his logic makes his conclusions appear inevitable. They are based upon a personal clinical experience of the most sophisticated sort. His special interest is any human illness. His care of the patient does not end with the correct diagnosis. His thoughtful management of the total problems of the sick person makes mere treatment of a disease or a symptom seem woefully inadequate. He is inexhaustibly capable of in-fusing into his patients insight, self-discipline, optimism, and courage. Those he cannot make well, he comforts. Versed in medical science, he also understands human nature and enjoys working with it. Analytical and logical, he is at the same time warm and charming, and although gentle, he is strong in his beliefs and ideals but never brittle. The things he works with are intellectual capacity, unconfined clinical experience, and the perceptive use of his eyes, ears, hands, and heart.

Chapter 7
The Hippocrates Myth
Martin Cherkasky, MD

The myth that doctors are somehow different from other men continues to flourish . . . but we must take cognizance of the fact that money, status, and power are the forces which strongly motivate people, doctors included, in this country today.

THE MYTH

In envisioning the doctor as a superhuman who would possess all virtues, Hippocrates created a myth that both physicians and their patients have willingly perpetuated. The myth is that at the core doctors are somehow different from other men. This has been highly acceptable to doctors who, understandably, are not reluctant to be looked upon as demigods. Laymen, who must place their lives in the hands of the doctor, want the physician to be godlike so that he can cure them and so that his devotion to their needs will not be sullied by the greed and self-service which they recognize in themselves and in others.

VIOLATIONS Even now the myth continues to flourish, although all around us there is evidence that the noble purpose and noble commitment of medicine are commonly violated. While doctors certainly cannot be blamed for

Editor's Note: Dr. Cherkasky is active in the field of social and community medicine and has made a career of service in the delivery of health care in the large urban centers.

all the ills of society, they have largely, by omission or commission, assented to medical abandonment of the thirty to forty million Americans who live in the culture of poverty. For these blacks, Puerto Ricans, Indians, Mexican-Americans, and poor whites, medical care either doesn't exist or, where it does, is crisis oriented, fragmented, and depersonalized.

The Hippocratic Oath says,

The regimen I adopt shall be for the benefit of my patients according to my ability and judgment, and not for their hurt or for any wrong.

Yet, where indemnity insurance provides coverage for specified procedures, we often find the doctor's interest in his pocketbook overriding what is truly to his patient's benefit. In some localities where there is third-party payment, you can't find a tonsil left in town. Since there is no evidence that those areas have suffered widespread epidemics of rare tonsil disease, we are quite right in believing that most of these tonsillectomies should more rightly be called "remunerectomies.'' In the United States the surgical rate for tonsillectomies is 637 per 100,000 males. In England, where there is no financial incentive for surgery, the rate is 322.7, or just about half that number.[1]

Unnecessary surgical utilization is a tragic manifestation of poor quality care, yet study after study shows that, for all too many doctors, the temptation to equate cash with care

---

Study after study shows that, for all too many doctors, the temptation to equate cash with care is too strong to resist.

---

is too strong to resist. A review of the hospital care received by members of the Teamsters Union[2,3] and their families found one-third of the hysterectomies performed totally unnecessary and questioned the advisability of another 10%. The surgical rate for patients covered by Blue Shield under the Federal Employees Benefits Program proved to be 70 per 1,000. However, for those federal employees who opted for care in a group practice, the surgical rate was only 39 per 1,000.

Are we to assume from this that group-practicing doctors[4,5] are better qualified or basically more honest than those in solo fee-for-service practice? Or is the difference rather clear evidence that, when the decisions of doctors in group practice are subject to the continuing scrutiny of their colleagues, it is peer monitoring that forces the doctor to put professional excellence above other considerations? There is also substantial evidence to show that, in the case of prepayment plans, unless supervisory measures keep doctors from turning patients away, the converse is true and underutilization occurs. In view of this, we can no longer pretend that doctors are so basically different from other men.

It is interesting to note that for considerable periods the doctor's social performance was often not far from the stated virtues and to wonder whether or not in the selection and education of medical students and their exposure to the Hippocratic Oath we had produced a special kind of man. Events have proved it was none of these but rather that social pressures to live up to established, accepted standards of behavior acted as a powerful control upon the doctor, forcing him to conform to society's expectations regardless of what his inner feelings might urge.

As pressures for conformity throughout our society have become less and less intense, impermissible acts have become permissible. Just as it is possible now for the nurse not to respond to the patient's call for a bedpan, so doctors have found it possible to gradually unmask the drives they have hitherto held carefully in check. In his desire to obtain an abundance of the materialistic ''things'' the society affords, and at the same time retain the special privilege and status accorded to the healer and servant of mankind, the doctor has bemused a people anxious to be misled. While professing commitment to the delivery of high-quality health care and selfless service, doctors individually pursue, and permit their professional societies to pursue for them, economic and self-protective goals that are absolutely counter in their effect to what the communal commitments require.

In a society dependent upon an undersupply of doctors, this double game has created a real life struggle for many physicians. Anyone with an eye can see that doctors are grievously torn, and often seriously damaged, by the conflict between the ideals of medicine and the irresistible blandishments of society. Listen to any group of practicing doctors today—when their earning capabilities are higher than ever, when the hated and bitterly opposed Medicare program has helped enormously to swell their purses. Listen, and you will hear their insecurity, and the fear that someone is going to take it all away from them. Every recommendation for change, for improving the accessibility and quality of care, for implementing the rhetoric of ''we are the servants of the people,'' scares the organized, practicing doctor half to death and triggers the knee-jerk reflex, ''Nyet!''

THE MEDICAL CARE SYSTEM

It is evident that reliance on the myth of the doctor as a human without frailties, coupled with the economic preoccupation of organized medicine and the general abandonment of moral for material values, has produced systems of medical care practice and reimbursement seemingly designed to encourage delinquency. These have been effective beyond the wildest dreams of the devil, if he had wanted to seduce doctors from paths of probity and humanity.

License to practice medicine is no assurance that the quality of care in this country is anywhere near what our present capability and knowledge permit. Given the licensing laws of our states and the laissez-faire attitude of professional medical organizations, it is possible that a general practitioner who graduated from medical school 30 years ago might not have read, in all that time, any of the professional journals in his field, attended refresher courses, or made any attempt to keep his knowledge and skill up to date. Given this situation, and since financial rewards are less often for quality and more often for quantity —quick, shoddy work and unnecessary services—it is clear that continued education makes only better doctors, not generally more affluent ones.

EDUCATION Medical education, in its own way, has helped to weaken the physician's commitment to patient care. The explosion of science in medicine has given us knowledge and capabilities for dealing with disease which are certainly extraordinary. Yet everyone is now aware that advancements in technology do not of themselves improve the quality of life and can, if not socially controlled, damage life. For some years, medicine was so captivated by the capabilities of science that all else became of lesser or little importance. In the best schools, science and research dominated the scene and unconsciously, but nonetheless effectively, downgraded patient commitment, clinical care, and even teaching. The clinician had to overcome incredible difficulties to achieve a promotion because his expertise in the care of patients and his ability as a teacher did not translate into ''academic excellence,'' which seemed instead to be synonymous with ''research papers.'' Young, impressionable students, during four years of medical school, get the message through verbal and nonverbal communication about what is important and what is not, what gets rewarded and what does not—and compassionate, clinical responsibility to patients and the community does not fare very well. That science is lifesaving and must be expanded does not mean that society can tolerate a choice between science or compassion; science everywhere, especially in medicine, must be pursued in the service of humanity. All aspects of medical education, including the teaching of basic science, should be so thoughtfully arranged that they foster the fragile qualities of concern, caring, and commitment, instead of reflecting the self-serving interests of powerful departmental chairmen as most medical curriculums do.

For thousands of students in their clinical years, the introduction to patient care takes place in institutions that primarily serve the poor. What happens to a young medical student in a big municipal or county hospital when he sees these unfortunates—people who already suffer from joblessness, inadequate housing, poor diet, and all the other stigmata of poverty, cared for in dilapidated hospitals, whose human and material resources are totally inadequate? He must either rebel or accommodate, and it is very tough for the student to rebel when his preceptors and other leaders seem to have managed so well.

But all is not lost in medicine. There have always been idealistic young men and women who have come to medicine only to find their models in medical school and medical practice prone to the seduction of socially non-constructive rewards. Everything in our society encourages success—as defined by real estate and stock market holdings. How can the idealistic overcome this? A new generation of young people—the best we have ever had —have seen clearly what discrimination, poverty, and war do to humans. They have recognized these as concomitants of avarice, greed, and inhumanity. This generation is demonstrating to us that man's self-serving drives can be controlled; that there are ways in which he can satisfy his own inner needs that do not require him to put others down; that deep personal rewards can be found in doing good and caring for humanity. The Pediatric Collective at the Lincoln Municipal Hospital in New York City, in its efforts to restructure both inpatient and outpatient services toward delivering comprehensive, dignified care, is a case in point.[6]

However, the medical care of a whole society cannot rest on so slender a reed as the internally generated idealism of some physicians. Inspired by the dedication and imagination of these new, young, committed doctors and galvanized by their energy and resourcefulness, we must devise a framework for medical care organization and financing that will actually meet the needs of the people, rather than purport to meet them, and we must develop a system of social pressures and rewards which will move all of medicine toward the patient and communal responsibilities envisioned in the Hippocratic Oath.

THE MEDICAL SCHOOLS The place to begin is in our medical schools. With new techniques constantly emerging as a result of the technological revolution in which we are living, it is foolish to suggest, as some have, that our doctors should be less well-trained in scientific medicine. The problem is not one of subtracting, but one of adding, reorienting, and reassigning priorities.

We must require of our incoming medical students a background in the humanities as well as proficiency in science. The medical

It is foolish to suggest, as some have, that our doctors should be less well-trained in scientific medicine. The problem is not one of subtracting, but one of adding, reorienting, and reassigning priorities.

school curriculum must place as much emphasis on the social and behavioral sciences as on the natural sciences. The student must be taught the underpinnings of human biology in such a way that he will clearly understand how these scientific facts relate to people and the ills which afflict them. We will produce doctors who are both compassionate and competent in an educational environment that humanizes rather than dehumanizes the student and rewards him for the thoroughness with which he evaluates the patient's "health" [7] just as it rewards him for the scientific excellence with which he diagnoses a disease.

While study after study over the past 20 years has attested to the growing shortage of physicians,[8,9] only very recently has organized medicine given up its fiercely protective stance as guardian of the doctor's economic security and begun to support the expansion of medical schools. Thus, the shortage of doctors, a crucial factor in our entire health care crisis, was artificially induced and is poignant evidence of the misuse of the public trust placed in medicine.

CHANGING LAWS To alleviate the shortage of physicians, we must double our educational capacity, providing 11,000 new places in medical schools by 1978. This would enable us to produce 100,000 new doctors by the early 1980s, so that a total of approximately 400,000 practicing physicians would be available to our society by that time. If we then continue to increase medical school admissions with an additional 1,000 students each year, by 1985 we will be producing 25,000 new physicians annually, or roughly double the number graduated each year in the mid-1970s.

Our experience in educating doctors during the emergency of World War II indicates that we could accomplish this end without a myriad of new schools, although we would probably wish to create some in those geographical locations where there is virtually a total vacuum in the medical care system. However, the bulk of the increased enrollment could be absorbed by the existing medical schools through expansion of the six-year college-medical school combination and, above all, by means of more effective utilization of all medical school facilities and faculties. This will require that academicians take a hard look at their practices and priorities in order to recognize and accept the fact that the *prime* responsibility of the medical school is producing physicians to meet the health care needs of the society.

There are those who say we will never have enough money to do this, but I believe they do not acknowledge the will of the people. The most liberal abortion law[10] in the country has now been enacted in the state of New York, whose position in this matter, until now, had been regulated by the religious beliefs of one highly vocal group. When a sufficient number of the residents of the state changed their views on abortion and decided that the law no longer reflected their beliefs, they changed the law.

Many separate proposals are now before the federal government on the subject of national health insurance.[11-15] Without question, this is an idea whose time has come, and we shall surely have some form of national health insurance within the next five years. This will happen—not because the politicians want to spend the money and not because the medical profession has shown leadership. It will happen because many Americans have suffered cruelly from the high cost of medical care. All Americans will soon be freed from the threat of medical pauperization because a significant number of them have decided that national health insurance is both desirable and necessary. And, when a significant number of people also decide that they are entitled to at least the same ratio of doctors to patients as prevails in other advanced nations,[16] I am convinced that the money for buildings, faculties, and tuition will be forthcoming.

MEDICAL CAREERS   While Hippocrates (in declaring that the training of future doctors should be provided by doctors for their own sons and the sons of teachers of medicine) hardly encouraged the idea of drawing medical school candidates from the broad spectrum of society, he also did not decree, as we do, that most candidates for medical education must come from monied families.[17] In the United States today, what really decides who

> *In the United States today, what really decides who will become a doctor and who will not is whether a candidate's family has between $40,000 and $50,000 to pay for his education.*

will become a doctor and who will not is whether a candidate's family has between $40,000 and $50,000 to pay for his education. Indeed, at the college level, well before medical school, we undoubtedly lose many of the young people who would become compassionate, insightful doctors and surgeons of great dexterity because they cannot pay college tuition costs. This is especially so among our lower socioeconomic groups who are also blocked by cultural differences and poor preparation at the lower educational level. Our scholarship programs are too inadequate to support many candidates from these groups, and so the privilege of being a doctor remains primarily an option open to the middle and upper-middle classes. This is not because these groups produce more young people who are dedicated, unselfish, noble, or intellectually gifted, but because they possess that ingredient which is the sine qua non in our society—money. Here, again, the medical profession's avowed commitment to provide society with the best, most qualified doctors possible is inconsistent with its silence—which has permitted this practice of exclusion to continue.

Careers in medicine should not be limited to just those who can pay. With tuition free and modest living expenses available, we could attract to the medical profession the very best young people our society has to offer. Not only would this increase the number of skilled professionals with a commitment to the needs of the poor, but this would also greatly diversify and enrich our understanding and approach to medical care—and it would make the medical establishment more truly reflective of the population as a whole.

Noting, as we have, the inadequacies of solo, fee-for-service medical care and the advantages of group practice, we will prepare future doctors to work as members of groups which are hospital-based or hospital-related. In so structuring medical care delivery, we will limit unnecessary hospitalization and we will ensure, by peer review as well as medical audit, high-quality care. By building neighborhood health centers and providing special rewards for doctors who serve in our less desirable urban areas or in remote rural villages, we will be able to provide comprehensive, family-oriented care to all Americans.

All of this is not only expedient, it is possible. The price is simply that we discard the myth of the doctor's natural superiority and base our actions upon a clear view of his human qualities and society's needs. Physicians, among others, are responsible for society's health. While we destroy the myths, we must also address ourselves to the fantasy that our society can long remain viable with affluence and abject poverty existing side by side. The conditions of diet, housing, sanitation, narcotics, crime, and education which prevail in the culture of poverty have a greater impact upon health than all of the services medicine can possibly render, and their impact is not limited by geographical or cultural boundaries.

Some will surely ask, ''Are these the re-sponsibilities of the doctor?'' The answer must be that if the doctor acts as a healer to the society he must concern himself with all the things that impinge upon health. Who knows better than the doctor that unheated apartments foster pneumonia and influenza; that rickety, unsafe stairways can cause accidents; that poor sanitation encourages the spread of disease; that being without a job engenders self-repugnance and despair; that alienation destroys emotional stability and breeds violence? Using the prestige and power that his profession confers upon him, the doctor must prod the political establishment to commit the resources necessary for eliminating these social sources of disease.

As George Bernard Shaw pointed out more than a generation ago, ''Such poverty as we have today in our great cities degrades the poor, and infects with its degradation, the whole neighborhood in which they live. And whatever can degrade a neighborhood, can degrade a country and a continent and finally the whole civilized world, which is only a large neighborhood. Its bad effects cannot be escaped by the rich. When poverty produces outbreaks of virulent infectious disease, as it always does sooner or later, the rich catch the disease and see their children die of it. When it produces crime and violence, the rich go in fear of both. When it produces bad manners and bad language, the children of the rich pick them up, no matter how carefully they are secluded. The saying that we are members one of another is not a mere pious formula to be repeated in church without any meaning; it is a literal truth; for though the rich end of the town can avoid living with the poor, it can not avoid dying with the poor.''

The time has come when we must relegate myths to the category of folklore, where they belong. As far as medicine is concerned, we must, with cool and practical vision, rearrange the ways in which we select and educate doctors, prescribing the mode in which they will practice, and designing a system of rewards and penalties that take cognizance of the fact that money, status, and power are the forces which strongly motivate people, doctors included, in this country today. We must do this to ensure the quality of our lives and our survival.

While fostering those conditions in the society, the home, and the family life which promote idealism and prompt progress, we must also be hardheaded enough to institutionalize progress. We must be prepared to examine, with tough-minded realism, every development in medicine, keeping in mind the plasticity of human beings and recognizing that the very characteristic that makes people fallible also makes it possible to encourage them to attain the most humane and socially productive activities and goals.

To my mind, truth is to be venerated above even ancient and beautiful words, because truth opens to man hitherto unseen pathways by which he can seek solutions to the problems that beset him and thereby enrich his own life and the lives of his brothers. It is his willingness to see the truth and act upon it, not a new version of the Hippocratic Oath, that will bring honor to the profession of medicine and compassionate, high-quality care to all people.

REFERENCES

1 Bunker JP: Surgical manpower. *New Eng J Med* 282:137.
2 Trussell RE: *The Quantity, Quality and Costs of Medical and Hospital Care Secured by a Sample of Teamster Families in the New York Area. A Report.* Columbia University School of Public Health and Administrative Medicine. New York, July 1962, 82 pp.
3 Falk IS: *Special Study on the Medical Care Program for Steel Workers and Their Families.* US Steel Workers of America. Pittsburgh, Sept 1960.
4 *Report of the National Advisory Commission on Health Manpower.* Nov 1967, vol 2, pp 197–228.
5 Message from the President of the United States Relative to Building a National Health Strategy, Section A: *Reorganizing the Delivery of Service.* US House of Representatives. House Documents, 91st Congress. Sup Documents, 1971, 19 pp.
6 Kaufman MT: Lincoln Hospital: Case history of dissension that split staff. *New York Times,* Dec 21, 1971, p 1.
7 "Health is a state of complete physical, mental and social well being—and not merely the absence of disease or infirmity." World Health Organization.
8 *Report of the National Advisory Commission on Health Manpower.* See ref 4, vol 1, also Feb 1967.
9 *Physicians for a Growing America.* US Dept of of Health, Education, and Welfare, 1959.
10 An Act to amend the penal law in relation to justifiable abortional acts by physicians in the course of their practice or medicine, New York State, effective July 1, 1970.
11 Report of the Committee of 100—The Committee for National Health Insurance, appointed by Walter P Reuther, Pres, United Automobile Workers, Nov 1968.
12 National Health Insurance, 1970 Fact Sheet no. 1, Legislative Department, AFL-CIO.
13 Introduction of the Health Security Act, S.4297, 91st Congress, Second Session, Aug 27, 1970.
14 Message from the President of the United States Relative to Building a National Health Strategy, Feb 18, 1971. See ref 5.
15 Kindig DA, Sidel VW: Impact of national health insurance plans on the consumer, in Eilers RD, Moyerman SS (eds): *National Health Insurance.* Homewood, Ill, Richard D Irwin Inc, 1971, pp 15–61.
16 *J Med Educ* 41:64, 1966.
17 *How Medical Students Finance Their Education.* Public Health Service Publication 1336-1, Health, Education and Welfare, National Institute of Health, Division of Health Manpower.

Chapter 8
Cloudy Trophies
Lawrence D. Grouse

*Every day I see people suffering; many of them will die while I watch.
Can I put so much love into an enterprise so full of death? That is the
constant question.*

*Ay, in the very temple of Delight
Veil'd melancholy has her sovran shrine
Though seen of none save him whose
strenuous tongue
Can burst Joy's grape against his palate
fine:
His soul shall taste the sadness of her
might
And be among her cloudy trophies hung.*
        John Keats: *"Ode on Melancholy"*

It is always a turbulent dream you remember, and as you bring the story through your mind, the threads of subplots shuttle for a moment into consciousness but then disappear again leaving perhaps a name or a location. For example, I dreamed last night about a group of men, myself among them, who wished to sleep with a beautiful young girl. I am suddenly aware as I stop to think that the dream took place in my childhood home. The girl was Nancy, a close friend of mine for many years. All evening Nancy chanted poetry, played

Editor's Note: Mr. Grouse wrote this fictionalized piece during his second and third years at the University of Washington School of Medicine in Seattle.

bluegrass music with her fiddle and Elizabethan madrigals on her recorder, while I dissected fingernails and memorized their structure. Finally I threw the sheet over the head of my cadaver, and the medical aphorism which I had invented, "Don't think of it as losing a patient, think of it as gaining a cadaver," went through my mind. With relief I picked up my guitar to join Nancy, and walked out of my parents' old bedroom. However, as I entered my old bedroom there were 20 or 30 other men crowded on the floor around Nancy, all with guitars. I noticed my guitar was strung, not with guitar strings, but with human muscles and their long ligaments. The room was silent. I plucked at the ligaments and sang "Melancholy Baby." With total seriousness I pointed at the lowermost ligament and said, "Flexor carpi ulnaris!"

Suddenly it was late at night. Nancy had been secretly sleeping with a boy named Ray. She would sneak out in the night to meet him in the bed where my sister used to sleep. Craftily, I padded down the hall and into the target bed. Soon she dived into my arms professing love and devotion. I could say nothing, obviously. The feeling of powerful lust mixed with terrible sorrow brought tears to my eyes. The love was not intended for me although I desired it. She felt my beard and, startled, suddenly understood my little ruse. With an irony uncharacteristic of Nancy she acidly remarked, "You must have forgotten to shave this morning."

I awake with an intense awareness of the weight of reality around me. I examine each emotion as it occurs, first fear that I am alone in a dark room, then sadness mingled with lust that I do not have a woman with me. I watch these passions appear and then decay out of consciousness; I hover in a state of awareness, marvel at how desires silently erupt into my thoughts. Then I grasp at the boundaries of my internal voice.

Words enter my consciousness and I write them down. I am not sure how they arise or how I control their appearance. The words "Joseph Kern" appear; I have come to know them as my name. I know, when I ask myself, that Joseph Kern possesses certain objects, among which are the typewriter I am using at this moment, a leather briefcase, and an array of books on a shelf in the corner. Joseph Kern also possesses unwritten but specified privileges in touching certain other humans. Joseph has a history and a future.

But there is a gap between this information that seems to be available to me and the objects that are external to me. What do I know? Other men and women are like other islands. I do know that I am meant to fall apart some day. This single fact used to frighten me and may still, but I don't dwell on it. During the few lucid moments of consciousness which infrequently occur, I concentrate on the "I" that arises so often in these words. What are the images and ideas which purport to describe him? A living man is more a miracle than an object. Unexplained and mysterious, he stands gasping on a huge solid, surrounded and infiltrated by the unknown.

Just as certain actors carry into a play a simple description of the character they portray to which they can constantly refer, I want to begin my story close to the actual data of decision because this story deals with the motivation for my choice to enter medical school and ultimately the decision to become a doctor. I have known Nancy for several years; she more than anyone has been a partner to these decisions. She was not present at the very beginning, and I can tell that this is the time for some musty history.

The South Minneapolis area where I grew up, like most suburbs then and now, was the American Dream in the uncomfortable period after people are forced to live in it. I suppose living in the solipsistic suburbs made me think the way I do; I don't know whether I am grateful or resentful. Ambiguity is another byproduct of my childhood. If we ever meet we can exchange stories about troubled, surreal childhoods.

It is not crucial that you know about my life; however, I am well acquainted with it, and it is one of the few ongoing enterprises in which I have an abiding interest. I seldom think of myself as Joseph Kern. I do not feel that I should be held responsible for my name. It was just the first of an endless series of givens which pattern our experience. We are pawns in a game which we would never have chosen.

With a careful questioning, I can remember watching bass jump on still, warm summer evenings as I rowed across Crystal Bay toward Enchanted Island on Lake Minnetonka, where I spent my summers as a child. I was another person then — isolated, full of anxiety, with secret terrors, and driven by a need for approval. Of course, these traits were regarded as virtues at that time. I reflect on this description and can find no evidence that I have changed.

This should not sound like a success story, but I came to a realization during my senior year at Washburn High School after a summer in Munich. It occurred to me that maybe it wasn't me that was unhappy, perverted, compulsive, and materialistic, but something outside of me. Further, I began to realize that my feelings and behavior were not obligatory but matters over which I could exercise personal control. When I attempted to make a decision about my goals in life, I discovered myself to be a dependent, derivative creature who needed to engulf himself in an outside structure. Of course, there were many opportunities for doing just that, and no other opportunities.

I read Beckett, Joyce, Shakespeare, and Eliot as if each moment spent in activity other than reading or writing would condemn me to eternal unconsciousness. As I wrote I discovered a self which I, in part, created. On the evening of the day that John Kennedy was killed I wrote feverishly for hours, sensed unseen presences, and felt a mystical concordance with the murdered president. Questions of meaning became paramount in my thoughts. I resolved on that occasion to become a physician. My image of a doctor was a man with control over life, a man who could defend the human spirit against the irrational, evil power of death. In retrospect, I suppose, it was just my means of reconciling the unknown with my anxiety through intellectualization, but I have come to identify the experience as my personal metamorphosis. Medicine became a symbol of reason that was always contraposed in my mind to a searched-for but undiscovered symbol of emotion.

Nancy and I were sophomores at Carleton College when we met. My roommate and I had gone to a rock dance in the old gymnasium one snowy Saturday night in January. He quickly found a girl in his chemistry class. I remember because they began to talk about thermodynamics. I was immediately bored, and I was even a chemistry major.

I left them and walked up a winding staircase to the balcony where I could sit and watch the dance from a distance. I tripped over planks and beer cans in the dark walking down near the railing. I watched my roommate who began dancing with the lady chemist. She had a fine body; I wondered why they spent all their time talking about chemistry, which they both probably hated. Suddenly a paper airplane whizzed past my head, and I turned to see a girl with a large face, her arms wrapped around herself, and smiling a huge conspiratorial smile. Amused, I stumbled over to her, and we had a wild, expressionistic conversation about the weight and shapes of imaginary snowflakes. Talking with Nancy was like taking part in a poem or entering an imaginary world. But what I considered fantasy, as I think back, was an extension of everyday experiences that brought our feelings into a new perspective. At one point that night she wrote a couplet that I still remember by heart, "Oh, happy mammals, the wonder of your reproductive apparatus terrorizes infants and mobilizes the meagre forces of the intellect." She initially disarmed me, but I came to depend on Nancy's questions to confide my feelings. Unpredictably she would stare at me and interrupt her fantasy with complete honesty. Once she told me sadly, "Friendship is a pile of shared experiences, but your friends leave you and you leave your friends and all the piles keep getting washed away. Hard, no?"

Nancy was just different from other girls. She might walk up to me excitedly with a new poem or jump down at me from a tree where she had been watching stars. One evening as I was about to enter a scene from Pinter's *The Birthday Party* in which I was playing McCann, Nancy handed me a scroll reading, "Pinter is the refutation of Sartre, consciousness is not a smooth-running process / But is like a train in a switching yard with few options." Usually she would accompany the note with a sketch. Often the pictures would be of thin-faced autistic children morosely contemplating porridge while a wicked queen would be standing over them with an eggbeater. The drawing might be labeled: "My dream doors are affronted by the gates of Sweden."

Nancy was not a verbal person. She disdained to limit the meaning of what she experienced to words, and expressed her feelings freely through movements, faces, and gestures. This is not to say that she found it hard to express herself in writing. She engaged competently in rhetoric and trod the narrow margin of lucid, uncomplicated explanation; only occasionally did she fall off into the abyss of what she actually experienced.

She loved my best friend, Mike James, who also happened to be my roommate that year. I remember one time when I was sleeping in my shorts during a warm spring night. Nancy and Mike ran in after their usual dash past the proctor's door. On a crazy impulse they took off their clothes and began to read from Blake's *Songs of Innocence*. Sitting in my shorts in the dark with only a candle to illuminate the book while both of them sat cross-legged in the nude, I had the strange feeling of being overdressed.

When I look back at my life during those years or any years, I am overcome with a sense of meaninglessness, just as I will be when I look back on my activities today in another five years.

When I look back at my life during those or any years, I am overcome with a sense of meaninglessness, just as I will be when I look back on my activities today in another five years. I follow the strings in my life forward and backward, but there is nothing at either end. All this concern about what I was and what I will become, how absurd! A man can decide to do any of a number of things and once the ritual of its performance is fixed in his head he will stay nestled in the routine like an oyster and build as elaborate a justification of his tiny occupation as is necessary to sustain him in its drudgery. We proceed, driven by necessity, supported by all the sharp, invisible hooks of expectation and emotion, all the while pretending that we exercise decision. I accept the feeling of free fall through my own life. What else is there to do?

But even in free fall there can be a glimpse of recognition. It is not in the hollow cycles of procreation and oblivion that my mind finds itself alive and unique, but in the mysteries of life and death. What work can a man do that

is not so meaningless that he will have to become a stranger to himself to continue?

I remember the day I decided to apply to medical school. It was during the fall of my senior year. Mike had broken up with Nancy and had a new girl, Bonnie, whose main asset was having lived for a year as the mistress of a state senator in New York City. This does not seem to me like the basis for a relationship now, but we were living what we thought to be an idealistic hedonism that arose from an existential view of the world. It was our way of protesting what we considered oppressive curtailment of our freedoms by indulging, usually beyond the limit of pleasure, in the proscripted areas. Mike once told me that he wished as his ultimate goal in life to become a symbol of wasted potential. It was as if he demanded to live, if only metaphorically, his world view. Although I aspired to Mike's goal, I was still driven to participate and succeed at each absurd, arbitrary game that was delegated for me to play.

We drank rum in some form that evening. Alcohol and glorious drunks were the only dignified ways of celebrating the chaos of the vacuum we inhabited and of rebelling against the puritanical authorities who planned our lives in their dusty archives. Tom Steele was telling me about his ardor for the poetry of Spenser.

"The man is a master of poesy," he said. He began to read to me:

. . . In that same shadie covert, whereas lay
Faire Crysogone in slombry traunce whilere:
Who in her sleepe (a wondrous thing to say)
Unwares had borned two babes, as fair as springing day.

Edmund Spenser:
"The Faerie Queen"

He explained how one section represented the synthesis of pagan and Christian myths in literature. I watched patterns of cigarette smoke. It occurred to me that I would teach

English eventually, perhaps this same poem. Was it all an exercise in poetic conventions and figures of speech that no one had enjoyed for centuries? I lit another Camel and smoked nervously, tried to listen.

I talked with Terry Werner and his wife Stacey. Terry was a poet who had published poems in several of the avante garde magazines in the country. He and his wife had graduated two years earlier. His gentleness always impressed me. I wanted to talk with him about my plans to hitchhike around the country and write short stories when I graduated, but he was preoccupied. Instead of his usual grin, he looked dejected. When I asked, he spoke without emotion about his frustrations since leaving college. To support Stacey and their new baby, all that was available for an English major, he felt, was to teach English. Few jobs were open, and the ones that he had held appeared to him to involve destroying minds and not opening them. He was pumping gas at that time, starting work each morning at 5:00 AM, an hour when most of the rest of us would not yet have retired for the night.

I told Terry that most of my old friends had sold out. They wrote advertising convincing people to consume things they didn't need, sold insurance by playing on fear, and became wage slaves. I told him that once money became the prime commodity they lost their own freedom since everything they did was figured in terms of dollars. It all seemed so simple.

Our whole group walked down past the TV room where couples sat to do their homework and drank chocolate syrup as a special treat on this Saturday night. We always received angry looks as we paraded by in our hunting jackets, cowboy boots, and old jeans like characters from a 1950 motorcycle epic. Their rejection pleased us because we had no desire to share their world with them even if we were not sure where we were. We stopped that night as we heard the announcement that President Johnson had committed 200,000 more troops to Vietnam. A local release by the Minnesota draft boards made it obvious that I would be drafted as soon as I left college.

After spending about an hour at the local bar with my friends, all of us silent and moody, I walked back to the dormitory alone, letting it sink in that my plans were destroyed.

I found Nancy in my room. She looked like she had just observed some ghastly traffic accident which only she could have imagined. Then she was crying in my arms, sobbing about her father who had died that evening in Winona. He had died slowly with emphysema. We sat on my bed holding each other until almost morning. She described her father's peculiarities and related his old stories about growing up during the years of prohibition. She told me his favorite jokes and early in the morning she tried to imitate the different duck calls he had taught her. At about 4:00 AM she lay down and whispered to me, "I would trust you with my life," and went to sleep.

I walked slowly past the sleeping dormitories toward an isolated bluff in the nearby arboretum that bordered on the campus. For a moment I imagined that I saw soldiers with bayonets rising from under dewy piles of leaves and darting behind the looming tree shapes. I ran up the little ridge and looked down on the path through the trees.

The wooden bridge over the Cannon River reminded me of a similar bridge over the Isar near Munich where I had often stood. I used to imagine all the people who had ever walked by that river, parading by in an endless array. Then all I could think of was a beerhall and hundreds of men and women drinking, singing songs. Sitting at the head table was John Kennedy with blood on his forehead and crying while I tried to cover up the wound with a handkerchief until he finally slumped over. As I watched, the word "death" emblazoned on a green plastic object was laid on his chest.

I had accepted and rejected the idea that I would enter medicine dozens of times. Again I weighed the choices. Perhaps I would be able to take care of people. Nancy had said, "I would trust you with my life." It suddenly appealed to me, the idea that I could relieve suffering, that I could comfort others. But I knew myself well enough to doubt that I could be so selfless, that I could sacrifice my beautiful nihilism on anything so positive as medicine. Although I was nominally a chemistry major, my plans had always revolved around writing, and the tedium of medical school was reportedly incompatible with creative activity, a truism which I have gone on to verify. A friend in medical school told me that medical students were compulsive drudges, possessed of large memories but no imagination.

It is possible that I had all these thoughts during that early morning walk. Perhaps I have just been thinking them now. About 5:00 AM I called my sister who lived in Seattle and worked at the medical school. I asked her to send me an application form.

She asked, "Who is it for?"

"For me!" I answered

The first two years of medical school are a haze of long, depressing nights. In some ways it was like reentering the unthinking rituals of high school, but mainly it was the shock of a totally new life. I memorized structures and processes whose significance to me as a prospective physician was never clear, much less to me as a person. The classes were mainly lectures with too many students to comfortably ask questions, not that I wanted to. As a medical student one does not stop living, though he is less alive.

As a medical student one does not stop living, though he is less alive.

At night I stared at a blank tablet, unable to concentrate. After studying I came home to drink beer and listen to records. I had no close friends. I lived in a house on Portage Bay in Seattle with three other medical students. I did not touch any of them deeply and they did not touch me. Often I would call my friends from college: Nancy in Minneapolis, Mike and Terry in Kansas City. Events in our shared past were more important to me than the events in my present life. The words I memorized had all the mystery of today's prices on the stock exchange. It seemed to me that scientific language deliberately excluded any glimmer of feeling and actively blocked consideration of the relevance of a fact to matters of human concern.

I wrote a letter to Mike during my first year which he recently returned to me. One part read, "The view from my window is a subject I can approach straightforwardly and without fear. When I want to be alone I simply go to find it. I pick out a nonthreatening book, read through a couple of pages, and stare out at the fascinating scene. The movement hypnotizes me. Sometimes it is the sunlight or a person just walking down the little road in back of my house. I used to write, but nothing meant much to me later. I try not to think about the day's lectures or to question an infantile assignment to build a scale model of a muscle fiber. The view from my window is no trouble. It is the view from inside my room that gives me trouble."

I was plagued with fears of death and somatic pains which came and went with anxiety. Typical of this period is a dream which I described one morning in the following way: "I was sitting in a third grade classroom decorated with bulletin boards with my fellow first-year medical students when a pedantic comment I was making was interrupted as I suddenly noticed my father who had been (squat and buried beneath layers of old plaid-patterned clothes and a tacky grey suit) listening to me from a corner of the room near the door. Shuffling, raising a mist of coal dust, he walked out of the door and I followed. I called to him as I walked down the Washburn High School corridor until he came to a stairway. I felt that something was wrong, that he was unhappy, or was it that his appearance always inspired that fear in me?

"'What's the matter?' I asked, and asked again, 'What's the matter?' He looked up worried and mumbled, 'You need money?'

'No, no!' I said, 'not money, what is the matter?'

"With the crisis of his anxiety and my inability to express myself to him, the dream, peculiar for its clarity, is terminated and I wake with a persisting, mild, substernal pain."

I learned what my life in medicine might become at a three-day rock festival held near Eatonville last summer. As the first day began I was sitting on the front porch of a deserted wooden house in Seattle with boarded windows and weeds that covered the yard. An old friend from Carleton had arranged to pick me up so that we could drive together to the rock festival. I worked in the Open Door Clinic at the festival, sewing up lacerations, distributing antibiotics, and giving tetanus toxoid. As I waited, I stared at an empty notebook on my knees and tried to write. Some lines began with paradoxes which bored me as soon as they appeared. I attempted to write what I felt, but was disgusted with the poverty of my honesty and clumsiness in writing. I had no idea how I felt. Cars sped past one by one on the freeway.

My mind turned to the research project I was doing during the summer with DNA-RNA hybridization studies. The thought that the mystery of humanness lay simply in a long linear code depressed me. What am I but cells and what are cells but little factories organized by protein molecules blindly repeating over and over their individual tricks? Where is the permanence of the I to whom these thoughts occur and what is that human permanence written in if not in these words only?

My friend finally pulled up in his 1954 Cadillac hearse decorated with surrealistic paintings that I recognized. Nancy was sitting in the back seat. She had hitchhiked out from Minnesota and was staying at a commune outside of town with people I knew. The first hour I just sat grinning and listened to Nancy bubble over about her past three years which I had only heard about sketchily in her few letters.

We were together most of those three days.

I once asked her to explain her poetry and painting to me.

"I just play with images, words, and—feeling, I guess," she said. "I express a feeling that I can share, something that's happening to me, like how happy I am being with you again, Joe. And how happy I could be staying with you."

"I could never be an artist now," I told her.

"Why not?" She seemed surprised.

"Spontaneity isn't possible for me now, if it ever was," I said.

I talked with her about the barrenness I felt as a medical student. I found myself explaining my feelings about doctors, medical school, and my patients, feelings I hadn't believed existed. Early the next morning I dreamed that several of my former patients who had gone on to die were alive, but as I stood watching they were shot and stabbed by some malevolent force, perhaps myself. There were reward posters for each of them although I knew them to be gentle men. One shouted to me, "Don't shoot, doctor!" as he was killed.

I walked to a long ambulance and went toward the rear. As I looked in the middle door I saw the grim reaper, old, long-bearded and thin-limbed, wearing a medieval costume. He sat looking at me. His garments were colorful; he resembled a hippie. Behind him in the next compartment were two or three other ancient, long-boned, thin people, two with white hair. Behind the ambulance was the shadow of a circular grouping of symbols which I could not look at directly but recognized as a sign of impending death. When I turned back to the ambulance the three old people had changed to beautiful young people with colorful tunics and gowns. There was a beautiful white-haired girl, a young athletic Norwegian boy, and Nancy smiling at me and playing with a large, red polished stone. I threw my arms up, silently screamed, then ran away from them. Almost immediately the ambulance passed me. I turned to see the shadows from the circular symbols and with relief turned back, leaping into the shadows.

I watched Nancy sleep peacefully, and I didn't want to disturb her. Perhaps I should have because I never found time to tell her about the dream.

More than ever I felt possessiveness and even love for Nancy, but seldom before or since have I controlled my emotions so well. She talked abstractly about poetry, and I lectured her about medicine.

Late the second night we delivered a baby, and Nancy stood petrified during the procedure. After the little girl was born, Nancy held her until the ambulance drove the baby and mother to a nearby hospital. When I went to talk with her she was crying.

"It was so beautiful," she said, "but so terrible and bloody and all the pain! How can you stand it?"

We talked about the goals of medicine. I read her the Hippocratic Oath. She seemed impressed that it advocated a united community of doctors caring for each other like members of a family. She saw this unity as a part of the future that young people wish to establish to counter the American, alienated individualism. Also, she admired an ethic of medicine oriented solely by concern for patients, a radical concept which she doubted could function in American medical practice.

She was probably right. We both disagreed with the specific policies relating to abortion and euthanasia proposed in the Oath, but I felt that it was not a disagreement with the ideals, only a different value judgment about what is considered most precious in life.

Nancy and I read through a histology textbook that night for fun, and she wrote stories to describe the adventures of blood cells, liver cells, and spermatozoa. She drew pictures and figure legends in her Gothic script. We talked until early morning; we watched the stars pose their questions.

The next morning she wondered if being a doctor would mean that I would be forced into a middle-class mold of exploiting people.

I said, "I suppose it probably will. It's true that most humanistic principles of medicine would dictate that disease be treated in all people. I also know it's true that medical care isn't available for large groups who suffer and are disabled needlessly. It may even be true that medicine is so expensive that it impoverishes its patients whether it cures them or not. I don't like to think about it."

"So you agree that all this is the result of the American obsession for money, the rich people depriving the poor of every opportunity and even life?"

"Probably," I said.

"Why in hell don't you try to change it?" she demanded.

"I'm an activist by default," I told her. "I don't believe in positive action. Back in the days when I had never worked up a patient I was very sincere about my fellow man. Now, I'm not sure that I have one. Who knows, maybe I am an activist. On weekends over beer my friends and I say revolutionary things. At 8:00 AM before Saturday classes we conspire while drinking our coffee."

She frowned. "Until the doctors are out in the streets nothing is going to happen. You know that. You tell me that you hate doctors' insensitivity and racism. You say more students with human concerns should become doctors. You tell me about your free clinics. Doesn't that mean something?"

"Okay," I said, "but I don't think in big terms. I think about my patients, that's all I can handle. I want to learn to be a decent doc. A doctor has to be a scientist gathering information, reasoning and acting on his decisions."

"But first he's got to be a man," she said angrily, "relating to another person who is sick and frightened and probably more frightened because your doctor is such a great scientist. Doctors hide behind their busy schedules to defend their inability to deeply relate to anyone!"

I agreed. To change the subject I added irrelevantly that it was the AMA that originally restricted the number of doctors who could be educated to tighten their monopoly.

"I suppose you'll be a member," she said with more resignation than anger.

"I don't think so," I said, "and I won't defend it, but the AMA just furthers the best financial interest of its members exactly as the other professions and industries do, at the expense of their customers."

"Customers!" she yelled. "So now life is a product like a TV set."

"Sometimes that's the only way I can stand to look at it."

She couldn't believe that I had said it. "I see, so because you can't find spiritual values you sell out to material values," she accused.

I tried to explain. "Medicine programs you for coldness. Medical schools are run by men who are scientists and nothing else. They don't care about emotional problems or what their patients are like as people."

"That's no excuse for you, Joe. You're trying to intellectualize, to justify accepting what you don't believe. Medicine is inhuman and unfair and you could help change it if you weren't so occupied with yourself."

"Perhaps I could," I said flatly.

She looked at me, but I couldn't meet her eyes. "You have always been alone, Joe. Maybe you like it, maybe you even need it, always talking about the nature of your soul."

"Perhaps I do."

She looked sad. "I care for you, Joe," she said, "and I know that I could always trust you to care for me, but I don't think I could ever love you—do you understand? I could never stay with you because—I couldn't live alone."

She did stay, though, for a week. We walked through the university district, talked about modern drama, bought books and records. One morning I woke up and she was gone. I fixed myself breakfast slowly. I noticed that she had left a drawing on my desk. It showed two children looking into what appeared to be a mirror or possibly a pond where several miraculous creatures peeked out and skated on the surface. Deep in the mirror one could make out a face with features that resembled mine and a shape like Nancy's. It looked sadly out of the mirror.

I tried to justify myself. I wrote letters to Nancy which I didn't send. "It's easy to become cold, Nancy. Every day I see people suffering, many of them will die while I watch. Can I put so much love into an enterprise so full of death? That is my constant question." But it is no longer an important point to make. They were not the relevant questions; they were not what mattered. A doctor's life merges with his patients' lives, filled as they are with little victories and little defeats. My dreams are filled with my patients' problems; they keep me busy.

I still remember that absurd argument with Nancy. What was it that I was saying to her? It was about the person I had become. It had nothing to do with medicine. Or did it? I feel that these years have changed me, but how have I changed?

I read about medical diseases on the medical ward late at night, and about biochemical processes. Sometimes I fantasize that they are taking place in this person in Nancy's drawing. I find myself curious even in the face of the endless reading. I must end this tedious monologue with myself. Most of my time is spent in rooms with no windows.

Chapter 9
Motivations and Satisfactions: Growing Up Needed
Michael J. Halberstam, MD

Listen to your patients—they are telling you your future.

There it is, unearthed from my dusty file at Boston University Medical School (why did they bother to save it, anyway?) and written in my painfully clear late-adolescent hand:

> *I grew up in a medical atmosphere (and) from what I have learned from my father and uncle medicine is a profession that is both intellectually and emotionally satisfying—intellectually because of its complexity and constant innovations, emotionally there is nothing because of more immediate definite good than the easing of human pain.*

So *that's* why I wanted to become a doctor—now I remember it all. And certainly the statement must have been true, because Boston University accepted me and I became a doctor and after God knows how many years finally had a practice of my own and it's been just as much fun as—maybe more than—I ever hoped it would be. So certainly the statement must have been true.

Editor's Note: Now in his late thirties, Dr. Halberstam is a practicing physician with special interest in internal medicine and cardiology.

It doesn't pay to be too cynical; the statement was true and yet, of course, it was incomplete. Boston University asked its applicants to limit their statements to 200 words, but that wasn't the major reason it was incomplete.

Take the part about growing up in a medical atmosphere. That was certainly true. Not only were my father and closest uncle physicians, but we lived in an apartment house in the Bronx where, in the depression years, the management had lured physicians by giving them a financial break if both their apartment and their office were in the building. The building was sort of a Mayo Clinic where all the doctors lived over the store. The elevators were crowded with neurologists' wives, pediatricians' children, and internists' patients. All the kids I played with were the children of doctors, and all of them were Jewish. Certainly for us boys medicine was the obvious career choice—it had to be ruled out first, before any other profession could be considered.

Many of us *did* become doctors; others did not. Why did I stay with this one ambition from age seven and never seriously consider anything else? Part of it, I suspect (although I didn't tell Boston University), was fear of death. I don't know that as a child or adolescent I feared death any more than my friends, but it did scare me, and I am sure I thought that by being a doctor I would keep it at bay a little longer. I think I still do.

Then, as my family followed my father from army base to army base in the early days of World War II, I became increasingly aware of the fact that we were Jewish and most other people were not. A great many others, it transpired, did not like Jews. Those were the days, remember, when if you went to a good restaurant or tried to make reservations at a good hotel, they might suddenly decide they were all filled up if your name was Goldberg or Halberstam. But doctors—doctors were always welcome. Rich gentiles came to them and asked them for help. Some were my father's patients. Doctors were not of necessity tied for life into the intensely loving, intensely demanding world of the Bronx, a world that appeared less and less happy to me. Alex Portnoy and I were born in the same year. . . .

Prurience fanned my desire to be a doctor (I certainly didn't tell *that* to Boston University). What did girls look like, feel like? What did they think about, talk about? I found out eventually, but by the time I did a new kind of curiosity plagued me. What about other people's sex lives? Their imaginations? Were they as baroque as my own? Remember, my friend Alex hadn't yet voiced his complaint. This kind of curiosity stayed with me until medical school itself. I was briefly tempted by psychiatry and part of the attraction of the field was, I think, talking about sex. When, as a student, I finally did talk to living patients about their sex lives, the subject turned out to be so anti-erotic that I felt kinship with a virginal but horny classmate whose initial encounter with female genitalia in GYN clinic was so traumatic that it made him doubt if the chase were really worth the effort.

I entered college intending to become a physician, and left with an acceptance in hand. Yet my college years were officially devoted to the study of history and unofficially to an obsessive love affair with the college daily newspaper. I became a journalist and, retrospectively, a good one. In the summers I worked as a reporter for a fine paper in Hartford and during the college year I earned money writing for the Boston papers, but this was small stuff compared to the college paper, where the standards were immeasurably higher, the criticism of one's writing, displayed so all one's colleagues could comment on it, infinitely more vicious and perceptive.

Journalism delighted me. It fed on some of those same quirks that moved me toward medicine—the desire to know all about people, what they thought, how they acted. Friends asked, naturally enough, if I were going into journalism. The college paper's alumni were scattered in powerful positions on papers and magazines all over the country. As undergraduates we knew just who they were, knew that we were of the same heroic mould. Why not join them at *Time* or *Life* or the *Times* or the *Post Dispatch*?

No, I wanted to be a doctor. In journalism you were forever the outsider, watching while others were doing. After a while, the thrill of the press pass would vanish and I would become like the 40-year-old reporters I worked with in the summers, loving their work but hating themselves for loving it. In a way, journalism was almost too easy. I wanted something that a kid like myself just out of college couldn't do, something arcane, hard. I had also been strongly influenced by Tolstoy's view of human events in *War and Peace*, his conviction that it was the ordinary activities of ordinary people which were the most significant, perhaps the only significant, human events.

Like my friends who also applied to medical school, I wanted to know more about people. We wanted to help the sick. There's no doubt about that. We were sincere and idealistic and not particularly neurotic. Reading now my statement to Boston University, I am struck by the fact that I saw the doctor's task as "the easing of human pain." I think I meant it then in the metaphorical sense, encompassing psychic as well as physical pain, but I'm not sure. Certainly the broader idea must have come upon me in medical school, because by the third year I was seriously considering psychiatry. I was good at it, just as I had been good at journalism, but when in my fourth year the late Dr. Ralph Adams of Wolfeboro, New Hampshire looked at me and said, "You will be a psychiatrist—I know it," my spirit rebelled.

Did I become an internist just to spite a fine man now 15 years dead? I doubt it. I didn't have the patience for psychiatry. I was interested in people's problems, yes, but I wanted quick people with quick problems. I had no talent for the ruminative work of psychiatry. And again I was suspicious of something that came so easily, where the sensitive lay person might by flashes of insight unearth psychic truths which escaped the specialist. No one could interpret electrocardiograms by intuition alone.

For a while it looked as though I wouldn't be able to interpret them at all, either by insight or by puzzling over cabalistic diagrams in whole series of texts. Medical school had been no academic triumph, and my internship was not much better. I made mistakes. I still went numb when acid-base balance was discussed. I had doubts about my ability, and again considered retiring to the quieter, safer shores of psychiatry.

The Public Health Service, however, assigned me directly after my internship to a one-doctor station in northern Alaska, an experience from which one emerges either completely shattered or remarkably self-assured. Amazing what one can do all alone if there is no other doctor within 500 miles to help. I delivered babies, set fractures, took x-rays, and learned to read cardiograms. Could there be a more satanic testing place for a semipsychiatrist two weeks out of an academic medical internship and one week married? A year in Barrow outdoes all the LSD, heroin, and other

drugs people take as a scarifying experience. I have always pitied the doctors who had their military experience in Bethesda, Maryland or Atlanta, Georgia.

And so, figuring (falsely) that if I could do Barrow I could do just about anything else, I went to Washington, DC by way of New Mexico and Vermont, hopefully learning as I went. In Burlington, E. L. Amidon bruised the egos and ruffled the rather bland liberalism of his house staff and, in retrospect, it did us some good. We glimpsed, perhaps, the extent to which the conventional liberalism of our Boston and Cambridge instructors was founded on a disdain for money that only a family fortune based on Fall River textile mills could give. Hard scrabble Vermont farm boys were different.

Two years as a cardiac fellow in Washington convinced me, if I needed any further convincing, that research was not my thing and in the spring of 1964, pressed by a need to tell the Yellow Pages what my office address would be, I decided to go into practice in Washington. Originally I planned to practice with a couple of friends, but through some trivial real estate mishap this fell through and I started work as a solo practitioner, and have so remained.

Why single practice, private practice in this era of conglomeration? In part, at first, just to see if it could be done—to see if at age 32 one could finally exist outside the corporate, institutional security blanket. As it progressed I enjoyed it and began to think to myself, "Free at last—Great God Almighty, free at last."

Finally being free of other people's plans for my immediate surroundings was a good feeling. The mistakes to be made would be my own but, so I told myself, I could always take off from the office on a lovely May day and go fishing. Sometimes I did.

Besides the satisfaction it gave me, my little womb of an office was good—is good—for my patients. My patients come to *me*. It's a neat feeling, knowing that these patients have braved the hazards of urban life to come to me. Contrast it to those afternoons when I used to do physical exams on government executives in a little Public Health Service-run office in a government building. The executives were nice enough people and I spent a fair amount of time with them, but damned if I could remember their names from one moment to the next, much less one year to the next. I knew that the reason they were coming to me was because my services were free and I was the doctor in the Health Unit. If I left, another doctor would be in the Health Unit and they would go to him. How different from the wisdom of my private patients, who track me down to my cottage industry office and insist on paying me for my time. What a noble group of people they are!

An ego trip, surely, but we are not saints and when we talk of "satisfactions" we must talk of ego fulfillment. But, though I would insist that for me and many others the private office, fee-for-service relationship becomes a mutually reinforcing transaction in which the best is obtained from both doctor and patient, this isn't true for all physicians or all patients. And certainly the satisfactions of a medical practice in a great city extend beyond the manner in which the practice is conducted.

For medicine gives us a hold on the past and a look to the future. The historical continuity of medicine, the knowledge that great minds have worked for centuries over the problems which baffle us on rounds each morning, becomes increasingly significant. No wonder computer programmers, advertising men, and industrial chemists are often seized with great doubts about their work. No wonder that a college graduate dropped into the world with an AB in English Literature worries about the "relevance" of his education, and suspects that the whole system is wrong. Physicians worry about the importance of their work and the relevance of their education (at least, they *should* worry), but in our worst moments we are sustained, not only by our patients, but by the sense of a long and honorable tradition. Rembrandt painted "The

Anatomy Lesson," not "The Media Brainstorming Session."

The past steadies medicine, but does not anchor it. In our offices, if we are alert, we catch the first scent of changing social patterns.

The past steadies medicine, but does not anchor it. In our offices, if we are alert, we catch the first scent of changing social patterns. That's part of the particular fun of a big-city practice, for the trends show up in the cities first, and they show up in strange ways. A couple of years ago I casually told a young male patient, "Just go into the examining room and take off everything but your underpants." He replied, "Sure, but I don't wear underpants." Okay, the first man like that was a freak, but the next few who didn't wear underpants meant a trend, and so I asked about it and discovered the underground community to be uptight about warm testes, sperm counts, and defective babies. In a similar way I found out about vegetarian diets, communes, drug addicts, hard-hats, and silent Americans, each discovery forcing me on to more reading and thinking.

Listen to your patients. They are telling you your future.

One thing my patients say is that the physician must remain the prime healer in our society. Sometimes this is admitted grudgingly. One young man with gonorrhea came to me after four days of symptoms. "I am a health nut," he said, "and I figured if I could eat the right herb, it would go away." He looked disconsolate about this, and I tried to cheer him up by saying that if the Indians had had penicillin, they no doubt would have used it.

But most patients, "straight" or "freak," don't have theoretical objections to physicians. Technicians may administer multiphasic screening exams and paramedics may ride shotgun on trauma teams, but people who

> *Technicians may administer mul-*
> *tiphasic screening exams and par-*
> *amedics may ride shotgun on*
> *trauma teams, but people who*
> *feel sick will still come to physi-*
> *cians—should still come to physi-*
> *cians, for the degree itself, that*
> *little MD, has wondrous healing*
> *power.*

feel sick will still come to physicians—*should* still come to physicians, for the degree itself, that little MD, has wondrous healing power (it doesn't even have to be an earned MD—unlicensed doctors also have a lot of grateful patients). And, if physicians are still going to be taking care of the sick, we will have to husband our precious bodily fluids and limit our responsibilities elsewhere. We need not renounce our civic and social duties, but we will have to limit them. Medical schools should teach the humanities, anthropology, and urbanology as they relate to individual health, which must remain the core concern of medicine. There is no sense in medical schools turning out second-rate city planners or overtrained social workers.

It is this anachronistic concern for the individual that remains one of the beauties of medical practice. "Freaks" as well as "straights" respond to the idea of working in a one-to-one relationship, strengthening the individual against the sometimes intolerable demands of state, community, and family. Certainly some of the future's best doctors will come from today's underground community. And I would predict that most of today's young radical doctors will be someday practicing in a manner closer to mine than to Kaiser Permanente. It may not be a single practice, fee-for-service office, but it won't be a Pediatrics Collective either.

We will see, too, a reaffirmation of professionalism. It is understandable that confused young people today overreact rebelliously to a concept that has often been synonymous with elitism, and that in their overreaction they have tried to pretend that the professions do not exist. But it is all pretending and the pretense is obvious to patients and other doctors alike. Brilliant young graduates of Exeter and Bronx High School of Science do not become blacks merely by interlacing their speech with "man" and "right on," nor do the children of Winnetka stockbrokers become simple country folk by wearing blue jeans and fringed leather vests. The pretense, painful as it is to me, is certainly much more tiresome to the blacks, chicanos, Puerto Ricans, and other decent people upon whom it is practiced. Neither in dress nor life style nor education can most doctors be honestly anything other than what they are—bright, slightly compulsive members of the middle class.

It is just as silly, however, for a physician to isolate himself from the cultures of his patients as to pretend that he is part of them. The doctor whose social life revolves around a country club where his wife, his children, his colleagues, and his patients meet informally seven times a week to reinforce their own views is as pathetic as little boy blue pretending to be black. Good country doctors have always known this. They respect their farmer-patients without condescending to them. They participate in all aspects of community life—school board, hog-butchering, deer-hunting—but when they have to get drunk they do it at Atlantic City. Is that elitism? Shouldn't a doctor be able to show his weaknesses as well as his strengths? In theory, yes, and someday perhaps, yes. In fact, over a period of time a physician may reveal his weaknesses and eccentricities to a small community and not suffer for it, for he has done so gradually, allowing the community to see his strengths as a physician first. I know of a doctor practicing happily in a small New England town where he lives with his male friend. His homosexuality is not flaunted, but it is there. There is less concealment about it now that his practice has grown. The townspeople say, "Oh sure, Dr. Smith's a homosexual, but he's a fine doctor—he comes when you need him." Smith had already shown as much sensitivity toward the community's prejudices as they have shown toward his.

Medicine, if it is well practiced, brings the physician outside the walls of the monastery or university and into the community. I have finally realized why my friends in New York and Cambridge quote with so much relish what they have been told by their taxi drivers. Those are the only people they speak to all day who don't have a college degree. The taxi ride and the garage stop are the academician's encounter with Middle America. We physicians have our finger on the pulse of Middle America much of the day, and we hear people when they speak of their deepest concerns. Only a fool would fail to be intrigued by the lives as well as the illnesses of his patients.

Clearly medicine has been good to me, as to most of my colleagues. It is honest work, honestly rewarded. In an age of megastructures, it has preserved the individual. In a nation of neophiles it has not forgotten the past. In a time of vague sentimentality it has honored fact. In a time of polarization it has provided an entryway to other cultures. It remains a great calling for young men and women if they are up to it.

Chapter 10
Hippocrates Revisited:
A View from General Practice
John H. Leversee, MD

Hippocrates' strictures on dying and abortion are at variance with current practice, but his appeal to logical and orderly thought in the practice of medicine is as valuable today as it ever was.

THE HIPPOCRATIC OATH

Seldom does one person influence a profession or a branch of science as Hippocrates has done in the field of medicine. His contribution has been very valuable. The Hippocratic Oath is the best known code of ethics or code of conduct presented to the medical profession.

These aphorisms of his times, as set forth in the Oath, have been very helpful and are fascinating to contemplate. The durability of his teachings are all the more remarkable when one realizes they were compiled 400 years before Christ. This kind of wisdom is needed as much now as it was then. How valuable it would be to have such a person give his interpretation of the ethical and moral dilemmas of today.

His was a time when superstition ruled men's minds, and yet Hippocrates believed only in facts. He believed man could discover the laws of nature by studying facts and reasoning from them.

Editor's Note: Dr. Leversee wrote his essay in 1970 at the age of 43. In his article he shows the reader something about the life and rewards of a thoughtful family physician by manifesting the depth and breadth of his ethical and philosophical concerns.

Life is short
And the art long;
The occasion fleeting;
Experiment dangerous
And judgment difficult.
            Hippocrates · *Aphorisms I*

His application of logic and reason made the practice of medicine workable.

And yet, one must place the Oath in perspective. Webster's dictionary tells us that an aphorism is a statement of principle, a terse formulation of a truth or sentiment. Just as it was important that Hippocrates set forth his statements, we must recognize that new knowledge broadens one's horizons—truth changes a person's sentiments and helps formulate new principles.

A literal interpretation of the Hippocratic Oath in the twentieth century would be contrary to the very principle of application of fact that was so important to Hippocrates. Time does change most, if not all, things. The passage of 24 centuries certainly changes the circumstances under which one must interpret facts. To recognize the necessity of change one merely has to recall that Hippocrates' favorite diet for ill persons was a barley gruel and his favorite medicine was honey: ''The drink to be employed should there be any pain is vinegar and honey. If there be great thirst, give water and honey.'' He admonished against performing surgery—''I will not cut a person who is suffering with a stone, but will leave this to be done by practitioners of this work''—and yet he repaired wounds, reduced fractures or dislocations, and bored holes in the skull.

Thus, it seems to me, we must see his principles in their broadest sense and not be bogged down by literal interpretations. Change is inevitable. As Paul Goodman stated, ''Human society does not let one be —it is too total—it forces one's hand.'' It strikes me that several sections of the Oath are particularly vulnerable and could be improved with reinterpretation in the light of present knowledge and the needs of this century.

REINTERPRETING THE OATH   ''A knowledge of the Art will be taught to his sons, the sons of his teachers and to disciples bound by stipulation and oath; according to the law of medicine, but to none others.''

The foregoing statement is not applicable to present-day medical education. Medical science is so immensely more complex in our times that teaching by apprenticeship or disciple is no longer possible. Health science educators and planners have greatly broadened their outreach to candidates for careers in medicine and related fields.

As never before, we are entering an era in which the health care delivery system is being reevaluated. New fields of medicine are developing. There is a growing recognition of the need to expand the number of persons involved in giving health care, and not only are numbers being increased. There is also a new emphasis on training paramedic personnel in broader areas of skills and responsibilities. The doors to training in the medical sciences have been opened or are being opened

to many persons previously denied entry. It is no longer a particular advantage to be a son or daughter of a doctor or teacher of medicine. Motivation and performance are more important than legacy. Thus, bright young persons from minority groups and others with no family connection with medicine are gaining entry to education in the health sciences. By moving in this direction, the Oath is perhaps being heeded more than we think, for these persons may be more highly motivated and more firmly ''bound by a stipulation and oath, according to the law of medicine.''

In the practice of medicine today one is faced with new dimensions of difficulty in interpreting life and death. The new methods and machines available to him pose a great

---

The new methods and machines available to him pose a great dilemma for the doctor: is he prolonging living or merely prolonging dying?

---

dilemma for the doctor: is he prolonging living or merely prolonging dying? Hippocrates inveighs, ''I will give no deadly medicine to anyone if asked nor suggest any such counsel.''

The basic premise of this admonition is undeniable. However, we have long since passed into an era of complexities unimaginable 24 centuries ago. In Hippocrates' time, life or death was measured by the presence or absence of perceptible pulse or respiration. This definition persisted until recent times. As a medical student, I can recall being called upon to determine if someone had died. I placed a stethoscope over the heart and listened and listened, making certain that there was no discernible heartbeat, and then made the pronouncement that the patient had indeed passed away. The nurses would cover the deceased and the relatives would be notified. It was quite simple; no heartbeat, no life.

THE QUESTION OF LIFE

It is no longer that simple. Now quite the opposite is often the case. When a patient's pulse is no longer discernible lifesaving measures may be doubled. A team of doctors and nurses especially skilled in resuscitation takes over. Numerous complicated machines are part of the team. A pulse may return and respirations continue, either spontaneously or with support.

WHEN IS A PERSON DEAD? This is well and good and as it should be—up to a point. However, the real dilemma soon begins. Is the patient dead or alive? How is this to be determined—and by whom? The physician has the heaviest and most immediate responsibility and needs answers urgently. For a long time he has had to make decisions about the patient who is in the process of dying, but only recently has he had much power to influence the outcome. In some instances he now has considerable control over the time of death and

---

We must learn to define death, or learn to define life so that the absence of life can mean death.

---

the nature of living or dying. We must learn to define death, or learn to define life so that the absence of life can mean death.

If one uses the legal definition for determining the time of death, this can be found in Black's Law Dictionary as, "The cessation of life; ceasing to exist; defined by physicians as the total stoppage of circulation of the blood and a cessation of the animal and vital functions consequent thereon, such as respiration, pulsation, etc."

However, respirations can be restarted or be carried on by machines and the heart can be restarted once it has stopped. We must therefore develop a new definition for death. New attempts to define death emphasize brain function as a major criterion. The most widely recognized new definition of brain death, "A Definition of Irreversible Coma," was set forth by an ad hoc committee of the Harvard Medical School.[1] The following points were established as criteria:

Unreceptivity and unresponsivity (ie, no response even to painful stimuli).

No muscular movement and no spontaneous breathing for at least one hour, or for three minutes if a mechanical respirator is turned off.

No elicitable reflexes, ocular movements, or blinking, and the presence of fixed dilated pupils.

A flat isoelectric electroencephalogram (EEG).

No change when all of these tests are repeated at least 24 hours later.

These criteria to be exclusive of two conditions: hypothermia (body temperature below 90° F) or central nervous system depression due to drugs such as barbiturates.

These criteria are helpful and are a step forward but are lacking in some important areas. New consideration must be given to time factors in the pronouncement of death because of the success of organ transplants. Various organs such as kidney, liver, lung, bowel, cornea, heart, and skin have been transplanted, all with varying success. These organs die at varying rates and too long a period of time in deciding that the "death" of a person has occurred may make certain organs unsuitable for transplanting. As these new definitions are worked out, some consideration for the legal protection of the medical team must be taken.

Certainly life has come to mean much more than the presence of circulation. An adequate level of brain function almost certainly must enter into the definition. There has to be some ability to respond to outside stimuli, to act and react to one's environment. The patient must be able to function as a person, not just register baseline responses on bedside machinery. In fact, this ability has to be considerably above animal responses and abilities for the patient to have a reasonable chance for a worthwhile and fulfilling life. The level of responses necessary for this will vary greatly between individuals and family groups. Very likely no hard and fast levels will ever be defined, but definition of life must include some reference to higher brain function.

In clinical practice a physician comes face to face with these difficult decisions and is more often than not the primary resource the family looks to for help in their dilemma. In addition to the presence of circulation, respiration, and brain function in the definition of life, one soon recognizes that there must be an evaluation of the extent of brain capability. One is inescapably drawn toward an evaluation of the meaning of life or the quality of life possible for that individual. It seems to me that being alive requires the ability to interact with another person, with a person's family or with society—in order to be able to function as a person. One would like the patient to retain the potential to be a responsible and responsive adult, maintaining some dignity and self-respect. The quality of the potential life left to the dying person must be a consideration. If our patient is old, infirm, limited, and uncomfortable, can we really make his remaining time fulfilling and productive for that individual or his family? And what about the younger person so grievously brain injured that future function will be almost meaningless? Prolonging "life" in this case might be counterproductive for all concerned. Perhaps we would only be adding to the unhappiness of an ever-increasing number of people.

One must consider the feelings and needs of the family. Perhaps they have emotional needs that are best met by prolonged care even if it is fruitless. If the patient is beyond suffering and is staying "alive" even with minimal function, he may be serving a useful purpose in life in meeting the needs of his family. On the other hand, a person who because of injury, disease, or aging has descended to a level of minimal function may be so foreign or re-

pugnant to a family or loved one that they will demand that no means be undertaken to prolong life. The family may prefer to remember the person as he once was. He will go on living for them in memory in a much more satisfying way than that which remains in the intensive-care facilities.

MORAL DECISIONS   In making these decisions, the physician is often torn between his obligation to preserve life and restore function or his obligation to relieve suffering and to allow the patient, if he must die, to die with comfort and dignity. Given a patient who, in the doctor's best judgment, has no chance for recovery, what should he do? To what lengths should he go to prolong life? The right to die in dignity is a problem more often raised by our successes in medicine than by our failures. Nietzsche has observed, "In certain cases it is indecent to go on living." It shows a lack of self-respect "to vegetate in a state of cowardly dependence upon doctors and special treatments, once the meaning of life, the right to life has been lost."

In pondering the moral questions raised in these difficult areas, some organized religions have been very helpful. Spokesmen for the Church of England and the Roman Catholic Church (Pope Pius XII, 1957) have taken the position that it is the moral duty of the physician not to prolong dying if life cannot be preserved.

The answer almost always involves making a value judgment. A doctor is not infallible; he may be wrong in his diagnosis and his prognosis. The patient's attitude, as well as that of the family, may change during a prolonged and difficult terminal illness. It is important for the doctor to maintain communication not only to help the family make decisions but to detect changes in feelings.

Society's attitudes about dying are changing. It is not uncommon for a family to come to my office and inquire about the attitudes toward death and dying. They may have reached an understanding among themselves and the infirm elderly member of the family in which no one wishes to employ unusual or overzealous treatment to prolong dying. They don't wish to come into conflict with me over terminal care. They may believe that death is good and acceptable and comes as a blessing to end the suffering when the will to live has gone, particularly after a full and fruitful life. They are reassured when I tell them I concur with their feelings in these matters.

Somehow we have to place death in its proper perspective. A majority attitude in America, it seems to me, has been that every problem has a solution. We should somehow be able to restore everyone. Death is just not acceptable. Even its inevitability is not accepted. Nevertheless death is inevitable and it does have a proper place and natural place in the total life process. The Society of Friends (Quakers)[2] believe, "Death should be viewed in proper perspective as a natural part of the process of life. We believe in its necessity and goodness as well as its inevitability."

One must realize in this discussion that the life span of man has not been appreciably lengthened in recent years and it is not likely to be lengthened in the foreseeable future.[3] Granted a higher percentage of persons will live until the later years of their life span, but this is not the same as prolonging the life span. If we are not making life longer, are we making it any better? Perhaps we are only adding to the unhappiness of an ever-increasing number of people. There must come a time when death is a reasonable or even preferable alternative.

There is no question that physicians need to spend more time in preparing for these decisions. Our current policies often show considerable ambivalence because we have not thought out our priorities. When faced with a difficult moral and ethical decision such as I have been discussing, it may be helpful to use a team approach and enlist the aid of religious, legal, social, and other medical advice. The doctor, the nurse, the minister, the patient, and the family should face this with insight, compassion, and intelligence.

Further consideration must be given to the realization that our health resources as presently constituted are not infinite. When we keep a patient "alive" with machines or infusions, we are doing this at an expenditure in terms of dollars and health resources that has to be subtracted from some other person's health care. Is the extra life span and the degree of rehabilitation possible worth the discomfort, the psychological hazards, the long stay in the hospital, the enormous cost, and the tying up of a large part of a hospital staff when other patients need care? The answers always involve difficult judgments. I believe we must more carefully think through our priorities and the mechanisms by which we reach our decisions.

WHEN DOES LIFE BEGIN? "I will not give to a woman an instrument to produce abortion." Hippocrates makes this statement without qualification or clarification. And yet, perhaps more than in any other issue in medicine, the attitudes and mores surrounding abortion have changed throughout the centuries and are changing dramatically in our present times. In case any of you have felt that Hippocrates' admonition has been observed inviolate throughout the centuries, this is just not the case. Even the ancient Greeks did not heed Hippocrates' dictum. Plato and his pupil Aristotle, who lived just after Hippocrates, differed from his views. Aristotle advocated abortion as a means of keeping population growth in bounds and Plato recommended abortion for all women over 40 years of age.

Most doctors in the United States favor liberalizing abortion laws. Polls have shown that as high as 87% favor some change. Organized religions have views that differ from one another and some have changed their own views over the years. Some religions approve terminating pregnancy if it is early but prohibit this after a certain state of fetal development. The time of ensoulment has been used as a limit beyond which pregnancy may not be terminated. However, religious opinion varies greatly as to the exact time of ensoulment. Within the same church (Roman Catholic), the timing pronouncement has changed from early to later and now all the way back to the moment of fertilization. For a period it held that the time of ensoulment varied between the sexes.

Scientists at the present time cannot determine the moment when life begins. Cinemicrographs have been taken of lower-animal embryo growth and one can observe the moment in development when the heart first contracts and circulation begins, but as we have discussed earlier, this is not necessarily synonymous with life. Many in the biochemical and biological fields believe that life is continuous, for it exists in the ovum and the sperm before conception and then has varying potential at every stage of development. There is a high percentage of loss at each stage of development. The majority of fertilized ova are rejected at an early stage because of developmental abnormalities; therefore preventing pregnancy or terminating early pregnancy may not be so dissimilar, and both probably have much more to do with life potential than with ending life. In any event, women have sought out and found ways of terminating pregnancies throughout recorded history. In the past this has been an extremely dangerous procedure. A disturbing number of women have lost their lives. In the nineteenth century an abortion done by anyone, even in a hospital, was a high-risk procedure because of the dangers of infection and hemorrhage. It was more dangerous to interrupt a pregnancy than to carry it to term. This situation and other contributing factors resulted in the development of restrictive laws pertaining to abortion.

New procedures have changed this risk. Abortions can be done much more skillfully and safely. Complications are few and can usually be effectively controlled. Now the risk from abortion is less than that of a pregnancy carried to full term. The laws that once protected the patient now often force her to accept a greater risk—by either continuing a pregnancy or sometimes seeking out a criminal abortion.

Even though some states have liberalized their abortion laws, the majority of states still have legal obstacles that make abortions difficult to obtain. Some indications for abortion are accepted medically and legally, but these vary from state to state and hospital to hospital. Because of severe infirmity and to protect the life of the woman, an abortion may be allowed. Such indications are rare. However, it is important to realize that this permission recognizes that in these instances allowing the pregnancy to continue carries the greater risk. Most psychiatric opinions hold that emotional stresses are greater in the pregnancy that is forced to go to term. Carrying an unwanted pregnancy a full nine months causes more psychic trauma in the vast majority of cases than does a prompt and safe termination. This has been true for women in and out of wedlock, even with the added guilt of breaking the law in seeking criminal abortion and the anxiety inherent in being treated by an unfamiliar, possibly poorly trained person, outside of accepted health care channels. Jerome Kummer, a Los Angeles psychiatrist, among others, has written extensively and convincingly about this. Rape, incest, and extreme youth have been accepted as reasons for terminating pregnancy. Recently, fetal indications have been added. Major genetic risks are sometimes predictable. Defective development can sometimes be determined in utero early enough so that a safe termination of pregnancy can be carried out. A good example of this is Down's syndrome (mongolism). This technique will undoubtedly become more refined and more available for widespread use.

The previously mentioned indications for abortion—physical and mental health of the woman, rape, incest, extreme youth, and fetal indications—have been fairly well accepted by the majority of persons in medicine. Two other indications are now being advocated. First, the rights of individuals have broadened considerably in modern times, particularly for women. It is now the opinion of many legal authorities that a woman should have the right to determine her own reproductive capacity and that the state does not have the right to force a woman to continue a pregnancy that she did not want and does not want to continue. There is reason to believe that the courts will soon invalidate the present restrictive laws. The second and perhaps more compelling reason for abortion is the runaway population growth being experienced throughout the world. Never before has our nation or the entire world faced such a threat. Prestigious medical leaders are now advocating that abortion be available for those who wish it as a temporary means of holding population growth to a manageable level, and that this be available until better means of pregnancy prevention are available to all who desire to limit family size. Dr. Duncan Reid, chairman of the Department of Obstetrics and Gynecology at Harvard University Medical School, recently advocated this use of abortion and urged that the medical profession hasten development of procedures and facilities so that abortions can be done on a large scale.

HIPPOCRATES REVISITED

In my opinion, Hippocrates' strictures on dying and abortion are more at variance with current practice and current needs of society than other sections of the Oath.

Even though portions of Hippocrates' teachings are not applicable to our present-day circumstances, he remains a giant in the history of medicine. The experiences and wisdom of the great men of the past can be very valuable if we choose to learn from them. Hippocrates' appeal to logical and orderly thought in the practice of medicine is as valuable today as it ever was. He developed and advocated a systematized approach to diagnosis and treatment. He also recognized the importance of dealing with the whole person in evaluating a disease.

As a general practitioner this appeals to me. Disease or lack of disease must be interpreted in the light of the patient's entire environment and personality. One must have some recognition of the patient's strengths and weaknesses and the important factors in his environment that may cause stress or protect him from stress. The ability to look at a patient as a functioning human being and not just as an isolated organ system with disease cuts across lines of specialization. A wise physician can ask the question or pick up the clue that identifies a patient's real needs and perhaps uncovers the factors which help create the organ system illness.

The personality of a physician may just happen to mesh with that of a patient so that he is in a unique position to understand and help that patient. This opportunity is not circumscribed by specialty. I have found referral physicians uncovering facets of a patient's being that the patient did not reveal to me. However, all too often, a presenting symptom is evaluated in terms of the specialty organ system only, and if no obvious pathology exists the patient is sent back to the referring physician as "OK." There may be no opportunity for the specialist to be like Hippocrates and deal with the whole patient and his overall needs, but I would like to enter a plea to make use of an opening if one comes along.

I am afraid that our health care delivery system is so fragmentary and organ oriented that the patient is figuratively torn apart. More and more, medicine in the United States moves in a direction that defines and protects what is good for a particular doctor or his specialty. If this pattern doesn't happen to fit the needs of the patient, then the patient just doesn't understand modern medicine or is neurotic or in some way a misfit.

Perhaps recruiting candidates to study medicine must change—as it is indeed changing. Applicants for medical schools have traditionally been selected for proficiency in the sciences and not for any knowledge of history, philosophy, or the humanities. Most persons delivering health care in our present system are primarily scientists and may or may not be humanitarians. In my opinion we need a more humanitarian approach to medical care.

I further believe it is easier to teach a humanitarian to be a scientist than it is to teach a scientist to be a humanitarian.

We need a more humanitarian approach to medical care.

The following quotation is from Thomas H. Huxley: "Men of science do not pledge themselves to creeds; they are bound by articles of no sort; there is not a single belief that is not a bounden duty with them to hold with a light hand and to part with it cheerfully, the moment it is really proved to be contrary to any fact, great or small. Our great purpose is the improvement of Man's estate and the widening of his knowledge. The moment a concept ceases to be useful for this purpose, away with it to the four winds; we care not what becomes of it." I think what Huxley says is somewhat applicable to the parts of the Oath that have been presented in this discussion. Medicine does change as do all things. Interpretations of Hippocrates' writings will also change. Much in medicine will always remain a dilemma. Those of us in medicine today can be thankful for Hippocrates' contribution.

REFERENCES

1 Beecher HK, Adams RD, Borger AC, et al: A definition of irreversible coma. Report of the Ad Hoc Committee of the Harvard Medical School to Examine the Definition of Brain Death. *JAMA* 205:337–340, 1968.
2 *Who Shall Live—Man's Control Over Birth and Death.* A report prepared for the American Friends Service Committee. New York, Hill & Wang, 1970.
3 Huxley J: The Future of Man—Evolutionary Aspect, in Ciba Foundation, *Man and His Future*, Gordon Wolstenholme (ed), Boston, Little Brown & Co, 1963.

Chapter 11
Affect or Fact
Ralph G. Victor, MD

Physicians and medical educators must also attempt to emphasize affective relationships and human values along with technical knowledge so that ultimately the whole person may benefit.

Recently, at one of the psychiatric teaching sessions arranged for first-year medical students, the professor interrupted his lecture. He then asked some students wearing open shirts without white coats to dress more properly for the occasion. The professor in question had arranged for some patients to be interviewed in front of the class and felt uncomfortable about the appearance of these students, who did not look the way medical students traditionally were supposed to look. Quickly, this matter became a major issue between the students and the professor. The students challenged their teacher to tell them why it should make any difference how they were dressed. They felt strongly that personal appearance has nothing to do with professional competence, and that particularly the doctor's white coat was more of a uniform than anything else and had no special im-

Editor's Note: Dr. Victor has had a vast and varied clinical experience both in the United States and in India. He is now Director of Mental Health Services, Fresno Community Hospital, Fresno, California.

portance. The students were not really interested in the professor's counterarguments, which included his thinking that professional appearance indeed facilitated certain professional relationships. By externally defining a role, the work of the physician was made easier.

On another occasion, in giving a series of lectures to an evening class, I was interrupted and challenged by a young man who objected to what was going on. The sessions had been set up to consist of a one-hour presentation of factual information, and a second hour in which this material could be discussed. This seemed reasonable to me. However, the objecting student expressed the point of view that the times had passed when professors could stand in front of a class and give lectures. All such material could supposedly be obtained from other sources, and besides, it was unimportant anyway. What was important to the objecting student was that his emotions be engaged. This should be the primary purpose of teaching. Facts are secondary.

TODAY'S STUDENTS

The new moral vision of modern students is both refreshing and challenging for the older generation. Before attempting to find some of the causes for the profound attitudinal changes, I will try to describe them. Essentially, there is a rejection of the subordination of emotional and sensory experiences to the rational faculties, to reason. A demand is often expressed that the dominant, almost exclusive position granted to cultivation of the intellect be modified to include more attention to developing affective and aesthetic capacities. This demand may be perceived by some as a form of anti-intellectualism. There is profound dissatisfaction that, in the academic setting, development is primarily thought of as development of rational faculties. Reason is suspect not because it is necessarily defective, but because teachers use it to the exclusion of other values. In a recent confrontation at one of our colleges, the leader of the militants accused one professor (who had actually been helpful to the student and understanding about the militant's viewpoint) of being a middle-aged, white liberal who tried to use reason to understand and settle issues. To most of us in the older generation, being liberal and rational seems highly desirable. Yet, in the mind of this student, these were among the worst insults to hurl at a teacher.

FEELINGS Feeling is especially important, just because it cannot be subjected to critical and rational analysis. Thus, it enables the young person to defend himself against the dominance of older people, and by elevating feeling as a special virtue each individual, especially young individuals, can live in the conviction that he is superior because he can feel more intensely. It is quite easy to agree that feeling indeed is important, but feeling, just like knowledge and learning, has to go through a process of maturation and learning from early infancy to adulthood. The feelings of a young adolescent or a young adult may

be genuine and profound; as a matter of fact, they usually are. Nevertheless, this does not mean that acting on these feelings will necessarily bring solutions to problems or make the world a better and easier place in which to live. What really matters is how these feelings are used.

HIPPOCRATES Do subjective feelings have a place in scientific endeavors, and particularly in the practice of medicine? If they do, is this a new phenomenon, or do we find any evidence that there is awareness and respect for affective interrelationships, apart from strictly systemic, usually descriptive approaches? Since in this volume we are more specifically concerned about Hippocrates, we might raise a specific question about how relevant he would find the values which he expressed or which were expressed by his contemporaries, if he visited us at this time. In the tradition of his time, he was deeply interested in the etiology of diseases and finding cures based on the established causes. He seems to have concluded that many diseases were self-limited, and required no active interference on the part of the physician. Was this a reaction against certain practices of his time (perhaps somewhat parallel to the present) in which there was an overemphasis on overtreatment and a mechanistic manner of approaching disease?

Perhaps this is paralleled by the uneasiness the present-day medical student feels about technical aspects of modern diagnostic methods and treatments. Much of modern medicine has become highly mechanistic. An attempt is made to find a cause for every symptom. Frequently the cause is identified by impersonal laboratory tests or physical means. Treatment to follow must be action oriented; something very tangible must be done. In this process the physician as a person may play a very minor part, casting himself or being cast into the role of the highly trained technician. There is no question that computerized blood tests, computerized data collection, and often dramatic surgical or pharmaceutical interference have produced worthwhile and highly significant advances in modern diagnosis and therapy. But Hippocrates today might be drawn more closely to the student concerned about affective relationships than to the allergist, cardiac surgeon, or biochemical professor, even if he had the technical knowledge to understand what they would be talking about. He and the student might agree that a vital element in patient care is undefinable and by present standards probably quite unscientific. To Hippocrates it might have meant "doing nothing" and waiting for the disease to run its natural course. To the student this might be restated to mean that the ingredient most needed for getting a person well often is in the affective relationship between the sick person and his physician.

TECHNICAL ADVANCES

Are many students, then, trying to stop technical advances? Are they trying to use violent means to accomplish this, just as the cotton pickers tried to destroy the new machines or the longshoremen's strikes attempt to delay using containerized cargo? Rollo May's formulations are of help in thinking about this conflict in values. He writes about the fact that the crisis of modern man is the crisis of "loss of significance." The population explosion, the computer, the nuclear bomb, the enormous power of the military-industrial complex—all combine to make the individual feel helpless, insignificant, and anxious. For the individual, this increased anxiety is dealt with by withdrawal, violence, and alienation.

Technical changes are occurring at an increasingly rapid rate. The rapidity of change leads to conflict with fixed values and results in profound effects on the individual, as well as society at large. The rate of change is increasing for mathematical reasons. New tools are invented all the time. Allen Wheelis has made an analysis of the shifting values of modern times. The more tools there are in existence, the more new tool combinations are possible. What is new is not the fact that

social character is changing—this has always been in process; what is new is the more rapid rate, and our awareness of the change as it takes place.

A recent ad by the Pacific Northwest Bell, part of the nationwide Bell system, commented: "We are trying to prepare children for a future in which some 60 percent of them will hold jobs which haven't been invented yet. When President Eisenhower was re-elected in 1956, there was not a single commercial jet airplane flying in America. Computers were exotic machines used only by a few rich companies . . . but the knowledge explosion is only beginning. Current estimates are that man will increase his fund of information by over sixty times in the next thirty-five years." As the Washington State Superintendent of Public Instruction, Louis Bruno, put it in 1968: "If half the future occupations of today's child do not exist, retraining of today's skilled workers will be required every 12 to 15 years—how can the graduate of 1985 store enough facts in 12 or 16 years of formal schooling to serve him for the next 40?" What is both predictable and essential is that children must be given the tools and methods to think; there is a whole new way of teaching. In fact, the word teaching is out; the key word now is discovery. The child must discover for himself. That is the true way to learn. Many present-day medical students are seriously reacting against the traditional methods of teaching. Their sense of irrelevancy may be an indirect response to the type of questions raised, as the advertisement quoted further emphasizes.

In his psychiatric writing, Harry Stack Sullivan talks about "security operation." He refers to the fact that, in the face of overwhelming anxiety, individuals tend to construct life situations in such a way as to experience the minimum insecurity. Obviously, this may result in very neurotic responses. Faced with the certainty that most facts learned now will be completely out of date a few years from now, or at best a decade or two from now, the modern medical student's emphasis on knowledge requires a new search for what the contents of knowledge should be. Obviously, a security operation in the face of all the facts presented would be a denial that facts are important at all, an attempt to seek refuge in purely affective relationships.

NEW VALUES   In challenging the professor, his facts, and definitions, and in rejecting his values, the student attempts to define a new set of values. But because there may be a rejection of the very basis of traditional scientific methodology, of the rational, measured, quantitated, defined approach, a meaningful dialogue may be quite difficult. It is almost as if the young person were saying, "I am not interested in your facts. I do not want to think of consequences, logical cause and effect, relationships, and long-term goals. Before I can use your facts, they will probably be totally out of date. Or maybe I will be dead, with most of mankind. The future is too uncertain for me to be thinking much about it. Life is *now;* I shall not worry about the tomorrow because I cannot influence what is to come. You may call me irresponsible, but living totally in the present indeed means that I do not feel responsible for the future."

Would Hippocrates have been able to relate to this attitude of modern students? It is likely that he would have been utterly shocked by the challenges the students present to their teachers, and by their views. The relationship between teacher and student in his days, and until very recently throughout the world, was a truly rigid one, controlled by standards of obedience and respect. It is true that students did rebel in particular cases, even as recently as in the late fifties. But their defiance was usually specific. Students defied authority without creating any theory that something else should be put in its place.

CONFRONTATIONS   As yet we have no historical perspective about our own time, of course. But it is quite possible that future historians will call this the "age of confrontation." Confrontation, per se, is not new, yet the essential

issues during the first half of this century were primarily economic. They were best exemplified by struggles between employees and employers, and the development of effective and powerful labor unions, particularly in Western countries. It is also true that ideological struggles between conflicting views, religious or national, have a history dating back thousands of years. But what seems new, certainly on a massive scale throughout the world, is the direct confrontation between teachers and students, parents and children, racial minorities and their alleged or real oppressors, priests or ministers and the church hierarchy, welfare recipients and public social services, and more generally, the consumers and the suppliers of goods and services. Some social analysts wonder if this phenomenon of the young rebelling against the old may not always have happened. Others wonder if the present generation of young people is not simply a bit more intense. To view the massive confrontations so superficially seems to ignore their true significance.

The historian H. Stuart Hughes comments on this. "Such a sudden shift to a revolutionary temper has occurred many times before in the history of Western nations, although it is unfamiliar to the American experience. What has been unusual about the insurgent mood of the past half decade has been its juxtaposition of anarchism and the peremptory silencing of opponents. Its peculiar blend of political puritanism and personal license, its cult of confrontation as a quasi-religious act of witness. Together this complex of attitudes suggests something quite different from the conventional revolutionary aim of seizing the means of production or the implements of power and redirecting them for the benefit of the masses. It suggests, rather, a basically unpolitical aspiration to see through, to unmask, to strip—literally as well as figuratively—down to total nakedness. The goal is psychological, or to use old fashioned vocabulary, spiritual, and marks the culmination of a quarter century of amateur psychologizing among the young. Such a characterization would doubtlessly surprise a great number of the unmaskers themselves. A sense of history is not their strong point. Indeed, in listening to them, one has the impression that in their minds history begins with the catastrophes of the mid-decade that shook them into awareness.''

PSYCHOLOGY Amateur psychologizing among the young is indeed a phenomenon characteristic of recent decades. The modern psychotherapist finds considerable sophistication in his patients, and the strictly interpreted and intellectual parts of therapy often meet with rapid understanding by the patient. He has been trained to think in psychological terms. As he wonders about who he is and where he stands, he has awareness about himself. Modern man has become more aware of "covert" motivations. Passivity, anxiety, disguised hostility, masochism, and latent homosexuality are not new with the present generation, but the awareness of them is new. This awareness is mostly a result of modern man's prolongation of psychological development. In earlier years, most men and women assumed adult responsibilities in childhood or at puberty. Extending education and postponing adulthood has opened new possibilities to millions of young men and women for developing a degree of emotional maturity, ethical commitment, and intellectual sophistication that was once only open to a tiny minority. Because of greater independence of thought, emotional development, and ethical commitment, men and women will be more complex, more finely differentiated and psychologically integrated, and will be more developed as people.

But the greater development in complexity also leads to greater vulnerability. It is another major cause of anxiety, and instead of being useful for a richer and more constructive style of living, may lead to withdrawal and a sense of hopelessness. The ascendancy of technological man may be bitterly resisted. It may create new humanistic countercultures devoted to all that technological man minimizes. It will emphasize feeling, intensity of personal relationships, fantasy, and the exploration and expansion of consciousness.

When Adlai Stevenson ran for the presidency against Eisenhower, he was described as an individual who was much tormented because he could always see two sides of a question. He supposedly stayed awake nights worrying about decisions. On the other hand, Eisenhower apparently had no difficulties about self-doubt after he had made a decision. The age difference between these two presidential aspirants was not more than a decade or two, yet in a way they represented two entirely different value systems. Eisenhower exemplified the value system of our grandparents, where character was supposed to be fixed and rigid, where ideas and principles were firmly established, and where nobody worried about being rigid. Stevenson seemed to be more closely related to the conflicts of modern man. Nowadays, all commitments are made more tentative: social, vocational, marital, and moral. The individual faces much uncertainty. He knows much about himself and his emotions, but it is difficult for him to establish his own sense of belonging, his own identity. Psychological sophistication gives both greater awareness and also leads to greater uncertainties and doubts.

When there is doubt about oneself—a feeling of insecurity, a sense of alienation, or at least a question about the significance of one's own life—it results in the challenging of all existing values. As the individual is less certain about himself and more aware of covert motivation, he doubts not only himself but others. Parents, educators, law enforcement agencies, and others base their authority on good reason, often given to the young person with careful explanations about the benefit this authority can extend to him. Yet the new knowledge of differentiating between overt and covert motivation not only gives the potential of greater psychological insight and vulnerability to the individual—it is also extended to others. Nobody is really to be trusted, either oneself or others.

The resulting confrontation may then take

on an irrational and extreme form. This confrontation has been disturbing to established medical institutions and some major professional associations. Yet the challenge the students present to the medical educators must not only be looked upon as a challenge of authority, though this is the result of the unrest, but also as a sincere search for new values, applicable to modern times. Because medical education is primarily in the hands of sober, intelligent, "sane" scientists and administrators, almost invariably individuals well grounded in the natural sciences, there is a real danger that alienation will increase, or that future doctors will be too much like their teachers, since the "rebels" will not be able to graduate. It seems that the real problem

---

It seems that the real problem presented is that too much value may be given to the accumulation and presentation of hard facts, while other values which may be so much harder to define are deprecated or even rejected.

---

presented is that too much value may be given to the accumulation and presentation of hard facts, while other values which may be so much harder to define are deprecated or even rejected. The argument is not in favor of an unscientific approach, but favors defining what is scientific. The old concept that aspects of health and disease, of emotions and personality must be fitted into a well-defined, essentially quantitative system bears continued critical observation. The most deliciously prepared meal in a restaurant can be spoiled by an unfriendly waiter. The most scientific concoction of remedies may fail to relieve an individual of his suffering if he is looked upon as a mechanism rather than a human being. But perhaps there is a need to really accept the fact that man is not a rational creature, and that in dealing with people or patients certain ill-defined components make up an

important part of communication. It seems trite to state this, since it has been said in one form or another many times before. Yet in most medical schools adequate teaching and discussion of man as an irrational, needful, lonely, anxious creature is only given lip service, or taught in a highly compartmentalized fashion in the department of psychiatry. There are so many "hard facts" to master

---

There are so many "hard facts" to master relating to medicine as a science that little time is left to look more closely at medicine as an art.

---

relating to medicine as a science that little time is left to look more closely at medicine as an art—allowing for some poorly defined boundaries, creative speculation, and a mixture of uncertain ingredients.

I believe I felt some of this restlessness and self-doubt when I undertook two major changes in my own medical work a few years ago. First, while practicing in a large city as a specialist in internal medicine, I accepted an assignment of several years' duration in rural India, working with the American Friends Service Committee in cooperation with the government of India as a medical volunteer in an Indian village. Following my return, I made two shorter trips to India. Secondly, some years ago I decided to completely abandon my medical practice and accept a three-year residency in psychiatry. At present I am active as a full-time psychiatrist. It is difficult to write about oneself and one's own motivations, particularly after having undergone some psychiatric training. Psychiatric training emphasizes skepticism and the ability to look for reasons behind reasons. Debunking becomes a habit, and idealistic motivation is quickly reduced to concepts such as exhibitionism or passive-aggressive drives. I am therefore reluctant to use noble terms such as service to mankind and sharing with the poor. Yet it is fair to say that one reason, even though not the only one, for accepting the great challenge of moving to a village in India was a direct result of feeling that I was turning utterly middle class, beginning to accumulate wealth, and that in many respects life seemed too easy—too early in life. I was about 38 years old at that time.

PRACTICE IN INDIA

On a personal level, the years in India taught me a great deal about myself, both in a positive and in a negative way. I was definitely cured of an "Albert Schweitzer complex"— trying to emulate the great philosopher, musician, and doctor. There was only limited enjoyment in practicing medicine under primitive conditions. I had been trained to be fairly thorough and detailed, and to use tests and procedures to back up diagnostic impressions. It was thus difficult to have a heavy volume practice with little follow-up and mostly symptomatic treatment. Yet there was also the satisfaction of really being needed at times and of being able to use dormant skills rarely brought into play in the practice of an internist in a large city. I did simple dental work, handled a few obstetrical emergencies, and worked with my hands, even though probably not with very great skill. There was the satisfaction of knowing that I had the physical and emotional capability to enjoy life under rather primitive conditions.

The actual practice of medicine, though devoid of most technical aids, was not more personalized than it is in the United States. The sheer number of people who had to be seen made them seem to be part of humanity rather than many individuals. The fringe benefits came mostly outside the practice of medicine. This is where the human adventures occurred: the poor weavers who had finally received commissions for work, yet found it most important not to let work interfere with meetings where religious and philosophical questions were discussed for days—the customers could wait; the surprise expressed by some

village elders when a distinguished American visitor insisted he had to leave in the midst of interesting talks and discussions which he seemed to enjoy greatly, and their comments to each other, "Americans measure time"; the ever-present nearness of birth and death with no skill or attempt at hiding the ugliness and tragedy of death, as is done in our own culture; the unusual loyalty and devotion of friends who would give all in time and love and attention. To the Westerner, many values were confusing and different. When we extolled the virtues of individualism, we had to learn that the clan or caste might be more important than the individual. When it seemed to us that the clear expression of opinions was an absolute value in our democracy and should be the basis of our relationships in the pilot project, we had to recognize that the primary values in that society were courtesy and respect, and that silence might not mean consent. Our co-workers might have strong feelings, but they would remain silent because it was not their place to speak.

All of this does not fit into a neat package of good on one side and bad on the other. Yet there is no question that my years in rural

---

There is no question that my years in rural India gave me new awareness of basic human values far removed from advanced technology.

India gave me new awareness of basic human values far removed from advanced technology. Relationships were intense; absolutes were determined on the basis of spiritual values rather than quantitative determination. Because death seemed so near, life assumed a more intense quality. Because poverty was so all-pervasive, there was a special joy and appreciation in the little pleasures.

There is a long tradition of American physicians doing missionary work abroad. They often served under great difficulties with a few tangible rewards. It seems that there now are many young Americans, including American physicians, who find satisfaction in working in other countries, even though their primary motivation is not religious. While they often bring special technical skills, they usually leave enriched by a new awareness of their own humanity revealed to them by the special quality of interpersonal, deeply affective relationships they encountered.

EMOTIONS Most physicians will agree that emotions have a distinct and often profound effect on body functions, and that body functions will also affect emotions. We even teach medical students that this is so. By example, we do not teach what we preach in actual practice. Medical students during their clinical years go through a rotation of services. They have to absorb an enormous number of facts. In most of the clinical services their performance rating depends on their mastery of the facts and their proper application to the specific problems found in that specialty. Little time is spent on emotional factors of disease, except in psychiatry and occasionally in internal medicine or pediatrics. Psychiatrists are called in as consultants when a patient does not get better or is troublesome. Again, in this technological age, the emphasis is on exact data. Emotions are not exact. Also, it takes time to establish interpersonal relationships with the patient in order to know and understand him.

Before entering the field of psychiatry I had done clinical teaching of medical students for many years. It seemed to me then, as it does now, that in general a second-year student is more imaginative about possible emotional factors in a patient's illness than medical school seniors. They have not been conditioned to concentrate on "facts." I cannot say at this point whether my intense interest in psychiatry and eventual change to that field was done primarily out of a sense of revolt against the practice of internal medicine. In many ways I enjoyed it. But there was a feeling that in the long run I would be out of step because I would not be sufficiently interested in the details of the impressive technological advances, or would feel unfulfilled because of the depersonalization of medical practice. This uneasiness presently is shared by a number of physicians and educators, as evidenced by the new specialty field of family practice and also by a relatively large number of older physicians who give up their practices and take on additional training in psychiatry. I feel that this is another attempt to emphasize affective relationships and human values rather than technological knowledge.

I am struck by the fact that psychiatry today is still more of an art than a science. Very little is proven or provable. Diagnoses are uncertain and often difficult to define. Treatment and treatment success are highly subjective. Pharmacologic effects can be predicted, but the factors of interpersonal relationships and of meaningful encounters defy quantitative measurement. Yet with all the uncertainty, there also is a frequent, joyful conviction that an individual's suffering has been lessened and that he has been enabled to resume a useful and active life. The uneasy feeling remains that this might have happened without the interference of the psychiatrist and that the patient, given enough time, might have done just as well.

This brings us back to Hippocrates. He realized the uncertainties of most remedies of his time and cautioned against self-deception of the physician with regard to his own therapeutic skill. I do not believe that the clock will be turned backward and that there will suddenly be a widespread revolt against depersonalization and technological advance. The technological advances obviously have been of tremendous importance in prolonging life, and often reducing suffering. Yet I do believe that there will be an important place in medicine for medical students and physicians who genuinely cultivate interpersonal, affective relationships. Because these are so difficult to measure and define, because they are not always reducible to facts, they still require a special kind of commitment and openness. Admittedly there is a thin line between sentimentality, quackery, or mysticism on the one hand and committed personalized care and caring on the other. But physicians and medical educators must give support and

encouragement to all aspects of therapy so that ultimately the whole person may benefit.

Note: Some of the ideas expressed in this article have been derived from reading a variety of writers such as James L. Green, David Riesman, Ashley Montague, Allen Wheelis, and others. A list of source references follows.

REFERENCES

Advertisement by Pacific Northwest Bell, *Seattle Times*, 22 Oct 1968.

Green JL: The new student morality. *Antioch Notes* 45, March 1968.

Harris TG: The young are captives of each other: A conversation with David Riesman and T. George Harris. *Psychology Today* 3:28–31, 63–67 passim, Oct 1969.

Hughes, H. Stuart: Emotional disturbance and American social change, 1944–1969. *Am J Psychol* 126:21–28, July 1969.

Keniston K: Does human nature change in a technological revolution? As quoted in *New York Times*, 6 Jan 1969, p 143, col 6.

May R: *Psychology and the Human Dilemma*. New York, Van Nostrand Reinhold, 1966.

Wheelis A: *The Quest for Identity*. New York, WW Norton & Co, 1958, 250 pp.

Chapter 12
The Evolution and Satisfactions of a Medical Career
J. Russell Elkinton, MD

What is it that gets all these older "established" people up early each Monday morning to return to work? Most of us would answer along the lines suggested by Dr. Lucas: Our work is useful to others and intensely satisfying to ourselves.

The happiest work, I think, must be creative—not in the narrow sense that we all should be painting pictures or writing odes, but in the sense that it calls on the individual for intelligent skill exerted in his own way. . . . Ideally, work should not only be interesting to the worker; it should also make him interesting to his intelligent fellow creatures. And it should be useful not only to the doer, but to others. It is this that makes, for example, the supreme good fortune of a good doctor.

A MEDICAL CAREER

These words of a wise and articulate Cambridge don epitomize what I would like to say about a career in medicine, about being a physician. It is indeed the intellectual and emotional satisfaction that comes from

Editor's Note: Dr. Elkinton has had a long and varied career. An outstanding clinical investigator with particular interests in renal disease and body chemistry problems, he has left an indelible mark on medicine through his research and thoughtful writing.

the challenge to develop personal skills and to extend professional knowledge to the end that others may be helped that makes "the supreme good fortune of a good doctor." And so it has ever been since Hippocrates practiced our profession under the plane tree on Cos so many centuries ago.

In a fictionalized account, *The Torch*, the story of Hippocrates has been told vividly by a famous member of our profession, Dr. Wilder Penfield.[1] This is a fascinating account himself and of his place in that world have changed since Hippocrates held his clinic. Although the human body and man's nature have probably remained much the same, the world around man and man's knowledge of himself and of his place in that world have changed by many orders of magnitude. With these changes, medicine has changed. Have the meaning and motivation for following the healing profession of necessity also changed? Presumably it is to answer this question that Dr. Bulger, as editor, has proposed this volume of essays.

The editor has charged his contributors with setting forth—for the benefit of the young men and women to follow—some of the many challenges and opportunities, motivations and satisfactions, that have given personal meaning to each of us as we have pursued our careers in medicine over the years. Dr. Bulger asks us to tell "what it is that gets all these older 'established' people up early each Monday morning to return to work." Setting aside the facetious reply that "the good wife wants to get me out of the house," or the mundane reply that "I have to earn a living," probably most of us would answer simply along the lines suggested by Dr. Lucas: Our work is useful to others and intensely satisfying to ourselves.

The ways in which a physician's activities can be useful to others and satisfying to himself are myriad. To convey to others one's personal experience with these many facets of a professional life, one perforce must write in an autobiographical vein. Yet no one physician achieves a totality of medical experience. Let the reader remember that each of us can provide only one small window on a wide and varied scene.

STAGES IN A MEDICAL CAREER   Assuming then the basic proposition that most physicians are motivated because their work is useful to others and satisfying to themselves, I would like to develop a further theme, namely, that the way in which a physician serves his fellows and satisfies himself evolves and changes over the span of his professional life. The paths of evolution and change are many and vary widely from physician to physician. Probably most doctors start their careers with the same sort of intense and total concentration on acquiring the technical knowledge and experience necessary to solve the medical problems of their patients. In this stage of a medical career all young physicians must find much the same satisfactions: the novelty of responsibility for the well-being of others who are ill and need help, the gratification when such help given is successful, the wonder at the multiplicities of ways in which the human body can function badly, and the

fascination with learning how to do something about it. The patients' illnesses on which he concentrates at this stage are usually acute, episodic, and often dramatic, and the therapeutic tools with which he meets them are intriguing and intellectually satisfying. This experience leads the young doctor to the next stage of his professional life, a stage in which he is occupied primarily in applying his skills to the care of particular patients and to the investigation of particular diseases. Here, the satisfactions come from seeing one's patients eased or cured and from the awareness that by acquiring new knowledge one can better control the progression of disease.

But many physicians go on to yet another stage in their careers in which they turn their attention to some broader aspect of the interplay of medicine with society at large. At this stage, their professional experiences and maturity motivate them to help to extend medical education, to implement measures designed to prevent disease, to improve and widen the delivery of health care, and indeed to apply where possible the insights of modern scientific medicine toward solutions of the great social problems of our age. In all these stages physicians function, of course, in many diverse ways with many different motivations and many different satisfactions; such is the subject of this book.

To illustrate this theme, there follows herewith the professional "pilgrim's progress" of one physician, namely, the author of this essay.

MEDICAL SCHOOL AND HOSPITAL YEARS

My own medical career has been spent primarily in academic medicine: in teaching, consulting, investigation, and subsequently medical editing. It began at Harvard Medical School, where the admissions committee took a chance on a candidate who was majoring in philosophy in college. I had decided that the field of philosophy was too abstract, and I turned to medicine as an antithetic activity that would combine generalities with the particulars of people and their problems. I have never regretted this choice.

At Harvard the arduous kind of medical school work that is so well remembered by all physicians began. In the mid-1930s I was fortunate to be exposed to some of the great teachers of the past—men like Walter Cannon, Hans Zinsser (without question one of the most dynamic teachers I have ever known), Henry Christian, Howard Means, Fuller Albright, James Gamble, Joseph Aub, as well as Hermann Blumgart and William Castle, both of whom are still actively teaching. These men were great teachers because each was a strong personality and each was a pioneer investigator on the frontier of medical knowledge. It was an exciting time to be training in medicine when so many new techniques from biochemistry and physiology were just beginning to be applied to clinical medicine.

But such general comment in retrospect conveys nothing of the flavor and excitement of being a medical student, intern, and resident in that most exciting of all institutions, the hospital. Some years ago I wrote an essay in an attempt to convey the flavor of that excitement:[2]

The hospital, of course, is the site of the young physician's first contact with the practicalities of his profession. Here, as a medical student, he meets for the first time the lame and the halt who are to be his main concern through life. Here he begins to realize that disease is more than a picture in a textbook, that disease is the wear and tear of flesh and blood, mind and body, of living human beings undergoing the biological rigors and vicissitudes of life. Here he learns that the results are often messy—to a degree he never dreamed of—and that his is the task to minimize the mess. My own medical school memories of this process take me back to the wards and clinics of many

Boston hospitals—Massachusetts General, Boston City, Peter Bent Brigham, Children's, Beth Israel, Boston Lying-In— legendary hospitals where I first learned that medical life was real, earnest, and absolutely fascinating.

It is as a house physician—intern and resident—that the young doctor really spreads his professional wings. These are his most formative years when he first assumes direct responsibility for his patients, the years of his closest sustained contact with acute illness in all its forms. These years of mine were spent in the Pennsylvania Hospital, the oldest hospital in the nation. I accumulated innumerable experiences and memories that have lasted a lifetime. On the old medical

---

I remember the young girl with the mycotic aneurysm of the abdominal aorta who stepped out of bed against orders and died on the spot, and the boy with typhoid fever who bled to death in a sea of blood and feces despite all the blood that we poured into his veins at the other end.

---

wards all sorts of things happened. I remember, for instance, the young girl with the mycotic aneurysm of the abdominal aorta who stepped out of bed against orders and died on the spot, and the boy with typhoid fever (we had eight or nine cases every summer) who bled to death in a sea of blood and feces despite all the blood that we poured into his veins at the other end. As a junior intern I used to sit up night after night with pneumonia patients, typing the pneumococci and administering antiserum, despite the vociferous opposition of the elderly head nurse who reiterated that the late chief (then just deceased) "said all that was nonsense." Happily for interns, not to mention patients, antibiotics were just about to arrive. Shortly thereafter we had an epidemic of meningococcal meningitis in 14 boys from a local reformatory and treated them with our first supply of the new English sulfonamide, M. and B. (sulfapyridine). Thirteen of the 14 boys recovered—an astounding result in a disease that heretofore had had a mortality of 90% to 100%! Death did not always win the contest.

Work in the receiving ward of the Pennsylvania Hospital was a unique experience. In my three months of daytime service on "receive" I calculated that I personally saw between 3,500 and 4,000 patients ranging from psychoneurotics to "DOA's" (dead on arrival). Here we had to learn to separate quickly the sheep from the goats, the acute abdomen from the dope addict, the comatose diabetic from the comatose alcoholic. Here was a continuous flow of people needing help for headaches, backaches, bellyaches, heartaches, for anything from inconsequential and minor upsets to life-threatening medical and surgical disasters.

Thus the hospital experience of an intern and resident is extremely varied and satisfying as well as intensely educational. But it is out of this experience that the next and more serious phase of a medical career springs, be it the setting up in practice or the training in a specialty.

SPECIALTY TRAINING: RESEARCH AND EARLY FACULTY YEARS

Not infrequently the young physician in his house-officer years becomes intrigued with some particular set of problems as seen in his hospital patients and hence is motivated to pursue further a special field of medicine. He begins to study and to care for many more such patients, he begins to explore the literature in depth, he begins to ask questions and to seek answers in the laboratory as well as in the clinic, he begins to share his interests and enthusiasms with like-minded peers as well as with younger students and physicians. And above all—if he is fortunate—he seeks and gains exposure to the skills, guidance, and wisdom of an able older physician who is a leader in his field. In a word, he becomes a research fellow or a junior staff member.

So it happened to me. In my years as intern and resident I became intrigued with the many practical problems of fluid balance and electrolyte abnormalities. Always, there were patients presenting diagnostic and therapeutic challenges: the patient who lost five liters of bile overnight through the tube placed in her common bile duct; the patient who died in shock, tetany, and metabolic alkalosis when his massive postoperative gastric fluid drainage was replaced only by glucose in distilled water; the unconscious hyperpneic patient in extreme uremic acidosis who subsequently survived to enjoy a reasonably comfortable existence for another 18 months on carefully calculated supplements of sodium bicarbonate; the patient with severe burns whose hemoconcentration and circulatory collapse seemed best treated with a then-novel infusion of plasma rather than of whole blood. These interests, as distilled in my first scientific papers, gained for me a National Research Council Fellowship in Medical Science that proved to be my springboard into academic medicine.

My fellowship began in the summer of 1940 at Yale in the laboratory of John P. Peters. Here, in the department of medicine chaired by an outstanding clinician, Francis Blake, and under the tutelage of Dr. Peters, a great medical scientist and physician, I spent the eight most formative years of my professional life. John Peters surely left an indelible mark on every man who studied under him. To convey some sense of his character and influence, I can do no better than repeat (in slightly modified form) part of a memorial that I wrote at the time of his death a decade later :[3]

John P. Peters was an able physician, but it was as a scientist and teacher that he left his major imprint on the medical profession. For 34 years at Yale he maintained a center dedicated to the application of physiological and biochemical knowledge to the diagnosis and treatment of disease in man. Quantitative clinical chemistry, in the broadest sense of the term, was nurtured here from a sturdy infancy to the maturity that it enjoys in medicine today. With Donald Van Slyke he wrote in 1931 the two-volume monograph Quantitative Clinical Chemistry *which has remained the classic in this field. A master of simple and lucid declarative writing, there flowed from his pen a number of books and chapters and many papers on a multitude of subjects, including water and electrolyte metabolism, acid-base equilibrium, renal disease, thyroid disease, diabetes mellitus and other endocrine disturbances, and the metabolism of proteins, fats, and carbohydrates. These constituted his major contributions to the science of medicine.*

At least as important as these written contributions was the influence which he extended to a host of physicians and investigators. Many young men were trained in his metabolic service and laboratory, invariably to have their knowledge enhanced and their intellectual curiosity stimulated. "Metabolism Rounds," held three times a week, were a famous institution at Yale—famous for their length and geographical coverage in the Hospital and even more famous for the interest they stimulated in the understanding and in the elucidation of disease processes.

The major weapon in Jack Peters' combat with disease was the chemical laboratory. His laboratory was an example of what a good laboratory of quantitative *clinical chemistry should be. There was no double standard between "routine" and "research" chemical techniques; the same procedures were applied to both, and duplicate determinations were performed without exception in all analyses. Every person who worked in his department went into this lab, be he medical student, research fellow, or staff member. Each investigator had to master each regular biochemical technique of the laboratory. And, at least prior to onset of the era of project research, each investigator performed with his own hands the chemical analyses required in his particular problem. The critical attitude toward laboratory values fostered by this experience was of inestimable value in the training of scientific workers.*

Thus the man, known affectionately to all of us as "The Boss." Perhaps it is harder to convey the excitement of being a research fellow in his stimulating department—of mastering new laboratory techniques, designing new experiments, eagerly analyzing the new data acquired, comparing results with those of other investigators working on the problem, and—above all—acquiring new insights and acting on them in an atmosphere of the highest laboratory standards and the keenest scientific criticism. With my colleagues, including especially A.W. Winkler and T.S. Danowski, many problems were attacked concerning the pathophysiology and chemistry of the body fluids including the abnormalities of intracellular water and electrolytes (especially potassium) in experimental dehydration, the measurements of fluid compartments by determining the volume of distribution of such substances as sulfocyanate, radioactive chloride, mannitol, and thiourea, the effects of various types of body fluid depletion on cardiovascular function, and—because we were at war—the physiologic sequelae of ingesting sea water and the role of diet in sparing the body water of thirsting men.

During World War II many men were cast away at sea or lost in the desert. Thirst and death from dehydration were not uncommon and irrational behavior and coma before death were reported in those who drank sea water. We and other laboratory groups were asking why and what to do. In one of my first sets of experiments as a research fellow (studying the effect of dehydration on the rate of secretion of gastric fluid) I had inadvertently stumbled on the hypernatremia resulting from water deprivation, and subsequently had characterized the loss of intracellular water and potassium in this condition. Applying these concepts to dogs given hypertonic solutions of sodium chloride as simulating sea water ingestion, we demonstrated the resultant shift of water from cells that in turn was associated with convulsions and respiratory failure. Conclusion: don't drink undiluted sea water. The nature of food under thirsting conditions also was critical; at the beginning of the war lifeboats and rafts were stocked with pemmican (dried meat). We and others quickly demonstrated that a dried meat diet with its high solute load was much more dehydrating than were diets of carbohydrate and fat. Could the ingestion of raw fish prevent dehydration? We fed raw fish to Air Force volunteers and to dogs deprived of water. The men became dehydrated while the dogs did not because of the superior concentrating abilities of the canine kidney. Raw fish alone was not the answer. And, I might add, it took 20 years for this investigator to be able to face a fillet of haddock again.

During this period new laboratory techniques were being developed including the first crude radioactive isotopes for tracer studies obtained from the university cyclotron across town, and the first flame photometer for analysis of sodium and potassium in body fluids. This latter instrument, replacing the tedious gravimetric and titrimetric chemical methods for measuring these ions, revolutionized the approach to studies of their abnormalities in experimental subjects and sick patients. In the pediatric laboratory on the next floor above, Daniel Darrow was exploring the vagaries of intracellular potassium in infants with acute diarrhea and in rats experimentally depleted of the ion. Under his urging we used our new flame photometer to find some of the first instances of the potassium depletion-metabolic alkalosis syndrome in adult patients. This phenomenon is old hat now but it was new and exciting then.

Throughout such a period as a research fellow and junior faculty staff member, one sees a host of patients with illnesses in the field of one's special interest. In my case, such patients were those with metabolic, endocrine, and renal diseases and with all the complications of body fluids gone awry. In addition, because most of our colleagues were away on World War II duty, those of us who remained behind attended wards for 11 months of each year on the general medicine and infectious disease services as well as on the metabolic service. Research was done in afternoons, evenings, and on weekends. The pace was heady and the results were satisfying beyond measure. And part of the work was writing up the results in scientific papers; work unpublished was work unfinished. John Peters was a keen critic of the written word: I remember one of our papers that we revised more than a dozen times before it gained his approval for submission to a journal.[4] This too is an essential part of the training of every medical scholar and academic clinician; good writing makes for good thinking and vice versa.

TEACHING, RESEARCH, CONSULTING: THE MIDDLE YEARS

Eventually there comes a time when education, training, and experience have prepared a physician to play a mature role in his profession. This period of maximum effectiveness may begin for some in the thirties, but surely covers the forties and fifties of a doctor's life. Admittedly, different attributes of a physician's character may mature at different times; creativity in research and ability to innovate usually reach a peak earlier in life, while balance, perspective, and the conscious and intuitive fruits of experience come later.

The physician in his prime may use his professional skills in many different ways, each of which is useful to others and satisfying to himself. He cares for patients (the major function of most doctors), he seeks new knowledge (research), he teaches colleagues and students, or he organizes and administers various aspects of these several functions. In doing so, the particular satisfactions that he gains will depend, of course, on the character of the man, but satisfactions will not be wanting. Throughout any or all of these professional activities, the wise physician recognizes that no knowledge or skill is static, that to be effective he must continue to grow, that education is a lifelong process.

The middle years of my own medical life have been spent primarily in teaching and in clinical investigation. Opportunities for private practice were opened to me and indeed were tempting in terms of human relations, patient care, and financial income. But academic medicine was more attractive in its intellectual challenge, scholarly milieu, and way of professional life. Furthermore, personal factors, which always must be considered in making any such decision, tipped the balance in this direction: academic medicine would give me more time for family life. In Philadelphia the academic opportunity came.

UNIVERSITY OF PENNSYLVANIA   So in 1948 I moved from Yale to the University of Pennsylvania. Here, Francis C. Wood, the newly appointed chairman of the Department of Medicine, asked me to set up one of the first full-time sections in the department, to be devoted to the care and study of patients with problems in electrolyte metabolism and renal disease. By the end of the first year this "chemical section" consisted of myself (supported in part as an Established Investigator of the American Heart Association), one research fellow, one secretary, one technician, and the country's second flame pho-

tometer (transferred from Yale). All these were established in a corner of the laboratory of William C. Stadie, the genial and able professor of research medicine. We attended the medical wards, taught medical students and house officers, and consulted throughout the University Hospital on electrolyte problems. The field and opportunities for the specialized interest were wide open at that time when the hospital and medical school were reorganizing in the aftermath of World War II.

To develop a laboratory and group for clinical investigation is a challenge to any young physician. In the 1950s the opportunities were great; postwar research support by the federal government was expanding at a tremendous rate through the extramural grant programs of the National Institutes of Health; interest in the part of young physicians returning from military service was high. Francis Wood, the chairman of the department and a wise and compassionate clinician, encouraged his section chiefs to develop their specialty groups and their laboratories to the utmost and yet at the same time to serve the patients of the hospital and to teach the students and the house staff. To achieve this triple function the young section chief inevitably was forced to take his first serious plunge into the murky waters of administration. Clinics and teaching conferences had to be planned, consultation services organized, fellowship applications processed, and budgets prepared along with grant applications and their unavoidable sequelae—progress reports.

Most important of all was the purpose for which this administration was undertaken, namely, the fostering of intellectual activity. This included the nourishing of ideas, the defining of problems and how to tackle them, the encouragement of research fellows, the mental digesting of one's own data and their interpretation in the light of other knowledge in the field, old and new. During these years we worked on many problems, including potassium depletion, whole body buffering in acid base disturbances, the electrolyte abnormalities of undernutrition, changes in body composition in, and the treatment of, renal failure, biochemistry of uremia, the etiology and pathogenesis of renal tubular acidosis, and the renal concentrating mechanisms in health and disease. Many patients helped us in these endeavors and were helped in return; some were unforgettable.

CASES There was Annie B., emaciated middle-aged spinster with anorexia nervosa, who time after time staggered back into the hospital with a serum potassium less than 2.0 mEq/liter, a serum CO_2 content above 50 mM/liter, and electrocardiographic U waves of alarming proportions. Recharged again and again on the metabolic ward with copious amounts in chloride, the mechanism of her ionic losses continued to puzzle us until she was caught surreptitiously disposing of her vomitus and bribing the newsboy to supply her with milk of magnesia. But there remained the question: does undernutrition alone lead to severe potassium depletion? Does potassium depletion alone lead to metabolic alkalosis? My research fellows, Edward Huth and Russell Squires, and I turned to the experimental depletion of normal human subjects and animals for answers to these questions: undernutrition leads only to mild potassium depletion relative to nitrogen; experimental potassium depletion is associated with intracellular acidosis.

There was Annie T., 30-year-old housewife admitted to my general medical ward hyperventilating and in coma. With an arterial pH of 6.97 (extremely low) but with normal levels of blood sugar and blood urea nitrogen, she was the first case of renal tubular acidosis to be recognized in our hospital. She went through an incredible course of alkali therapy with tetany and barbiturate and paraldehyde addiction leading to recurrent acidosis. Where did all the acid come from and where did her body store it? Richard Singer, John Kapp Clark, Earl Barker, and I experimentally induced acute acid-base disequilibria in normal

human subjects and demonstrated the resultant extensive buffering of the extracellular disturbances by the intracellular phases of the body fluids.

There was Marian C., housewife, mother of five children, referred to me for severe calcification of both kidneys and the passing of many stones in her urine—a classic case of adult renal tubular acidosis. Faithful adherence to an adequate regimen of alkali therapy eliminated much of her nephrocalcinosis and prevented further deterioration of her renal tubular and glomerular function over the subsequent 15 years. Did her children inherit the defect? This question and others led to extensive studies with Ed Huth, George Webster, Donna McCurdy and Vardaman Buckalew (as well as with R.A. McCance in England) on the diagnosis, pathogenesis, and nosology of this interesting disease.

There was Ida C., school teacher, who went baby-sitting one icy night, broke a leg, received a mismatched blood transfusion, and was sent into our hospital in acute renal failure. Threatened with a rising serum potassium level toward a lethal value (this was before the day of our artificial kidney), it occurred to us that exchange resin put into the intestinal tract might help. She received the first reported resin enemas—and her potassium came tumbling down. But potassium was only one of many components requiring treatment in renal failure. Subsequently, with Lewis W. Bluemle, an artificial kidney unit was established that for a period of years was the only one in operation between Boston and Washington. Still later, the program was expanded by Lee Henderson with Bill Bluemle and others to include chronic dialysis and renal transplantation.

OTHER STUDIES Many other patients and many other normal subjects were studied in relation to electrolyte disorders and renal disease. Prominent among these studies were those to elucidate the renal mechanisms for concentrating and diluting the urine and the effect thereon of various diuretic drugs; for these latter studies Martin Goldberg was primarily responsible. Repeatedly, the pattern was to carry our quest from patient to experimental human subject or dog or rat and back again to the patient. One result of all this activity was the publication of many papers and a book on the body fluids; one reward was the achievement of new understanding of the pathophysiology and pathochemistry of these diseases to the end that patients might benefit.

For the leader of a group engaging in this kind of professional activity there is another, and even greater, satisfaction. It is to see the young men developing their professional, scientific, and intellectual potential. The new research fellow comes from his hospital years, at home or abroad, full of enthusiasm and intellectual curiosity and eager to go. Just where he wants to go is usually not clear to him at first. It is the chief's role to help the new fellow work his way into the literature and into the interests and programs of the group, and to develop his own ideas (grassroots nourishment is better than authoritarian assignment to a project). Once embarked on his intellectual safari, the young physician-investigator's enthusiasm leads him forward and in turn stimulates the group. Beyond the many critical group discussions comes the exchange of ideas with other investigators at local and national scientific meetings. The acme of such experience, of course, was and is the occasion of the "spring meetings" held in Atlantic City. Here, in the first week of May, are held the annual meetings of the Association of American Physicians, the American Society for Clinical Investigation, and the American Federation for Clinical Research. At these gatherings of the "old Turks," the "young Turks," and the "young, young Turks," the country's medical teachers and clinical investigators present the cream of the year's research activities and examine the state of academic medicine. As I have written elsewhere,[5] these occasions have a unique character.

This cold cataloging of organization, however, gives little hint of the stirring and delightful potpourri of new ideas and old friends that is the essence of these four days. The formal meetings are held in Haddon Hall or (in the past) the Steel Pier Theater, and the opening presidential address in each organization is always a star occasion with its offering of wisdom and penetrating analysis. The scientific sessions each year become more stimulating as one's interests broaden or more frustrating as the accelerating rate of basic science leaves one floundering in a particular bay of personal ignorance. But the informal meetings are the ones that count the most; these are held in rooms over drinks, and across memorable repasts of raw oysters and broiled lobsters that are being conducted to their predestined goal. And on the boardwalk hospital-bound workers bask in the sunlight, breathe in the brisk salt sea winds, and discuss the intellectual fare offered during these four days.

To all these stimulating occasions the young men in my section were exposed. The weekly luncheon discussions of our own group were vigorous, stimulating, and sometimes ended closer to dinnertime than to lunchtime. Travel to and participation in scientific meetings were regular parts of our activities. The outlook of our group was broadened by including research fellows from foreign shores; we were particularly indebted to Theo Chalmers of England, Hiroshi Sasamoto of Japan, Andrzej Wojtczak of Poland, and Muel Ramirez of Peru.

In addition to the prime satisfaction of seeing young men develop into able investigators and academic physicians, the leader of a clinical investigation group has the delight and privilege of associating in his own institution with a host of men who share his interests and professional enthusiasms. This, of course, is one of the great satisfactions of any professional career and is the reason why any meaningful account of such a career must talk about particular people.

In my own institution, the University of Pennsylvania, in addition to my contemporaries too numerous to list completely, were the older associates whose competence and wisdom were drawn upon without stint. Besides Francis Wood and William Stadie, already mentioned, these included especially Isaac Starr, Joseph Stokes, and that presiding genius of the medical school, Newton Richards. Isaac Starr, cardiovascular physiologist and father of ballistocardiography, for many years had his office and laboratory next to mine; to me the benefits of his erudite medical scholarship were frequently and generously given. Joseph Stokes, pediatric professor, Quaker physician, protector of children as the creator of vaccines (and incidentally my uncle), bestowed on me kind and keen avuncular advice throughout my professional career; with him it has been my privilege to participate in various Quaker medical activities with the Friends Medical Society and the American Friends Service Committee. As for Dr. Richards, he was in a class by himself; for a picture of his life and character the reader is referred to the memorial monograph edited by Isaac Starr.[6] In the preface to that volume I wrote:

I had the privilege of many personal meetings with Dr. Richards during the last two decades of his life. . . . Two or three times each winter Francis and Molly Wood would invite to their home a group of younger staff members of the department for a convivial dinner and evening in the company of Dr. Richards. . . . These evenings were priceless occasions because of the exposure to the wit and wisdom of Newton Richards. The conversation ranged from the latest jokes to Dr. Richards' earlier experiences in pharmacology, to grouse shooting in Scotland, to the history and source of Chartreuse, to the story of how Joseph Wearn and he, over a bottle of beer, had dreamed up the idea of micropuncturing

the renal tubule, to the desirable future of medicine and how to get there, and to many other subjects, serious and otherwise.

"The wit of old age has a matchless quality, when it comes—a hardbitten saltiness that penetrates without hurt"; thus the biographer Catherine Drinker Bowen has written of one of her subjects, Justice Oliver Wendell Holmes. So it was with Dr. Richards. Even in his ninth decade his clear mind and rapier-like wit, exercised with a twinkle in his eye and a liberal sprinkling of mild oaths, gave him the pixie-like character of a small boy's mischievous spirit encased in the body and mind of a sage.

OTHER UNIVERSITIES Outside my own university, friends and associates were to be found in many institutions, communities, and countries; they were met on individual travels or at meetings of the organizations just mentioned above and of others such as the Interurban Clinical Club and the American College of Physicians, or during work sessions of the Metabolism and Nutrition Study Section of the National Institutes of Health. Of particular interest in my professional life were the physicians whom I came to know in Great Britain. Many trips to England were undertaken to see my English wife's family and friends and during these trips I visited medical schools, hospitals, and research laboratories. I made cordial professional friends, especially in the medical schools of the universities of Birmingham, Manchester, and London, and in the Royal College of Physicians of London. This process reached a peak in 1957 with a sabbatical half year spent in the research laboratory of Professor R.A. McCance at Cambridge. Here, during a halcyon interlude of relief from telephones, clinical duties, and administrative pressures, I began working with the unique team of McCance and Widdowson and their associates— eminent for their ability to design and carry out definitive experiments. More than a decade later, at the time of Professor McCance's retirement from the chairmanship of the MRC Department of Experimental Medicine at Cambridge, I tried to characterize my experience during that period :[7]

In my mind's eye I can see so well again the dinner table set out each day in the middle of the lab in the old quarters of the Path building. . . . There is the Professor at the head of the table nursing his tall lone cup of coffee, and Elsie Widdowson and the others ranged below him. . . . Those lab dinners were unforgettable occasions to me; Mac would fix his penetrating eye on each of us one by one and pin us down as to what we had been doing. We had many fascinating foreign visitors and Mac kept a very tight control on how the visiting went. His system was simply Machiavellian—fifteen minutes with himself immediately before dinner, then public extraction of the visitor's relevant information, then pass him off for successive post-prandial interviews down the Departmental totem pole. . . .

I have another memory of Mac which often comes back to me. Occasionally he would accompany me on his bike as I rode back to the house in which we were living. I remember one very hectic afternoon when we were riding down Trumpington Street in the middle of the evening rush traffic: Mac riding along serenely next to the gutter, I riding between him and the swiftly passing lorries and trying to keep from being annihilated by them on one side and from bumping the Professor into the ditch on the other—and all the time he was quietly discussing the tubular reabsorption of bicarbonate! . . .

Working with Mac and Elsie in their laboratory was a great scientific experience. When I arrived in January 1957 he was already studying a small child on the pediatric ward in Addenbrooke's who had a peculiar form of acidosis apparently of renal origin. . . . The study of this boy with his very low ammonium excretion and normal ability to acidify his urine set us off on a long course of investigating the mechanisms of the kidney for the excretion of acid and the effects of these mechanisms of renal disease, studies that have gone on over the succeeding decade in Mac's laboratory in Cambridge and in my own laboratory in Philadelphia.

And so it went—mature and fascinating professional years with patients to care for, diseases to investigate, young men to encourage, and old friends to enjoy.

MEDICAL EDITING: YEARS OF BROADER INTEREST AND WIDER OUTREACH

At certain times in a mature professional life the opportunity may present itself to change the direction of one's activities, to do something new and different. For some physicians this may mean the chance to practice in a new community, to practice a different kind of medicine, or to use one's professional experience in a different way such as in administering a department in medical school or organizing a medical mission overseas. Often such a change is associated with a desire to apply one's professional experience to a broader field of social need or action. In my own case such a change came with the opportunity to become a medical editor.

In 1960 the Board of Regents of the American College of Physicians offered me the editorship of the *Annals of Internal Medicine*. The former editor, Dr. Maurice Pincoffs of Baltimore, was retiring and the regents wanted an editor who lived in Philadelphia, the home of the national headquarters of the college. Thus the opportunity came my way. I began as a part-time editor while continuing to administer the chemical section of the Department of Medicine at Penn. As the subsequent decade wore on I retired from this latter post and progressively gave more time to editing. During my entire editorship I have been fortunate in having an extremely able associate editor, Dr. Edward J. Huth, who has shared with me the burdens and the delights of bringing out the *Annals* each month.

The reason for undertaking the editing of a medical journal is not hard to state: it is to contribute to the continuing education of physicians, on a national and international scale, to the end that doctors everywhere may become better doctors. This no doubt is the principal motive of most medical editors.

The reason for undertaking the editing of a medical journal is not hard to state: it is to contribute to the continuing education of physicians, on a national and international scale, to the end that doctors everywhere may become better doctors. This no doubt is the principal motive of most medical editors. In addition I had other personal reasons. Editing a medical journal would allow me to play a major role in the profession without undertaking the oppressive administrative burdens of a departmental chairman; editing would be less demanding physically; editing the *Annals* would allow me to continue to live in my home town of Philadelphia; a higher salary would be welcome at a time when my children were reaching college age and the time to pay high tuition fees was approaching; and I like to write.

The physician who becomes an editor enters a new kind of life. On the procedural side he must master many facets of the processes of printing and publishing, organize the flow of manuscripts, learn to oversee the copy editing and proofreading of papers in press, and—most of all—learn how to select critically those papers that he believes will best serve the in-

terests of his readers. The interaction between authors, readers, and himself is always uppermost in the mind of an editor; to explain, I can do no better than to present part of an editorial essay that I once wrote on the subject:[8]

Between each would-be author and his hoped-for reader stands an editor. His is the job to distinguish, in the flow of words, the worthwhile message and to help to get it through to the reader—loud and clear. . . . And he may dream—even as the author and the reader may dream—of medical writing, not as it is, but as it should be. Perhaps the dreams of these three protagonists are worth analysis. This way the couch.

AUTHORS, READERS, EDITORS *The author dreams that his manuscript is recognized by the editor as a paragon of medical wisdom that will be quickly accepted and rapidly published; he dreams that in the process each word is preserved in its perfection and that no single datum (so hardily won) is eliminated. . . . How sweet the dream, and, alas, how ethereal the achievement! . . . It comes as no surprise that one detects a steady undertone of complaints by authors about editors. . . .*

The medical reader, quite simply, dreams that he has read everything in the medical literature and knows all. . . . Alas, the poor reader! Buried in the avalanche of medical literature, flattened by the blast of the "information explosion," he appears to be beyond the help of even the most sophisticated electronic retrieval systems. . . . Beyond his own struggles the chief hope for the reader is the energetic editor—the man in between.

An editor, quite simply, dreams of receiving and publishing good papers. By "good" he means papers that contain worthwhile information presented clearly and succinctly, papers that meet the needs of his readers. He dreams . . . of authors whose grammar is impeccable, whose style is lucid if not elegant, whose manuscripts without blemish. . . . In short, the editor dreams of getting the best papers.

The editor is servant to both reader and author. For the reader, as his first care, he must choose the most useful and stimulating fare and see that it is presented in most readable form. For the author he must combine the functions of critic, judge, and compassionate physician to ailing manuscripts. The editor must insist on clarity of expression yet be tolerant of honest, less-than-perfect efforts to present work of integrity. The editor yearns for the author to write well . . . to appreciate that the very effort of putting one's ideas into clear succinct prose contributes to the clarity of those ideas. These are dreams that the editor dreams for the author.

To realize these editorial dreams a medical editor needs to be someone akin to "a man for all seasons." He must know what is going on in the nonmedical as well as in the medical world. He must read widely and get to know many people. He no longer applies medical skill in depth to particular patients but deals with the field of medicine in general; he tends to become a physician whose medical knowledge is a mile wide and an inch deep. If he can keep in touch with some particular branch of medicine or make ward rounds and teach over particular patients, he has some chance of keeping his medical feet on the ground. But of necessity an editor's horizons must be broad if he is to edit his journal well. And he must be alert to the changing conditions of the world of modern communications in which new ways are proposed for getting information to the physician.

During my eleven years as a medical editor many of these experiences have come to me and with them great satisfaction. I have come to know many more able physicians and medical scientists, writers and leaders in our profession. Editors of other medical journals have become my friends.

At the beginning of my editorship I was encouraged by Sir Theodore Fox, then editor of the *Lancet*, and by Joseph Garland, then editor of the *New England Journal of Medicine*, through personal discussions of their own experiences. Irving Page of *Modern Medicine* supported my early editorials on ethical issues; William Bean of the *Archives of Internal Medicine* set a personal example of the wide and erudite use of all English literature in medical editing. In more recent years at an annual luncheon meeting in Atlantic City during the "spring meetings," Alexander Gutman of the *American Journal of Medicine,* John Talbott of the *Journal of the AMA,* Franz Ingelfinger of the *New England Journal of Medicine,* and other editors have joined with Ed Huth and myself in trying to surmount certain common problems such as standardizing references and discouraging duplicate publication. During these years of editing the *Annals* I have had the privilege of a continuing association and friendship with the official family of the American College of Physicians—with the officers, regents, governors, and staff. I have known the excitement of seeing at an early stage new work and new ideas and the pleasure of helping authors by providing sound peer review and editorial criticism. I have had the satisfaction of assisting readers by providing material that not only is worthwhile professionally but is in readable form (as, for instance, new format and typography for easy reading, duplicate summaries and individual first pages for easy filing). I have had the fun of writing editorials, supplementing them with thoughts and quotations from literature outside as well as inside the field of medicine, and receiving the response from readers pro and con. I have had the interest of hearing periodically from authors rejected or disgruntled, if not eccentric, who remind me how delicate is the proper exercise of responsible editorial power and how varied are the foibles of the human race. For instance there is:

The author who requests a preliminary scan before submitting his paper officially, oblivious of the fact that the editor already has manuscripts running out his ears.

The author who encloses, inadvertently, the letter of rejection from the editor to whom he had submitted his paper previously, thus relieving this editor from his usual speculation on this point.

The author who practically rewrites his paper in galley proof.

The author who defends his Henry Jamesian style to the last subordinate clause.

The author who resubmits a second version of his paper before the first submitted version has been returned from the outside reviewers.

The author who, after a whole series of rejected papers, writes an 80-page polemic damning the entire medical establishment including especially its editors—and labels his magnum opus (also rejected) as the present-day "Flexner report."

Quite a few funny things happen to manuscripts on the way to the forum.

MEDICINE AND SOCIETY   The overall view of medicine as it relates to society presents itself repeatedly and forcefully to a medical editor. We live in a time of rapid social change and turmoil that involves our profession as well as all society. The major issue before the medical profession today is how to improve the delivery of health care to an inadequately cared-for public imbued with rising expectations, beset with soaring costs, and faced with a progressive diminution of medical facilities and personnel relative to the expanding population. A generation ago most young physicians gave little thought to this subject;[9] today many young doctors are in the vanguard of those citizens (physicians and laymen) who are pressing for better systems of delivering medical care. No one can be oblivious to this great problem that confronts American medicine today.

There are other problems, moral and ethical, that have developed with the rapid advances of medical science, problems that have been of particular interest to me during my editorship. Because of the experience in my section with a hemodialysis program I had been impressed with some of the moral problems posed by the use of borrowed organs, artificial and transplanted. In 1964 I wrote an editorial that apparently helped to precipitate extensive discussion of the subject.[10, 11] But the

---

The dilemmas of right and wrong go well beyond the fields of dialysis and transplantation.

---

dilemmas of right and wrong go well beyond the fields of dialysis and transplantation :[12]

The issues of life and death are no strangers to the practicing physician. Daily he confronts them in the persons of his patients—endeavoring to detect and diminish disease, to promote health, to relieve suffering, to confound death. Sooner or later "death comes to all men," as he well knows, but his is the task to put off for his patient that day. The patient, whether he cherished life with gusto or clings to life with despair, looks to his physician for all the help and hope that one human being can give another in a time of need. In this mutual relationship of trust and compassion lies the major glory and the satisfaction of our profession.

But—and life being what it is there is always a "but"—this relationship between doctor and patient has become more complicated in recent years. The rapid accumulation of scientific knowledge and techniques has given the doctor much greater power to actively influence the life and health of his patient, and this power in turn has forced upon him ethical judgments that in former times he did not have to make. Some of these judgments concern the question of whether or not to artificially prolong a life that has become hopeless as well as burdensome to the patient and his family. Some concern the question of aborting a potential life because of the likelihood of developmental defect in the child or risk to the mother. Some involve the choice of which patients shall receive the benefit of a life-prolonging procedure (such as hemodialysis or kidney homotransplantation) when the availability of the procedure is limited. Some involve the decision whether and under what conditions to subject a patient to an experimental procedure that is not for his own benefit but is for the sake of new knowledge for the benefit of others. All such judgments pose moral problems that transcend the boundaries of the medical profession and cut across the general fields of law, philosophy, and religion.

Beyond the technical, economic, social, and ethical issues inherent in the interface of medicine and society, there are larger problems facing humanity to which the physician may make a special contribution:[13]

Every physician is first a citizen, a citizen of his country and—in this age of rapid travel, intercontinental rocketry, and instant communication—a citizen of the world. Like other men he must share to a greater or lesser extent the burdens and problems of humanity. Yet the physician as a citizen and member of human society has certain special responsibilities that devolve upon him because of his professional training and occupation. In his capacity as a healer or preventer of human illness and with his knowledge of human biology he is especially equipped to contribute to the resolution of some of the national and international issues of our day. . . .

The first of these great problems is that of pollution of the environment—the atmosphere, the water supplies, wilderness areas. . . . Inextricably bound up with this problem is that of the rapid expan-sion of the world's population. The central fact is the accelerating rate of increase in the number of births over the number of deaths. . . . Thus, a vicious cycle now exists that poses great problems to the statesmen of the world. No one is in a better position than the physician to appreciate the importance of solving these problems in order to stabilize the world's population and so to preserve at a decent level the quality of human life.

Finally we come to the major threat to the human race that lies in nuclear, chemical, and biological warfare. . . . Thermonuclear disaster (all too often euphemistically labeled "exchange") cannot possibly be dealt with medically after the fact; it can only be managed by preventing it from happening. . . . Chemical and biologic weapons are now being intensively developed and stockpiled. . . . No activity of society can present a more direct ethical challenge to the physician and his profession than the preparation for, and possible use of, nuclear, chemical, and biologic weapons.

Man is indeed "born into trouble as the sparks fly upward," as one of Job's comforters put it. . . . Can homo sapiens rise to the challenge of the intensifying "troubles" of the world today? . . . What to do is often very difficult to know . . . the physician is especially well-fitted to contribute to the public opinion that inevitably must underlie any effective social and political action. As such he is an important citizen of the world.

One of the chief satisfactions of a medical career is its evolution to the point where this truth is borne home, namely, that the physician is indeed an important citizen of the world.

EPILOGUE

So much for the evolution and satisfactions of a professional medical career, as illustrated by the pilgrim's progress of one particular physician, who seems, incidentally, to have traveled a full circle in his flight from philosophy. Whatever one's achievements may have been (and certainly mine have been modest compared to those of many of my contemporaries), one is left with a sense of opportunities unseized and potentialities unfulfilled. There are always higher mountains to climb and bigger giants to slay. But personal satisfaction and fulfillment come at least as much from the journey as from the destination, from the struggle as from the goal attained; most men have to settle for less than the highest peak or the complete victory.

Many factors condition a man's sense of fulfillment and satisfaction with life beyond his primary work and occupation. The qualities of his personal life, character, and beliefs play a critical role. The physician who has a full family life with the love, comradeship, and interest of his wife and children is fortunate indeed, as I well know. Fortunate is the physician who has recreative avocations in areas such as art, literature, athletics, travel, nature. Fortunate is the physician who takes opportunities to serve his church or community and fortunate the physician who has his health or, if ill health, the ability to live with it and to rise above it. Indeed, the physician who himself has been a patient has an opportunity to learn something about illness that will serve him well in understanding and caring for his own patients. And finally, the physician who is able to cultivate within himself that serenity of spirit that permits him to face calmly not only himself but the world and his work in it, has an essential ingredient for the abundant life—medical or otherwise. He is ready for the creative work, useful and interesting to others as well as to the doer, that constitutes "the supreme good fortune of a good doctor."

REFERENCES

1 Penfield W: *The Torch*. Boston and Toronto, Little Brown & Co, 1960, 367 pp

2 Elkinton JR: That hospital smell, in *Footnotes on the Sands of Time*. Unpublished essays, 1957–1965.

3 Elkinton JR: John P. Peters. Unpublished memorial from the *Minutes of the Interurban Clinical Club*, 6 April 1956.

4 The subsequent history of this paper also taught me something. In the paper Winkler, Danowski, and I presented data from many of our studies on dogs and men showing significant and unaccounted-for discrepancies between balances of water and balances of sodium plus potassium. As the explanation we postulated changes in the osmotic activity of intracellular electrolytes that were not the result of transfers across cell membranes. The paper was first submitted to the *Journal of Clinical Investigation* whose Editor, James Gamble, rejected it; it was then accepted by, and published in, the *Yale Journal of Biology and Medicine*. Some time later Dr. Gamble told me that he regretted his decision. By then he had observed similar discrepancies in his own studies of dehydration on liferafts. Thus I learned that the fate of the submitted paper is somewhat subject to chance and that editors sometimes change their minds.

5 Elkinton JR: From boardwalk to bedside—clinical research in American medicine (editorial). *Ann Intern Med* 66:437–440, 1967.

6 Starr I (guest ed): Alfred Newton Richards: Scientist and man. *Ann Intern Med* 71: suppl 8, 1–89 (Nov) 1969.

7 Elkinton JR: Greetings to the professor. *Cumberland Lodge Proceedings:* Record of a Weekend Gathering of Past and Present Members of the Department of Experimental Medicine, Cambridge University, held in honor of Professor RA McCance, at Cumberland Lodge, Windsor Great Park, 20–21 July 1966. Unpublished, compiled Oct 1967, pp 70–72.

8 Elkinton JR: Authors, readers, and editors—dreams of medical writing (editorial). *Ann Intern Med* 59:410–413, 1963.

9 During my research fellowship at Yale, my chief, Dr. John P. Peters, as secretary of the Committee on Physicians for the Improvement of Medical Care, was working actively for a greatly liberalized system of health care in this country. As a young investigator intensely occupied with my scientific work, I could not have paid less attention to this problem than I did.

10 Elkinton JR: Moral problems in the use of borrowed organs, artificial and transplanted (editorial). *Ann Intern Med* 60:309–313, 1964.

11 Elkinton JR: Letters and comments: Moral problems of artificial and transplanted organs. *Ann Intern Med* 61:355–363, 1964.

12 Elkinton JR: Life, death, and the physician (editorial). *Ann Intern Med* 67:669, 1967.

13 Elkinton JR: The physician as a citizen of the world (editorial). *Ann Intern Med* 65:611–615, 1966.

Chapter 13
Philosophy and Practice
Eugene A. Stead, Jr., MD

A knowledge of the biologic basis of behavior allows the doctor to develop a high degree of tolerance for the frailties of man and to enjoy to the fullest the triumph of individuals.

THE PURPOSE OF LIFE

Each person must sooner or later face up to the question, ''What is the purpose of life?'' The answer will have a great deal to do with the way one lives and one's relationship to others. I have never had a clear understanding of the purpose of life. I have, however, defined certain limits within which I think the answer must lie and, in this way, excluded a number of possible answers which lie outside these limits.

The purpose of life can hardly lie in the past. That period of time is over and will never recur. The purpose of life can hardly be to achieve something in the future, because the future has too little reality. In some way, the purpose of life must relate to the present. The

Editor's Note: Dr. Stead is presently the Florence McAlister Professor of Medicine at Duke University and the Director of the Regenstrief Foundation for Research in Health Care. He was for many years the Chairman of the Department of Medicine at Duke. By unofficial count, he has trained more chairmen of academic departments of medicine than any other man.

present is real and tangible. It belongs to you; it cannot be taken away from you.

The realization that the returns from living are collected each day does modify one's behavior. One is unwilling to sacrifice everything in the present for something in the future. As a doctor, I have taken care of many parents who over many years gave everything to their children with the expectation that the children, when they were grown, would return this devotion in kind. In fact, as the children matured they developed their own worlds, had their own lives to live, and their own children to care for. They resented their parents' dependence on them and wished the parents had developed interests to supply pleasure from living independent of them.

Because of our belief in the present, we did not give up everything for our children. We kept some time for ourselves and always spent some part of each year away from the children. What resources we had, we shared. We had our share of the free money; the children had theirs. We enjoyed our children each day and, when we put them to bed each night, the books were balanced. We had cared for them and we had enjoyed them. They owed us nothing. As the children grew older, we made it clear to them that we would support them until they were able to support themselves. After that time, we would expect to see them and their children, if all of us enjoyed the venture. When they were capable of independence, we owed them nothing and they owed us nothing. We had collected our pleasures as we went and there were no debts.

Many young men have talked with me about their plans for the next year or years. My answers have always reflected my belief in the importance of the present. If the young man is contemplating a program that he may wish he had not taken unless he achieves a particular position in some hierarchy, I advise against it. If the program pays dividends in satisfaction and pleasure while it is being pursued, he cannot lose. No matter what happens in the future, the fun of the present belongs forever to him.

THE DOCTOR

I have been surprised at how rarely the young doctor, engaged in planning his career, asks the question that I judge to be of the greatest importance: "How do I plan my educational program to help me gain the greatest satisfaction out of each day of my life?" His great concern is to become technically competent, and he assumes that out of this happiness will flow. Experience shows that this may be too simple an assessment.

A doctor cannot treat diseases alone. He must care for the patient who has the disease. The doctor who wakes each morning with zest for the adventures of the day is at peace with his patients. He knows the limits which the structure of the nervous system puts on the behavior of persons. He does not expect all things from all men. He can comfortably make demands on persons capable of rising to these demands; he can comfortably make fewer demands on persons who, because of genetic

The doctor who enjoys the day develops a high degree of tolerance for the frailties of man and enjoys to the fullest the triumph of individuals.

background, unfavorable environment, ignorance, fear, or prejudice, have lower ceilings of performance. The doctor who enjoys the day develops a high degree of tolerance for the frailties of man and enjoys to the fullest the triumph of individuals. The course of education selected by the young doctor should be one which teaches him to enjoy the people who have the illnesses he has learned to treat. This is the only way to assure that the work of each day will bring true satisfaction.

To keep one's perspective on the problems of living, one needs to have some sense of the geological time scale. The most famous men of recorded history occupy very few moments in our thoughts. How few of us spend any time thinking about Alexander the Great or Julius Caesar! Within a few million years, all traces of them could disappear from the thoughts of any living man. The purpose of life can hardly be to obtain fame, because it is too impermanent. Events which add to the enjoyment of the day may bring distinction and fame. The achievement of fame and distinction at the expense of the enjoyment of the day does not bring happiness.

The knowledge of the uncertainty of the future does influence the direction of one's life. A doctor knows that he or anyone else may die before a new day dawns. The wise man is not disturbed by this. He does each day what he wants to do and, if the date of his death were known to him, he would not need to change his plans. He has planned his life with the knowledge of its impermanence. If he lives in the present, he need have no fear of the future.

A doctor's philosophy does have an effect on his practice. I believe that young people can be "insurance poor" and give up too much of the present in caring about the future. I am not enthusiastic about burdening my patients with too many *dont's* when I have no way of knowing what will remove them from this earth. All preventive measures are wasted when the patient dies from another cause before the diseases which were being prevented would have actually interfered with his way of life.

Many persons will come to doctors complaining of certain ailments. The doctor often does not find, in any of his testing, disturbances in function great enough to account for the complaining. He will frequently find asymptomatic diseases which may at some future time cause symptoms. Obesity, hypertension, abnormal blood lipids, elevated uric acid, and an abnormal glucose tolerance test are common findings. In his search for a solution to the complaints of the patient, the doctor may institute a regime of preventive medicine in a person who sought medical help in the first place because he was barely able to keep his nose above water. The preventive measures cost money, require energy from the patient, and in no way relieve the situation which drove him to the doctor. A doctor with an eye to the present would never initiate programs aimed at the future until the patient was back on an even keel.

I have had little enthusiasm for the annual physical examination which is strongly test and x-ray oriented. It is a kind of negative medicine which puts me to sleep. On the other hand, I am keenly aware that our bodies are undergoing continual change, and that our behavior and our interaction with our environment change with the years. It is worthwhile for one to have an evaluation of his body and how he is using it to determine whether he is getting as much as possible out of each day's living.

Department heads should work harder to devise social systems that recognize certain biologic facts. They do not appreciate fully that all manifestations of behavior are a function of the structure of the nervous system. The structure is a mixture of nonreversible and reversible units. The number of reversible units decreases with age. Every five years, enough change occurs in each of us that, from the viewpoint of body-environment interaction, we can be considered to be a new person. This new person will have different perspectives, different aptitudes, a different interaction with the environment. The returns from the day will decrease unless we are allowed to change our activities as our bodies change. No one knows the direction or the magnitude of the changes that will occur in a young faculty member as he grows older. All we know is that change will occur, and we should structure our affairs to profit by the change. Many times the social structure is so tight that only penalties accrue as change occurs. A young man starting his career may be able to offer many contributions before he retires. He may begin as an excellent teacher of beginning students and in time he may evolve into an excellent bioscientist. Later, clinical interest becomes stronger and he becomes an increasingly important clinician; he now gives up a large part of his laboratory space to a younger person and takes a more prominent role in advanced graduate training. In due time he becomes an outstanding leader in his area of clinical specialization and devotes more time to national affairs. This type of evolution requires a flexible system of funding so that the man can be supported from different sources as his functions change. In time, the teaching and research dollars are replaced by patient-care and administrative dollars.

Each intern, resident, or fellow has some particular environment with which he can interact best. The head of a large educational program has the responsibility for identifying this circumstance. He must guide the young men to recognize their potentialities and limitations so that they can live comfortably with these realities. False notions that one kind of work is more honorable than another must be stripped away. Young men must be persuaded

Young men must be persuaded to determine the personal satisfactions—the returns of each day—which will come from a variety of different careers.

to determine the personal satisfactions—the returns of each day—which will come from a variety of different careers. Each career, however different, may be equally honorable. The returns to different persons in satisfaction may be widely different. The career which has been completely satisfying to the mentor may be a disaster for his pupil. An instructor interested in the joy of the present will not try to mold in his own image the young men whom he encounters.

Part IV
Some Philosophical and Ethical Considerations

Chapter 14
Toward an Expanded Medical Ethics:
The Hippocratic Ethic Revisited
Edmund D. Pellegrino, MD

The Hippocratic ethic is one of the most admirable codes in the history of man . . . but even its ethical sensibilities and high moral tone are insufficient for the complexities of today's problems. . . . An evolving, constantly refurbished system of medical ethics is requisite in the twentieth century.

MORE IS NEEDED

Custom without truth is but the seniority of error.
Saint Cyprian, *Epistles LXXIV*

The good physician is by the nature of his vocation called to practice his art within a framework of high moral sensitivity. For two millennia this sensitivity was provided by the Oath and the other ethical writings of the Hippocratic corpus. No code has been more influential in heightening the moral reflexes of ordinary men. Every subsequent medical code is essentially a footnote to the Hippocratic precepts, which even to this day remain the paradigm of how the good physician should behave.

The Hippocratic ethic is marked by a unique

Editor's Note: Dr. Pellegrino is an accomplished clinician and respected medical investigator. He contributed to the development of the innovative Hunterdon Medical Center in Flemington, New Jersey and the University of Kentucky School of Medicine. He is Professor of Medicine, founder and Director of the new six-school Health Sciences Center at the State University of New York at Stony Brook.

combination of humanistic concern and practical wisdom admirably suited to the physician's tasks in society. In a simpler world, that ethic long sufficed to guide the physician in his service to patient and community. Today, the intersections of medicine with contemporary science, technology, social organization, and changed human values have revealed significant missing dimensions in the ancient ethic. The reverence we rightly accord the Hippocratic precepts must not obscure the need for a critical examination of their missing dimensions—those most pertinent for contemporary physicians and society. The need for expanding traditional medical ethics is already well-established. It was first underscored by the shocking revelations of the Nuremberg trials. A spate of new codes has appeared which attempt to deal more responsibly with the promise and the dangers of human experimentation; the inquiry is well under way.[1-3]

More recently, further ethical inquiries have been initiated to reflect the change in moral climate and medical attitudes toward abortion, population control, euthanasia, transplanting organs, and manipulating human behavior and genetic constitution.[1-5]

In actual fact, some of the major proscriptions of the Hippocratic Oath are already being consciously compromised: confidentiality can be violated under certain conditions of law and public safety; abortion is being legalized; dangerous drugs are used everywhere; and a conscious but controlled invasion of the patient's rights in human experimentation is now permitted.

This essay will examine some important dimensions of medical ethics not included in the Hippocratic ethic and, in some ways, even obscured by its too rigorous application. To be considered here are the ethics of participation, the questions raised by institutionalizing medical care, the need for an axiology of medical ethics, the changing ethics of competence, and the tensions between individual and social ethics.

An analysis of these questions will reveal the urgent need for expanding medical ethical concerns far beyond those traditionally observed. A deeper ethic of social and corporate responsibility is needed to guide the profession to levels of moral sensitivity more congruent with the expanded duties of the physician in contemporary culture.

THE HIPPOCRATIC ETHIC

The normative principles which constitute what may loosely be termed the Hippocratic ethic are contained in the Oath and the deontological books: *Law, Decorum, Precepts,* and *The Physician.* These treatises are of varied origin and combine behavioral imperatives derived from a variety of sources—the schools at Cos and Cnidus, intermingled with Pythagorean, Epicurean, and Stoic influences.[6,7]

The Oath[8] speaks of the relationships of the student and his teacher, advises the physician never to harm the patient, enjoins confidentiality, and proscribes abortion, euthanasia, and the use of the knife. It forbids sexual commerce with the women in the household of the sick. The doctor is a member of a select brotherhood dedicated to the care of the sick, and his major reward is a good reputation.

Law discusses the qualities of mind and the diligence required of the prospective physician from early life.[9] *The Physician* emphasizes the need for dignified comportment, a healthy body, a grave and kind mien, and a regular life.[9(pp 311-313)] In *Decorum,* we are shown the unique practical wisdom rooted in experience which is essential to good medicine and absent in the quack; proper comportment in the sick room dictates a reserved, authoritative, composed air; much practical advice is given on the arts and techniques of clinical medicine.[9(pp 279-301)] *Precepts* again warns against theorizing without fact, inveighs against quackery, urges consideration in setting fees, and encourages consultation in difficult cases.[8(pp 313-333)]

Similar admonitions can be found scattered throughout the Hippocratic corpus, but it is these few brief ethical treatises which have formed the character of the physician for so many centuries. From them, we can extract what can loosely be called the Hippocratic ethic—a mixture of high ideals, common sense, and practical wisdom. A few principles of genuine ethics are often repeated and intermingled with etiquette and homespun advice of all sorts. The good physician emerges as an authoritative and competent practitioner, devoted to his patient's well-being. He is a benevolent and sole arbiter who knows what is best for the patient and makes all decisions for him.

There is in the Hippocratic corpus little explicit reference to the responsibilities of medicine as a corporate entity with responsibility for its members and duties to the greater human community. The ethic of the profession as a whole is assured largely by the moral behavior of its individual members. There is no explicit delineation of the corporate responsibility of physicians for one another's ethical behavior. On the whole, the need for maintaining competence is indirectly stated. There are, in short, few explicit recommendations about what we would today call "social ethics."

These characteristics of the Hippocratic ethic have been carried forward to our day. They are extended in the code of Thomas Percival, which formed the basis of the first code of ethics adopted by the American Medical Association in 1847.[10] They were sufficient for the less complex societies of the ancient and modern worlds but not for the contemporary twentieth-century experience. The Hippocratic norms can no longer be regarded as unchanging absolutes but as partial statements of ideals, in need of constant reevaluation, amplification, and evolution.

Without in any way denigrating the essential worth of the Hippocratic ethic, it is increasingly apparent that the ideas conveyed about the physician are simplistic and incomplete for today's needs. In some ways, it is even antipathetic to the social and political spirit of our times. For example, the notion of the physician as a benevolent and paternalistic figure who decides all for the patient is inconsistent with today's educated public. It is surely incongruous in a democratic society in which the rights of self-determination are being assured by law. In a day when the remote effects of individual medical acts are so consequential, we cannot be satisfied with an ethic which is so inexplicit about social responsibilities. Nowhere in the Hippocratic Oath is the physician recognized as a member of a corporate entity which can accomplish good ends for man that are more than the sum of individual good acts. The necessity for a stringent ethic of competence and a new ethic of shared responsibility which flows from team and institutional medical care are understandably not addressed.

It is useful to examine some of these missing ethical dimensions as examples of the kind of organic development long overdue in professional medical ethical codes.

THE ETHICS OF PARTICIPATION

The central and most admirable feature of the Oath is the respect it inculcates for the patient. In the Oath, the doctor is pledged always to help the patient and keep him from harm. This duty is then exemplified by specific prohibitions against abortion, use of deadly drugs, surgery, breaches of confidence, and indulgence in sexual relations with members of the sick person's household. Elsewhere, in *The Physician, Decorum,* and *Precepts,* the physician is further enjoined to be humble, careful in observation, calm and sober in thought and speech. These admonitions have the same validity today that they had centuries ago and are still much in need of cultivation.

The central and most admirable feature of the Oath is the respect it inculcates for the patient.

But in one of these same works, *Decorum,* we find an excellent example of how drastically the relationship between physician and patient has changed since Hippocrates' time. The doctor is advised to, "Perform all things calmly and adroitly, concealing most things from the patient while you are attending him." A little further on, the physician is told to treat the patient with solicitude, "revealing nothing of the patient's present and future condition." [9(pp 297, 299)] This advice is at variance with social and political trends and with the desires of most educated patients. It is still too often the modus operandi of physicians dreaming of a simpler world in which authority and paternalistic benevolence were the order of the day.

Indeed, a major criticism of physicians today centers on this very question of disclosure of essential information. Many educated patients feel frustrated in their desire to participate in decisions which affect them as intimately as medical decisions invariably do. The matter really turns on establishing new bases for the patient's trust. The knowledgeable patient can trust the physician only if he feels the latter is competent and uses that competence with integrity and for ends which have value for the patient. Today's educated patient wants to understand what the physician

Today's educated patient wants to understand what the physician is doing, why he is doing it, what the alternatives may be, and what choices are open.

is doing, why he is doing it, what the alternatives may be, and what choices are open. In a democratic society, people expect the widest protection of their rights to self-determination. Hence, the contemporary patient has a right to know the decisions involved in managing his case.

When treatment is specific, with few choices open, the prognosis good, and side effects minimal, disclosing the essential information is an easy matter. Unfortunately, medicine frequently deals with indefinite diagnoses and nonspecific treatments of uncertain value. Several alternatives are usually open; prognosis may not be altered by treatment; side effects are often considerable and discomfort significant. The patient certainly has the right to know these data before therapeutic interventions are initiated. The Nuremberg Code and others were designed to protect the subject in the course of human experimentation by insisting on the right of informed and free consent. The same right should be guaranteed in the course of ordinary medical treatment as well.

So fundamental is this right of self-determination in a democratic society that to limit it, even in ordinary medical transactions, is to propagate an injustice. This is not to ignore the usual objections to disclosure: the fear of inducing anxiety in the patient, the inability of the sick patient to participate in the decision, the technical nature of medical knowledge, and the possibility of litigation. These objections deserve serious consideration but will, on close analysis, not justify concealment except under special circumstances. Obviously, the fear of indiscriminate disclosure cannot obfuscate the invasion of a right, even when concealment is in the interest of the patient.

Surely, the physician is expected by the patient and society to use disclosure prudently. For the very ill, the very anxious, the poorly educated, the too young, or the very old, he will permit himself varying degrees of disclosure. The modes of doing so must be adapted to the patient's educational level, psychologic responses, and physiologic state. It must be emphatically stated that the purpose of disclosure of alternatives, costs, and benefits in medical diagnosis and treatment is not to relieve the physician of the onus of decision or displace it on the patient. Rather, it permits the physician to function as the technical expert and adviser, inviting the patient's participation and understanding as aids in the acceptance of the decision and its consequences. This is the only basis for a mature, just, and understandable physician-patient relationship.

DEONTOLOGIC VERSUS AXIOLOGIC ETHICS

The most important human reason for enabling the patient to participate in the decisions which affect him is to allow consideration of his personal values. Here, the Hippocratic tradition is explicitly lacking, since its spirit is almost wholly deontological, that is, obligations are stated as absolutes without reference to any theory of values. Underlying value systems are not stated or discussed. The need for examining the intersection of values inherent in every medical transaction is unrecognized. The values of the physician or of medicine are assumed to prevail as absolutes, and an operational attitude of "noblesse oblige" is encouraged.

A deontologic ethic was not inappropriate for Greek medicine, which did not have to face so many complex and antithetical courses of action. But a relevant ethic for our times must be more axiologic than deontologic, that is, based in a more conscious theory of values. The values upon which any action is based are of enormous personal and social consequence. An analysis of conflicting values underlies the choice of a noxious treatment for a chronic illness, the question of prolonging life in an incurable disease, or setting priorities for using limited medical resources. Instead of absolute values, we deal more frequently with an intersection of several sets and subsets of values: those of the patient, the physician, sciences, and society. Which shall prevail when these values are in conflict? How do we decide?

The patient's values must be respected whenever possible and whenever they do not create injustice for others. The patient is free to delegate the decision to his physicians, but he must do this consciously and freely. To the extent that he is educated, responsible, and thoughtful, modern man will increasingly want the opportunity to examine relative values in each transaction. When the patient is unconscious or otherwise unable to participate, the physician or the family acts as his surrogate, charged as closely as possible to preserve his values.

The Hippocratic principle of *primum non nocere*, therefore, must be expanded to encompass the patient's value system if it is to have genuine meaning. To impose the doctor's value system is an intrusion on the patient; it may be harmful, unethical, and result in an error in diagnosis and treatment. Further, the concept of "health" as a positive entity is as vague today as in Hippocrates' time. Its definition is highly personal. The physician's view of health may be quite at variance with that of the patient or even of society. The doctor understandably tends to place an ideological value on health and medicine. Society should expect this from him as an expert, but his view must not prevail unchallenged. Indeed, society must set its own priorities for health. The amelioration of social disorders like alcoholism, sociopathy, drug addiction, and violence can have greater value for a healthy human existence, for example, than merely prolonging life in patients with chronic disabling disorders. Indeed, the patient and society now demand to participate in making the choices. The configuration of value choices each of us makes defines concretely our uniqueness and individuality. Hence, each patient has a slightly different definition of health. The physician is also a person with a set of values which invariably colors his professional acts. His views of sex, alcohol, suffering, poverty, race, and so forth can sharply differ with those of his patient. His advice on these matters, as well as his definition of cooperation, often have a strong ideologic or moralistic tinge. The physician must constantly guard

> *The physician must constantly guard against confusing his own values as the "good," to which all must subscribe if they desire to be treated by him.*

against confusing his own values as the "good," to which all must subscribe if they desire to be treated by him.

Disclosure is, therefore, a necessary condition if we really respect each patient as a unique being whose values, as a part of his person, are no more to be violated than his body. The deontologic thrust of traditional medical ethics is too restrictive in a time when the reexamination of all values is universal. It even defeats the very purposes of the traditional ethic, which are to preserve the integrity of the patient as a person.

INDIVIDUAL VERSUS SOCIAL ETHICS

Another notably unexplored area in the Hippocratic ethic is the social responsibility of the physician. Its emphasis on the welfare of the individual patient is exemplary, and this is firmly explicated in the Oath and elsewhere. Indeed, in *Precepts*, this respect for the individual patient is placed at the very heart of medicine: "Where there is love of one's fellow man, there is love of the Art." [8(p 319)]

As Ford has shown, today too the physician's sense of responsibility is directed overwhelmingly toward his own patient. [11] This is one of the most admirable features of medicine, and it must always remain the central ethical imperative in medical transactions. But it must now be set in a context entirely alien to that in which ancient medicine was practiced. In earlier eras the remote effects of medical acts were of little concern, and the rights of the individual patient could be the exclusive and absolute base of the physician's actions. Today, the growing interdependence of all humans and the effectiveness of medical techniques have drastically altered the simplistic arrangements of traditional ethics. The aggregate effects of individual medical acts have already changed the ecology of man. Every death prevented or life prolonged alters the number, kind, and distribution of human beings. The resultant competition for living space, food, and conveniences already imperils our hope for a life of satisfaction for all mankind.

Even more vexing questions in social ethics are posed when we attempt to allocate our resources among the many new possibilities for good inherent in medical progress and technology. Do we pool our limited resources and manpower to apply curative medicine to all now deprived of it or continue to multiply the complexity of services for the privileged? Do we apply mass prophylaxis against streptococcal diseases, or repair damaged valves with expensive heart surgery after they are damaged? Is it preferable to change cultural patterns in favor of a more reasonable diet for Americans or develop better surgical techniques for unplugging fat-occluded coronary arteries? Every health planner and concerned public official has his own set of similar questions. It is clear that we cannot have all these things simultaneously.

This dimension of ethics becomes even more immediate when we inquire into the responsibility of medicine for meeting the urgent sociomedical needs of large segments of our population. Can we absolve ourselves from responsibility for deficiencies in distribution, quality, and accessibility of even ordinary medical care for the poor, the uneducated and the disenfranchised? Do we direct our health care system to the care of the young in ghettos and underdeveloped countries or to the affluent aged? Which course will make for a better world? These are vexing questions of the utmost social concern. Physicians have an ethical responsibility to raise these questions and, in answering them, to work with the community in ordering its priorities to make optimal use of available medical skills.

It is not enough to hope that the good of the community will grow fortuitously out of the summation of good acts of each physician for his own patients. Societies are necessary to insure enrichment of the life of each of their members. But they are more than the aggregate of persons within them. As T. S. Eliot puts it, "What life have you if you have not life together? There is no life that is not in community." [12]

Society supports the doctor in the expectation that he will direct himself to socially relevant health problems, not just those he finds interesting or remunerative. The commitment to social egalitarianism demands a greater sensitivity to social ethics than is to be found in traditional codes. Section ten of the American Medical Association Principles of Medical Ethics (1946) explicitly recognizes the profession's responsibility to society. But a more explicit analysis of the relationships of individual and social ethics should be undertaken. Medicine, which touches on the most human problems of both the individual and society, cannot serve man without attending to both his personal and communal needs.

This is not to say that medical codes or physicians are to set social priorities. Clearly, the individual physician cannot quantitate the remote effects of each of his medical acts. Nor should he desert his patients to devote himself entirely to social issues. He cannot withhold specific treatment in hope of preventing some future perturbation of human ecology. Nor can society relegate solely to physicians such policy questions as how and for whom the major health effort will be expended.

In these matters the physician serves best

as an expert witness, providing the basis for informed public decisions. He must lead in pointing out deficiencies and raising the painful matter of choices. At the same time, each doctor must honor his traditional contract to help his own patient. He cannot allow the larger social issues to undermine that solicitude. The ethically responsive doctor will thus find himself more and more at the intersection of social and individual ethical values, impelled to act responsibly in both spheres. The Hippocratic ethic and its later modifications were not required to confront such paradoxes. Today's conscientious physician is very much in need of an expanded ethic to cope with his double responsibility to the individual and to the community.

THE ETHICS OF
INSTITUTIONALIZED MEDICINE

The institutionalization of all aspects of medical care is an established fact. With increasing frequency, the personal contract inherent in patient care is made with institutions, groups of physicians, or teams of health professionals. The patient now often expects the institution or group to select his physician or consultant and to assume responsibility for the quality and quantity of care provided.

Within the institution itself, the health care team is essential to the practice of comprehensive medicine. Physicians and nonphysicians now cooperate in providing the spectrum of special services made possible by modern technology. The responsibility for even the most intimate care of the patient is shared. Some of the most important clinical decisions are made by team members who may have no personal contact at all with the patient. The team itself is not a stable entity of unchanging composition. Its membership changes in response to the patient's needs, and so may its leadership. Preserving the traditional rights of the patient, formerly vested in a single identifiable physician, is now sometimes spread anonymously over a group. Competence, confidentiality, integrity, and personal concern are far more difficult to assure with a group of diverse professionals enjoying variable degrees of personal contact with the patient.

No current code of ethics fully defines how the traditional rights of the medical transaction are to be protected when responsibility is diffused within a team and an institution. Clearly, no health profession can elaborate such a code of team ethics by itself. We need a new medical ethic which permits the cooperative definition of normative guides to protect the person of the patient served by a group, none of whose members may have sole responsibility for care. Laymen, too, must participate, since boards of trustees set the overall policies which affect patient care. Few trustees truly recognize that they are the ethical and legal surrogates of society for the patients who come to their institutions seeking help.

Thus, the most delicate of the physician's responsibilities, protecting the patient's welfare, must now be fulfilled in a new and complicated context. Instead of the familiar one-to-one unique relationship, the physician finds himself coordinator of a team, sharing with others some of the most sensitive areas of patient care. The physician is still bound to see that group assessment and management are

---

The physician must especially guard against the dehumanization so easily and inadvertently perpetrated by a group in the name of efficiency.

---

rational, safe, and personalized. He must especially guard against the dehumanization so easily and inadvertently perpetrated by a group in the name of efficiency.

The doctor must acquire new attitudes. Since ancient times, he has been the sole dominant and authoritarian figure in the care of his patient. He has been supported in this position by traditional ethics. In the clinical emergency, his dominant role is still unchallenged, since he is well trained to make quick decisions in ambiguous situations. What he is not prepared for are the negotiations, analysis, and ultimate compromise fundamental to group efforts and essential in nonemergency situations. A whole new set of clinical perspectives must be introduced, perspectives difficult for the classically trained physician to accept, but necessary if the patient is to benefit from contemporary technology and organization of health care.

THE ETHICS OF COMPETENCE

A central aim of the Oath and other ethical treatises is to protect the patient and the profession from quackery and incompetence. In the main, competence is assumed as basic to fulfillment of the Hippocratic ideal of *primum non nocere*. In places, more specific admonitions are to be found. Thus, in *Law*, "Medicine is the most distinguished of all the arts, but through the ignorance of those who practice it, and those who casually judge such practitioners, it is now of all arts by far the least esteemed." [9(p 263)] The author of this treatise thus succinctly expressed the same concerns being voiced at greater length and with more hyperbole in our own times. In the treatise on fractures, specific advice is given to prevent curable cases from becoming incurable, to choose the simpler treatment, to attempt to help, even if the patient seems incurable, and to avoid "unnecessary torment." [13] Consultation is clearly advised in *Precepts*.[8(pp 323, 325)] In *Decorum*, frequent visits and careful examination are enjoined.[9(p 295)]

The Hippocratic works preach the wholly admirable common-sense ethos of the good artisan: careful work, maturation of skills, simplicity of approach, and knowledge of limitations. This was sound advice at a time when new discoveries were so often the product of speculation untainted by observation or experience. The speculative astringency of the Hippocratic ethic was a potent and necessary safeguard against the quackery of fanciful and dangerous "new" cures.

With the scientific era in medicine, the efficacy of new techniques and information in changing the natural history of disease was dramatically demonstrated. Today, the patient has a right to access to the vast stores of new knowledge useful to medicine. Failure of the physician to make this reservoir available and accessible is a moral failure. The ethos of the artisan, while still a necessary safeguard, is now far from being a sufficient one.

Maintaining competence today is a prime ethical challenge. Only the highest standard of initial and continuing professional proficiency is acceptable in a technological world. This imperative is now so essential a feature of the patient-physician transaction that the ancient mandate, "Do no harm," must be supplemented: "Do all things essential to optimal solution of the patient's problem." Anything less makes the doctor's professional declaration a sham and a scandal.

Competence now has a far wider definition than in ancient times. Not only must the physician encompass expertly the knowledge pertinent to his own field, but he must be the instrument for bringing all other knowledge to bear on his patient's needs. He now functions as one element in a vast matrix of consultants, technicians, apparatus, and institutions, all of which may contribute to his patient's well-being. He cannot provide all these things himself. To attempt to do so is to pursue the romantic and vanishing illusion of the physician as Renaissance man.

The enormous difficulties of its achievement notwithstanding, competence has become the first ethical precept for the modern physician after integrity. It is also the prime humane precept and the one most peculiar to the physician's function in society. Even the current justifiable demands of patients and medical students for greater compassion must not obfuscate the centrality of competence in the physician's existence. The simple intention to help others is commendable but, by itself, not only insufficient but positively dangerous. What is more inhumane or more a violation of trust than incompetence? The consequence of a lack of compassion may be remediable, while a lack of competence may cost the patient his chance for recovery of life, function, and happiness. Clearly, medicine cannot attain the ethical eminence to which it is called without both compassion and competence.

Within this framework, a more rigorous ethic of competence must be elaborated. Continuing education, periodic recertification, and renewal of clinical privileges have become moral mandates, not just hopeful hortatory devices dependent upon individual physician responses. The Hippocratic ethic of the good artisan is now just the point of departure for the wide options technology holds out for individual and social health.

The one-to-one patient-to-physician relationship so earnestly extolled for centuries makes the patient almost totally dependent upon his physician for entry into the vast complex of potentially useful services. We cannot leave to fortune or statistics the possibility that the patient's choice of a physician might impede his access to all he needs for optimal care. We must surround this one-to-one relationship with the safeguards of a corporate responsibility in which the whole profession dedicates itself to protecting the patient's right to competent care.

TOWARD A CORPORATE ETHIC AND AN ETHICAL SYNCYTIUM

The whole of the Hippocratic corpus, including the ethical treatises, is the work of many authors writing in different historical periods. Thus, the ethical precepts cannot be considered the formal position of a profession in today's sense. There is no evidence of recognition of true corporate responsibility for larger social issues or of sanctions to deter miscreant members. Indeed, in *Law,* there is a clear lament for the lack of penalties to restrain or punish the unethical physician:

". . . medicine is the only art which our states have made subject to no penalty save that of dishonor. And dishonor does not wound those who are compacted of it."[9(p 263)] Again, in *Precepts:* "Now no harm would be done if bad practitioners received their due wages. But as it is, their innocent patients suffer, for whom the violence of their disorder did not appear sufficient without the addition of their physician's inexperience."[8(p 315)]

The Greek physician seems to have regarded himself as the member of an informal aristocratic brotherhood, in which each individual was expected to act ethically and to do so for love of the profession and respect of the patient. His reward was *doxa,* a good reputation, which in turn assured a successful practice. There is notably no sense of the larger responsibilities as a profession for the behavior of each member. Nowhere stated are the potentialities and responsibilities of a group of high-minded individuals to effect reforms and achieve purposes transcending the interests of individual members. In short, the Greek medical profession relied on the sum total of individual ethical behaviors to assure the ethical behavior of the group.

This is still the dominant view of many physicians in the Western world who limit their ethical perspectives to their relationships with their own patients. Medical societies do censure unethical members with varying alacrity for the grosser forms of misconduct or breaches of professional etiquette. But there is as yet insufficient assumption of a corporate and shared responsibility for the actions of each member of the group. The power of physicians as a polity to effect reforms in quality of care, its organization, and its relevance to the needs of society is as yet unrealized.

Yet many of the dimensions of medical ethics touched upon in this essay can only be secured by the conscious assumption of a corporate responsibility on the part of all physicians for the final pertinence of their individual acts to promote better life for all. There is the need to develop, as it were, a functioning ethical syncytium in which the actions of each physician would touch upon those of all physicians and in which it is clear that the ethical failings of each member would diminish the stature of every other physician to some degree. This syncytial framework is at variance with the traditional notion that each physician acts as an individual and is primarily responsible only to himself and his patient.

This shift of emphasis is dictated by the metamorphosis of all professions in our complex, highly organized, highly integrated, and egalitarian social order. For most of its history medicine has existed as a select and loosely organized brotherhood. For the past hundred years in our country, it has been more formally organized in the American Medical Association and countless other professional organizations dedicated to a high order of individual ethics. A new stage in the evolution of medicine as a profession is about to begin as a consequence of three clear trends.

First, all professions are increasingly being regarded as services, even as public utilities, dedicated to fulfilling specific social needs not entirely defined by the profession. Professions themselves will acquire dignity and standing in the future, not so much from the tasks they perform, but from the intimacy of the connection between those tasks and the social life of which the profession is a part. Second, the professions are being democratized, and it will be ever more difficult for any group to hold a privileged position. The automatic primacy of medicine is being challenged by the other health professions, whose functions are of increasing importance in patient care. This functionalization of the professions tends to emphasize what is done for a patient and not who does it. Moreover, many tasks formerly performed only by the physicians are now being done by other professionals and nonprofessionals. Last, the socialization of all mankind affects the professions as well. Hence, the collectivity will increasingly be expected to take responsibility for how well or poorly the profession carries out the purposes for which it is supported by society.

These changes will threaten medicine only if physicians hold to a simplistic ethic in which the agony of choices among individual and social values is dismissed as spurious or imaginary. The physician is the most highly educated of health professionals. He should be first to take on the burdens of a continuing self-reformation in terms of a new ethos— one in which the problematics of priorities and values are openly faced as common responsibilities of the entire profession. We must recognize the continuing validity of traditional ethics for the personal dimensions of patient care and their inadequacy for the newer social dimensions of health in contemporary life. It is the failure to appreciate this distinction that stimulates so much criticism of the profession at the same time that individual physicians are highly respected.

PROBLEMS AND RESPONSIBILITIES What are some of the ethical problems and social responsibilities which are best assured by a corporate posture? We mention but a few as examples, especially those outlined earlier in this essay.

ASSURING COMPETENCE In a technical society with knowledge increasing exponentially, all members of a profession cannot attain the same degree of competence. The whole body of physicians must assume responsibility for guaranteeing to society the highest possible competence in each member. A most effective way to assure this is for each professional group to require, as some already have, the periodic demonstration of continued proficiency as a first condition for continuing membership in the profession. Physicians should take leadership in requiring relicensure and recertification, set the standards of performance, and insist on a remedial and not a punitive approach for those who need refurbishment of their knowledge to qualify for recertification. Implicit in this idea is the possibility that at some point each of us may fail to qualify for reasons such as age, illness, or loss of interest. A profession sensitive to

---

A profession sensitive to its ethical responsibilities cannot tolerate fading competence, even for reasons beyond the physician's control.

---

its ethical responsibilities cannot tolerate fading competence, even for reasons beyond the physician's control. Instead, it must provide opportunities for remediation or for alternate, more suitable functions within medicine. Surely, the wide range of uses of a medical education will assure a useful place for almost all physicians.

A most potent way to assure competence is to insist that all physicians practice within a context of competent colleagues and peer surveillance. It is an ethical responsibility of the whole profession to see that every licensed physician is a member of a hospital staff. The privilege of using a hospital is primarily a privilege for the patient, not the doctor. To deprive any licensed physician, because of training, economics, race, or other reasons, of hospital privilege is to deprive his patient and to perpetrate a social injustice. We also thereby lose the best chance to help the physician improve himself by contact with his colleagues and with institutional standards, as well as the informal network of teaching that links physicians together when they can discuss their cases with one another. No rationalization based on economics or professional prerogatives can excuse our profession from its ethical responsibility to enable every practitioner to participate in the mainstream of medical care, in the hospital and the medical school as well. This responsibility should extend to the osteopathic, as well as the allopathic, physician.

Once every physician is on a hospital staff, there is much the profession can do to develop a context within which competence becomes

a value of prime importance. Some institutional mechanisms for review of certain aspects of competence already exist in tissue and utilization committees, though these first steps are not universally applied with sufficient vigor. A well-functioning drug information center in every hospital, a rigorous pharmacy and therapeutics committee, critical reviews of diagnostic accuracy and work-up, comparison of practices against national standards—these are examples of further institutional devices we should insist upon as ethical imperatives. Ultimately, each physician should have available for his own edification a computerized record of his diagnostic acumen, therapeutic practices, complications, and autopsy correlations. The essential matter is not the specific mechanisms used, but acceptance of the dictum that the competence of each member of the group is, in some real sense, the responsibility of all.

These measures can easily be discounted as repressive, regimentalizing infringements of professional freedom. Or, in a more enlightened ethical view, they can be the practical expression of corporate acceptance of the necessity of workable mechanisms to ensure competence in a technological society. Is there a real ethical choice? The patient, after all, has no means whereby he can judge the com-

---

Individual physicians and the profession owe the patient every possible safeguard.

---

petence of the services rendered. Individual physicians and the profession owe the patient every possible safeguard. When these are not forthcoming, they will be imposed by a public demanding more accountability in medicine and every other sphere of life.

One of the gravest and most easily visible social inequities today is the maldistribution of medical services among portions of our population. This is another sphere in which the profession as a whole must assume responsibility for what individual physicians cannot do alone. The civil rights movement and the revolt of the black and minority populations have punctuated the problem. Individual physicians have always tried to redress this evil, some in heroic ways. Now, however, the problem is a major ethical responsibility for the whole profession; we cannot dismiss the issue. We must engender a feeling of ethical diminution of the entire profession whenever there are segments of the population without adequate and accessible medical care. This extends to the provision of primary care for all, insistence on a system of coverage for all communities every hour of the day, proper distribution of the various medical specialties and facilities, and a system of fees no longer based on the usual imponderables, but on more standardized norms.

Fulfilling such ethical imperatives is sure to cause discomfort for the doctor, as well as some loss of privileges and even of remuneration. But unless there is corporate concern translated into corporate action and self-imposed responsibilities, restrictive legislation to achieve these ends seems certain. To an ethically perceptive profession, such legislation should not only be unnecessary, it should be a scandal. It is intrinsic to the very purposes of medicine that physicians exhibit the greatest sensitivity to any social injustice directly related to their mandate in society. The lack of this corporate sensitivity has been acutely perceived by some of today's students and has seriously disaffected them with medical education and practice.[14] We hope, when they assume leadership of the profession, that they will feel these ethical discontinuities as clearly as they do now. If tomorrow's physicians practice what they now preach to their elders, they will indeed expand the ethical responsibilities of our profession into new and essential dimensions. To do so, they will need to supplement traditional medical ethics with a corporate ethical sense as we have just described it.

There are, perforce, reasonable limits to the social ills to which the individual physi-

cian and the profession can be expected to attend *qua* physician. Some have suggested that medicine concern itself with the Vietnam war, the root causes of poverty, environmental pollution, drugs, housing, and racial injustice. It would be difficult to argue that all of these social ills are *primary* ethical responsibilities of individual physicians or even of the profession. To do so would hopelessly diffuse medical energies and manpower from their proper object—the promotion of health and the cure of illness. The profession can fight poverty, injustice, and war *through* medicine.

A distinction, therefore, must clearly be made between the physician's *primary* ethical responsibilities, which derive from the nature of his profession, and those which do not. Each physician must strike for himself an optimal balance between professional and civic responsibilities. This will depend upon his energy, capabilities, the nature of his specialty, his family responsibilities, and other factors. The extremes of this choice are dangerous: a narrowly technical life, or a free-floating social concern which at best is neurotic and ineffectual and at worst can seriously compromise competence. Ever present is the seductive hubris to which physicians are especially susceptible—the assumption of some special authority or capability in the resolution of all social issues.

THE ORDER OF ETHICAL RESPONSIBILITY

It becomes a matter of prime ethical concern for each physician consciously to establish some hierarchy of values and priorities which

---

It becomes a matter of prime ethical concern for each physician consciously to establish some hierarchy of values and priorities which will define his individual and social ethical postures.

---

will define his individual and social ethical postures. The ethical responsibilities of the professional group should be broad; those of the individual may of necessity be narrow. Is there some reasonable order of values in the maze of conflicting duties thrust upon physicians today? We will examine this question from the point of view of the clinician.

Surely, the first order of responsibility for clinicians must remain with the patients he undertakes to treat. Here, the moral imperatives are clear: competence of the highest order; integrity; compassion.

These are contained in traditional medical ethics and can be made more relevant to our times by extension in some of the directions indicated earlier in this essay. To fail in this realm is to violate the trust underlying the personal relationship which characterizes medical care. Nothing is more unconscionable or socially unacceptable.

Only when this first order of ethical requirements has been met may the individual physician address himself to a second order of responsibilities. These are generally of two kinds: those which arise from medical progress—like human experimentation and genetic and behavioral modification—and those which bear directly on the condition of life of the community—population control, eradicating malnutrition, assurance of accessibility, comprehensive health care for all citizens, abortion, drugs, and so on. Of the two sets, the latter are more directly related to the daily work of the practitioner and pose ethical issues of an immediate nature, since they flow so directly from his first-order responsibilities.

In these matters, the physician can indeed act as a leader, a sensor of unmet needs, and an expert witness in constructing feasible solutions. He can mobilize his county and state society to assume corporate responsibility for distributing physicians, for mandating coverage of all communities, perhaps experimenting with use of nonphysicians. The physician can use his authority as a clinician to underline needs for improvement of services and facilities in his community. If he clearly focuses on patient and community health and not on his own prerogatives, there can be no more effective voice in initiating reforms.

The third order of responsibilities—those more properly related to the physician as a citizen than as a physician—are among the most crucial for modern man. Yet they are usually outside the physician's prerogatives and distant from his direct function in society. Important as they are, these issues—poverty, war, racism—require knowledge the doctor must acquire. If these are his major concerns, he should make no pretense at also being a clinician, or he will become one in the most limited sense. Medical education and experience make a legitimate base for service in new fields or social and political action, but they do not legitimatize the neglect of clinical competence in individual medical acts. This distinction needs careful scrutiny by those who would have the physician cure the accumulated social ills of our times and who upbraid him for his failures to do this and to maintain professional competence as well. "If you try to act beyond your powers, you not only disgrace yourself in it, but you neglect the part which you could have filled with success." [15]

THE INTERPLAY OF INDIVIDUAL AND CORPORATE ETHICS

The individual physician can, and indeed should, limit his ethical pretensions. The profession as a body can but should not. Physicians as a group must assume ethical responsibility for all three orders of responsibility which may bind each physician. The profession, as we have shown, must attempt to do as a body what individuals cannot do by themselves—namely, span the full range of ethical imperatives. The profession is bound to assume responsibility for the ethical behavior of its members, for setting the context which best guarantees good behavior and taking sanctions against members who fall from their high estate, while at the same time effecting their rehabilitation. Physicians as individuals may eschew certain responsibilities as inappropriate, but the profession cannot.

Herein, then, lies the final guarantee for the patient and the community: the interplay of ethical responsibilities for each individual physician and of the whole body of physicians. Each physician must consciously define on several levels his personal moral responsibilities. The profession simultaneously must call for deep involvement of its members at all levels of ethical responsibility—the individual clinical medical transaction, the social consequences of medical acts and medical progress, the quality and availability of medical services, and the duties of its educated group to engage in the larger social issues confronting contemporary man. This reinforcement of the ethical perspective of the individual physician by a heightened ethical perception of the community of physicians is an essential ingredient of any professional ethical framework which hopes to cope with the current flux in values and goals afflicting modern society.

ETHICAL TENSIONS IN AN EXPANDED ETHIC

What will happen to the conscience and the values of the individual physician if the claims of society and the profession are given new ethical force? The law can insist that confidences be revealed in the interest of justice; if abortion is legalized, the physician as agent of society will be expected to provide this service; the same is true if euthanasia, personality and behavioral modification, and chemical sterilization should become public mandates. How shall we balance social and public mandates against the conscience of the individual physician? How will we safeguard the integrity of the physician's own values?

We have a terrifying example of the inability of physicians to withstand social pressures in the acts of unmitigated evil perpetrated by the physicians in German prison camps. These physicians abdicated conscience and choice so thoroughly that they participated in the most reprehensible acts—convinced that they were innocent bystanders. The individual conscience simply ceased to exist, and the individual physician became a mindless cipher. They were willingly conscripted into that "auxiliary bureaucracy" which Gabriel Marcel so scathingly deplores in *Man Against Mass Society*.[16]

The very horror of this possibility should underscore how essential is the defense of the mind, conscience, and values of the individual physician and his patient in any system of medicine, ethics, or political organization. This is all the more reason for an axiologic approach, which always calls for an orderly analysis of the values underlying moral choices. The highest ethical call is still that of the conscience of an individual human person, a conscience which must be prepared at all times to take issue with social directives, corporate agreements, and political pressures. The dignity and the worth of the human being he treats must still remain the beacon that guides the physician's conscience in the ethical night before us. Marcel pinpoints this duty so peculiar to our times: "It is within the scope of each of us, within his own proper field, in his profession, to pursue an unrelaxing struggle for man, for the dignity of man against everything that today threatens to annihilate man and his dignity."[16(p 241)]

SUMMARY

We have attempted a brief analysis of some of the limitations and omissions in traditional medical ethics as embodied in the Hippocratic corpus and its later exemplifications. These limitations are largely in the realm of social and corporate ethics, realms of increasing significance in an egalitarian, highly structured, and exquisitely interlocked social order.

The individual physician needs more explicit guidelines than traditional codes afford to meet today's new problems. The Hippocratic ethic is one of the most admirable codes in the history of man. But even its ethical sensibilities and high moral tone are insufficient for the complexities of today's problems.

An evolving, constantly refurbished system of medical ethics is requisite in the twentieth century. An axiologic, rather than a deontologic, bias is more in harmony with the questions raised in a world society whose values are in continual flux and reexamination. There is ample opportunity for a critical reappraisal of the Hippocratic ethic and for the elaboration of a fuller and more comprehensive medical ethic suited to our profession as it nears the twenty-first century. This fuller ethic will build upon the noble precepts set forth so long ago in the Hippocratic corpus. It will explicate, complement, and develop those precepts, but it must not be delimited in its evolution by an unwarranted reluctance to question even so ancient and honorable a code as that of the Hippocratic writings.

REFERENCES

1 American Academy of Arts and Sciences. *Proceedings*, vol 98, no. 2, 1969.

2 Pellegrino ED: The necessity, promise and dangers of human experimentation. *Experiments With Man*. World Council Studies, no. 6. New York, World Council of Churches, Geneva and Friendship Press, 1969.

3 New dimensions in legal and ethical concepts for human research. *Ann NY Acad Arts Sci* 169:293–593, 1970.

4 Torrey EF: *Ethical Issues in Medicine*. Boston, Little Brown & Co, 1968.

5 Pellegrino ED: *Medical Progress and Human Values: The Changing Dimensions of Medical Ethics*. Cambridge, Mass, Harvard University Press (in press).

6 Sigerist HE: *The History of Medicine*, vol 11. New York, Oxford University Press, 1961, pp 260, 298.

7 Heidel, WA: *Hippocratic Medicine: Its Spirit and Method*. New York, Columbia University Press, 1941, p 149.

8 Jones WHS (trans-ed): *Hippocrates*. Cambridge, Mass, Harvard University Press, 1923, vol I, pp 299–301.

9 Jones WHS (trans-ed): *Hippocrates*. Cambridge, Mass, Harvard University Press, 1923, vol II, pp 263–265.

10 Leake C (ed): *Percival's Medical Ethics*. Baltimore, William Wilkins, 1927, p 291.

11 Ford et al: *The Doctors Perspective*. New York, Year Book, 1967.

12 Eliot TS: ''The Rock'' in *The Complete Poems and Plays*, 1909–1950. New York, Harcourt & Brace, 1952, p 101.

13 Michler, M: Medical ethics in Hippocratic bone surgery. *Bull Hist Med* 12:297–311, 1968.

14 Truett C, Douville AW, Fagel B, et al: The medical curriculum and human values. *JAMA* 209:1341–1345, 1969.

15 Oates W (ed): *The Stoic and Epicurean Philosophers*. New York, Modern Library, 1957, p 480.

16 Marcel G: *Man Against Mass Society*. Chicago, Henry Regnery, 1962, p 180.

Chapter 15
Social and Medical Contracts: Explicit and Implicit
Richard M. Magraw, MD

I am asserting that what has come to be called the system of medical care may be better understood as a series of contracts or understandings rather than an array of facilities, trained professionals, and instruments.

DIFFERING VIEWS ON MEDICAL CARE

With a view to enhancing our understanding of our professional work, I wish to draw attention to a circumstance so commonplace in medicine that it goes unnoticed, that is, to the widely differing understandings of what medicine is, what medical care consists of, and what is the real work of a doctor. There are marked individual differences in what people consider properly medical or why they go to a doctor. Were these differing views about the nature of medical care confined to the general public—which we once rather quaintly called "the laity"—we might dismiss this phenomenon as being due to ignorance or to a lack of sophistication in technical or medical matters. But, as may be noted at almost any medical gathering, the diversity is also apparent among physicians, and this is harder to get around.

The fact that doctors have differing views about the nature of medical care and about the essence of a doctor's work might suggest that they see different kinds of patients, or else that individual doctors (and necessarily also the patients that severally consult them) perceive such medical matters as symptoms, illnesses, and prescribed treatments differently, or at the very least that, because of the nature of their special work, they emphasize different aspects of the same clinical realities. There is, to be sure, somewhat less diversity in the way physicians in the same specialty view medicine than is so for physicians generally. Of course, the scope of a given specialty or its procedures or mode of relating to patients may occasion a kind of uniformity in patients. But it is also true that individual doctors often attract a more or less homogeneous kind of patient, and hence literally do see a different kind of patient from that seen

Editor's Note: Dr. Magraw is both an internist and psychiatrist who for many years served on the full-time faculty at the University of Minnesota Medical School. In 1969 he left a position in the Department of Health, Education, and Welfare to participate in the development of four new medical schools in the University of Illinois system.

by their colleagues. When all this is taken into account, however, it remains inescapable that there are different understandings about what medical care is. This means that the ways doctors and patients come together to accomplish their tasks must vary greatly now and suggests that achieving a standardized and uniform approach in the future would be both difficult and undesirable.

At a time when there is an increasing tendency to plan for and deal with medical care as though it were a concrete commodity or a uniform and readily predictable kind of process or operation, I believe insufficient consideration has been given to the implications of this diversity. Before I get into these implications as they relate to medical care organization, let me cite one special reason for beginning by emphasizing how these fundamental differences in views about our professional work contribute to a central problem in our relationship with American society. I refer to

---

I refer to our present inability as doctors to agree on where we are and to speak with any unanimity in advising our society on what needs to be done in medical affairs.

---

our present inability as doctors to agree on where we are and to speak with any unanimity in advising our society on what needs to be done in medical affairs. As everybody knows, there are rancorous and unproductive divisions in our profession. These are readily understandable, but it would be helpful to us as individuals, as a profession, and to our society as well, if physicians could come closer to a common understanding of what is going on and what needs to be done. We could, perhaps, paraphrase Francis Bacon and state that if we begin by acknowledging diversity, we may end in unity, whereas if we insist on beginning in unity, we are likely to end in division.

WHY SO MANY DIFFERENT VIEWS?

The different understandings about what medical care is and what is the real work of a doctor partly derive from what we doctors individually understand to be the social role of the physician, and this in turn is based on our own understandings of what patients need and what we are trained to and able to provide them. The differences can be easily demonstrated in the process which we call diagnosis, since that often involves a kind of negotiation between patient and doctor in which offers (of a symptom) and counteroffers (of an explanation, diagnosis, or treatment) are made and some sort of an agreement between the two parties is reached. There are many forces acting in such transactions to shape (or distort) the definition of the trouble or the illness and to determine what therapy is agreed upon. Thus, alcoholism might be defined as "cirrhosis" or as "gastritis." Emotional problems in parents may be only defined as the "battered child syndrome." Is it the doctor's proper job to take care of the cirrhosis, the alcoholism, or both? Is it his job to care for the battered child, is it his job to care for the disturbed family, or should he be doing both?

As we have said, doctors diagnose these problems differently. One doctor defines medical responsibility for these things differently from another. There are great individual variations of expectations about medical care and acceptance of intrusion by diagnostic inquiry among patients and families as well as variations among physicians. Up until now, there has been only a murky social consensus on these matters and the agreement negotiated has been a private matter. Now, with changing circumstances, that simple transaction is changing. New complexities require new understandings and conventions to maintain the individual character of personal service in a more complex and highly organized or industrialized context.

HOW WE HAVE COPED   The medical convention for coping with this diversity up to now has been deceptively simple. We have merely emphasized the primacy of the relationship between patient and doctor in medical care. This is about as precise as we have been in describing the idiosyncratic character of much medical care and the understandings between patient and doctor on which it is based. Unfortunately, the concept of the doctor-patient relationship as a central ingredient to effective medical care has become an unconvincing cliché in our society at this point.

Nonetheless, it is important to remind ourselves and our society (or at least our legislators) that since medical care is still largely a matter of one man who feels ill asking another for help, the relationship is obviously important. But we are not here citing the fact that often doctors, among themselves and with the public as well, cannot agree on what medical care is (is it primarily to reemphasize the human dimensions of medical service or to reassert the unique and private character of the transactions of medicine?). Rather, we here cite this diversity as a first step toward a clarification of the new understandings or, as I stated in the title, the new medical and social contracts (implicit and explicit) which the evolving arrangements for medical care require.

Before we undertake such a clarification, we should remind ourselves that since Hippocrates the social roles involved had been almost unchanged until well into the twentieth century. It really is only in the lifetime of doctors now living that significant modifications of these roles have been and are being required. To understand these new arrangements we first need to look at the contracts or understandings which had been present prior to now.

THE BASIC MEDICAL CONTRACT

The hundreds of thousands of small transactions and human confrontations which daily make up medical care in this country are best conceived of as individually negotiated two-party contracts. Much of what we have called the doctor-patient relationship is more accurately described as a medical contract. It is probable that a great deal of mischief has been done by our persistence in using the relatively inexact and easily misunderstood term, "the doctor-patient relationship," and our corresponding failure to think in terms of the contract between each doctor and patient. This is so partly because the concept of a special relationship between doctors and patients has come to be understood by the public and our co-workers as bolstering a claim by the medical profession to elite status, rather than as a commitment to serve the person who is the patient; but it is so even more because the concept of a preeminent doctor-patient relationship has not been sufficiently flexible for the larger and more complex arrangements for personal health services which are now developing. As medicine now becomes more complex, more systematized or industrialized, changes in and supplementation of the basic two-party contract have been occurring. Some of these have already taken place and are explicit, while others are only now evolving and might be said to be implicit.

Some authorities feel that the basic two-party contract between doctor and patient should be and will be supplanted. My own

---

My own view is that the two-party contract, wherein two individuals negotiate an agreement about what is wrong and what is to be done, remains central in medical care and is essential to its regular effectiveness.

---

view is that the two-party contract, wherein two individuals negotiate an agreement about what is wrong and what is to be done, remains central in medical care and is essential to its regular effectiveness. That is not to say that things will stay the same. The two-party contract is now being widened in scope and is being complemented by other understandings or contracts coming into being in our developing system of medical care.

In effect, what has come to be called the system of medical care may be better understood as a series of contracts or understandings (or arrangements) rather than an array of facilities, trained professionals, instruments, and so forth.

THE DOCTOR'S JOB Before getting into an analysis of the understandings or contracts now developing, I wish to consider the divergent ideas about what the doctor's job is and to point out that lurking beneath the seemingly philosophical issue of this remarkable diversity are some very real and practical matters. Unless we can reach consensus on what the doctor's job is, how can we agree on what it is that the patient, and specifically the third party, pays for,[1] what the doctor collects a fee for, and what that fee should be? It should be further pointed out that the presence of any third-party payer in this two-party contract inevitably tends to "regularize" and make more uniform the externals of the agreement (the contract). Obviously, such "distortions" in the contract as may be introduced by the presence of any third party do not meliorate the underlying human differences and individual needs that gave rise to the diversity in the first place. To avoid misunderstanding at this point, let me emphasize that I am not suggesting any retrogression away from third-party insurance or prepayment mechanisms in the financing of medical care. These mechanisms or some variant of them are here to stay. Rather, I am suggesting that instead of seeing such agencies as "third parties" intruding into a two-party contract, we may need to view them as having contracts in their own right. We must see these separate contracts as complementary to the two-party doctor-patient contract and

revise our concepts to consonance with the actual practices. Indeed, these are not the only such complementary contracts which come into the picture.

But I am getting ahead of the story. Before going on, I want to review a few points.

First, the basic transaction of medical care is an individually negotiated two-party contract. Moreover, keeping the contractual nature of medical care in mind will facilitate the flexible adaptation required in medical care organization without loss of the human dimensions of care.

Second, the thousands of relationships between doctors and patients (that is, the doctor-patient contracts) are extremely varied and diverse. Despite the fact that there are a relatively limited number of diseases (that is, a finite number), the number of variations of contracts between individual patients and doctors is almost infinite. This is so because the disease seldom fully defines the patient's illness, and also because there are individual differences among doctors as well as patients. The point is that the human dimension of medical care is maintained and individual differences are accommodated by those very features of the process, the individual medical contracts, which give it a handmade, personally tailored character and which have been disparagingly referred to as keeping medicine a cottage industry.

Third, I have also stated that as medical care has become more organized, systematized, or institutionalized this two-party contract has been subject to a kind of homogenization or standardization. The variations which celebrate the humanness of the patient are likely to be trimmed off by the cookie cutters inherent in institutionalization or bureaucratic organization.

Moving beyond these assertions, it is obvious that it would have been folly to assume that this basic two-party contractual arrangement would not be altered, given the sweep of change in medical care.

The factors which have played a major part in that alteration include:

The progressive change in the scope of the individual physician's responsibility for patients and families which has resulted from changing public expectations regarding care and specialization.

The increasing presence of third parties in the financial part of the transaction.

The increasing amount of care provided by health workers other than physicians.

The changing role of the hospital.

The changing public attitudes about the hospital.

What is occurring is not so much a change in the two-party contract per se (although this has been modified somewhat), but the basic two-party contract is being complemented by other contracts or at least other social understandings and agreements. The complementary character of what is occurring is obscured somewhat by the tendency of various partisan groups (hospitals, physicians, third-party insurers) to each exclusively claim the central or pivotal function for their role instead of make the less pretentious claim to one of a series of complementary functions.

In the balance of this essay we will consider these alterations in the contracts of medicine and their implications for doctors and patients.

THE HOSPITAL'S CONTRACT WITH THE PATIENT

One of the most obvious and concrete of the new contracts relates to the hospital's position or role. (I refer here primarily to the community hospital, since the public hospitals—city, county, or VA hospitals where doctors have traditionally been employed to provide medical care as part of the hospital's service—have a different role and mode of functioning.) It is now clear beyond any question that the community hospital has a contractual obligation to any patient who comes to it or is sent to it by the doctor (indeed, there are indications that this obligation may soon be

widened to contractual responsibilities for a defined population, as we will consider later).

THE DARLING CASE   The legal precedent in this regard first came to widespread notice in consequence of the Darling case in Illinois in 1965.[2] It is worth any physician's while to read the transcript of the testimony in that case in order to understand the irresistible logic behind the judge's decision holding that the hospital (and its trustees) had a contractual responsibility for the patient's well-being. It is impossible to read that transcript without concluding that, aside from the medical malfeasance involved, the hospital owed the young boy who lost his leg more protection than it provided.

The decision in the Darling case has had far-reaching implications. It has held up to public view, and particularly to the notice of hospital administrators and boards of trustees, the contractual reality of their responsibility to patients.

The decision in the Darling case has had far-reaching implications. It was held up to public view, and particularly to the notice of hospital administrators and boards of trustees, the contractual reality of their responsibility to patients. We would make a serious mistake, however, if we were to think that the Darling case or the earlier New York and California cases were what established that contractual responsibility. They only crystallized into legal precedent a significant social change in our system of medical care which had been gradually developing over a generation or more and which had actually come into being during that time in scores of changes in our professional work and in the expectations of the public. I emphasize this point because, if we get the idea that the Darling decision established that contract rather than simply confirmed what was happening in society, we will be likely to miss the significance of other developments now fully underway in our professional work.

When people talked about medical care at the time I started in medical practice, almost 30 years ago, they spoke in terms of "doctors and nurses." A little later, after World War II, they began to use the phrase "doctors and hospitals." Now they usually speak of "hospitals and doctors." These shifts in phrasing may be subtle, but they are not trivial. They reflect a widespread change in expectation and understanding as to how service is provided. They express the public's understanding and agreement on the role of the institution versus the physicians' role. These are the changed views which the Darling decision documented.

It is sometimes said (particularly by those who might be said to have a "hospital" view of things) that the Darling decision made the hospital trustees totally responsible for the care of individual patients provided within the hospital walls. The promulgators of this view suggest that the hospital holds the super ordinate responsibility for all medical care provided within it. While there is some truth that hospital trustees have such a responsibility, it is not strictly accurate to leave it at that. Certainly the public is not of a mind to entrust medical care to the hospital trustees. In fact, medical responsibility (that is, the basic contract) is clearly retained in the physicians' hands. However, there is no gainsaying that we have, as a society, turned a corner in this and have sanctioned something akin to what doctors have always feared—namely, the corporate practice of medicine. What society has recognized is that medical care by a physician now occurs in a more or less tightly organized system. I believe it is a more realistic and accurate portrayal of actual social expectations to say that the hospital's responsibility in such a system is a "back up" responsibility or a "fail-safe" device. In the terms used in this essay, the two-

party contract between the individual patient and the doctor remains and is fundamental; the hospital's contract to patients is complementary to that.

THE HOSPITAL'S IMPLICIT OBLIGATION TO ITS COMMUNITY

We have considered here the hospital's contract to individual patients—the only binding obligation the hospital has. It is appropriate to comment here on another set of hospital obligations or a public trust of the hospital which is increasingly mentioned. This has to do with the hospital's responsibility for coordinating care or insuring the availability of care to a defined population or community. As yet this is mostly in the thinking and talking stage, although more and more hospital administrators and trustees are doing their long-range planning in terms of regions, networks of service, and defined populations. However, it is precisely by means of such conceptualizing and planning that expectations in medical care have been progressively redefined over the past generation. The public trust which the hospital holds in regard to personal health services is now evolving toward an implicit social contract, that is, an unwritten understanding existing in society concerning the community's support of the institution and the institution's obligation to the community.

THE HOSPITAL MEDICAL STAFF AND THE COUNTY MEDICAL SOCIETY: PHYSICIAN'S COLLECTIVE OBLIGATIONS TO PATIENTS AND COMMUNITIES

Turning now from the basic doctor-patient contract and the recently explicated hospital-patient contract, I would like to discuss the largely implicit understandings of various physician groups about professional responsibilities to patients. It is striking to me that in most parts of the country no crystallized social understanding yet exists concerning the level of responsibility to the patient (or the community) intermediate between the responsibility of the individual practicing physician and that of the hospital corporation. I believe I can make my meaning clear in this by asking a series of questions.

Is there an expectation that physicians collectively have responsibility for providing required medical services for a given population? Does a county medical society, for instance, collectively have a responsibility for the care any member of that society provides a patient or patients? As another example, does the medical staff of a hospital have collective responsibility for the care provided individual patients in that hospital? I believe that physicians would answer "yes" to at least this last question. Would the general public answer "yes" as well? That is less certain. County medical societies and hospital staffs up to now have not in fact acted collectively in these matters. At least they have not been visible to the community as active agents in the medical scene and correspondingly are not part of the public's understanding or expectation.

There are such social understandings and expectations in those parts of the country where the individual physician is ordinarily perceived as functioning in the context of a balanced group of his medical colleagues (as in Minnesota where almost 70% of physicians practice in such balanced multispecialty groups). We may correspondingly assume that contractual obligations of a formal and binding kind may develop there.[3] If so, this would be another kind of complementary contract to that two-party contract between the individual physician and patient.

Social understandings have not yet crystallized regarding the implications of the fact that each physician now carries out only a portion of the generic medical function and that it is only when doctors are recombined into a balanced medical group or linked in some kind of formal network that a genuine synthesis of medical skill is available to the patient. We have not as a profession fully recognized or accepted this fact ourselves nor formalized the professional usages involved. Those usages will develop further, and patients (and society) may come to fully expect that obtaining the services of a single physician implies the dependable availability of a balanced group of various medical experts as a regular extension of that doctor's knowledge and skill. At such a time a social understanding will have developed and the patients will in effect have an implicit contract with the group of which a particular physician is a part.

Some medical groups, particularly but not exclusively those providing prepaid care, now make contracts directly with the patient or perhaps with groups of "consumers." Unfortunately, in such instances unless specific provision is made for maintenance of a defined individual medical responsibility for specific individuals or families, there may be an avoidance of or an alteration in the basic two-party contract between individual doctor and patient. The patient, in effect, while gaining a contract with the group, may lose a contract with a primary physician, resulting in risk of disorganization, incompleteness, and lack of continuity in care. In such groups the phenomenon of "easy disengagement" of the doctor from the patient or the doctor's careful adherence to a 9-to-5 workday or a 5-day workweek are the hallmarks of arrangements for care which lack the basic doctor-patient contracts.

Until now, the responsibility which doctors collectively might have—either for the care of individual patients or for the availability and quality of care to the community—has not been well understood or at least not clearly stated by either the medical profession or the public. Now the contractual responsibility which hospitals have for care has been legally defined and physicians are feeling the threat of progressive hospital "control" of their professional work. Because of these things, the collective responsibility of physicians for the care of individual patients, that is, as a hospital medical staff or perhaps as a county society or group practice, will be explicitly defined.

Formalizing such arrangements into contracts may not be far off in some parts of the country because of the pressures to link defined population groups in some formal or contractual way to the providers of care by a variety of organizational devices, for example, a health maintenance organization or health care corporation.

FINANCIAL OR "THIRD-PARTY" CONTRACTS

To round out the catalog of contracts or arrangements which now comprise the system of personal health services, we need to return to another kind of contract which was mentioned earlier in the chapter, that is, the fiscal contract involving third-party payers. The tendency (reflected in the name "third party") to regard the fiscal contract as an intrusion in the two-party contract rather than as a separate and complementary agreement was noted earlier in this chapter. Such separation is in fact being achieved in actual practice, but there are major unresolved problems. These regard the cost of care, particularly providing primary care, and relative overemphasis on those elements of care most visible and best remunerated under the third-party system of payment.

Some third-party payers want to refer to themselves as "purchasers of medical care" or "purchasers of health care" rather than as "third-party payers." Up to the present time, these agents have functioned primarily as disbursing agents and have indeed been payers, that is, fund dispersers, rather than purchasers, obtainers of service. This is an important distinction and has a bearing on the nature of the contract involved. It might be said that insofar as the care of the individual patient is concerned, third parties, for

example Blue Cross and Blue Shield, act primarily as payers. However, for the whole group of potential patients they serve, they may be more nearly purchasers. Persons having deductions taken from their paychecks when they are not sick may be thought to have more of a "consumers'" economic and psychological orientation than when they become patients. Again, in this matter, social understandings have been gradually crystallizing and new expectations are likely to be built into the fiscal contracts. Thus, it will be remembered that the leaders of Blue Cross and Blue Shield were sharply castigated in congressional hearings in 1971 for not acting more clearly in the interests of those paying for care or receiving care. In effect, they were scolded for a conflict of interest in being agents for hospitals (or doctors) as well as for their subscribers. They were chided for not acting as purchasers or negotiators on behalf of their subscribers in obtaining the most advantageous terms and conditions and for not concerning themselves more directly with the quality of service rendered their subscribers.

It seems quite likely that, in the time immediately ahead, if third parties continue to have any role their responsibilities will change from relatively passive disbursement or reimbursement of funds to a much more active concern for cost and quality of care provided, that is, to serving as purchasers.

Up to this point we have primarily been considering the arrangements and transactions involved in providing care to individual patients. We have focused primarily on the explicit medical contracts, and we have also noted the understandings and arrangements which are developing as the complexity of the medical care system inexorably increases. I have emphasized the complementary and mutually supporting character of the individual doctors, or groups of doctors' responsibilities, and the hospital as parts of the system. I have also pointed out that the idea of complementary contracts not only reflects what has in fact developed in medical care, but also permits accommodations to further elaborations of the system.

IMPLICIT SOCIAL CONTRACTS

Before concluding, we need to take another perspective for a moment and briefly consider the understandings among these various parts of the medical care system and the community or society.

Earlier we alluded to the fact that the scope of medical care has been widened by changing attitudes in society. Now it will be useful to examine the gradual process by which each new generation redefines the unacceptable and stakes out wider areas as the proper domain of medicine and the doctor.

It is easy for us to understand how the field is enlarged and expectations of service are changed by significant technological breakthroughs which result in specific treatments where none existed previously. What is more subtle and harder to perceive (and may be harder for us to be reconciled to) is another process by which expectations—in regard to medical care and health—are raised and responsibilities of the various parts of the system increased.

We need to keep firmly in mind the fact that the medical care system is a subsystem of a larger social system. When changes occur in the kinds of understandings which exist between the medical profession and society, what we might define as the "social contracts" of medicine (with apologies to Rousseau) also change.

Of course, there are no such things as legally binding social contracts, and except for purposes of emphasis "social understanding" is doubtless a better way of describing the less specific and implicit agreements which in loose and pervasive ways surround our work. As a prime example of what is involved here we may reflect on the change and scope of a doctor's responsibility implicit in the trend to remove or modulate any barriers to care (financial, social, and the like) which may ex-

ist, thus making every person in society some doctor's medical responsibility. Concurrently, there is a trend to adopt the perspectives for providing a balanced spectrum of care to an entire community as well as considering a patient's needs, one at a time.

The issues of the availability of care in the community and particularly of the medical profession's responsibility for making care available are nowhere more manifest than in the problems which cluster around medical service in hospital emergency rooms. It is common knowledge that 80% or more of the medical service provided in the emergency rooms is nonemergent ordinary office care. Does the corporate entity of the hospital (ie, board of trustees) have responsibility for providing what amounts to the office practice of medicine to those persons in the community who lack it, or is it rather a responsibility of the physicians of the community collectively? The answer would appear to be that if the trustees have such a responsibility, they got it only after the physicians had collectively defaulted. In some communities the assumption of such responsibility by the hospital corporation implies that doctors there agree that the basic contract for providing readily available service lies with the institution rather than the profession.

Society appears to be saying first to physicians (and if they don't respond, to hospitals) : "Concern with the individual patient and concern with the community's care are inseparable parts of a whole. We recognize that doctors have been doing a fine job caring for the individual sick patient with whom they have an established contract. We now wish to widen that contract to involve a continuing relationship with a prorated portion of the population (so medical care is more on tap), and with a defined population of persons (so no one is left out)."

Of course, that is an interpretation of a trend. No such statement has been expressly made in our legislatures, but the long-term trend appears to be unmistakable. Another example of changed expectations tending to lead to a wider area of responsibility is the expectation that physicians will now more effectively assist in the preventive maintenance of health. Again, although the rhetoric of health maintenance far outruns the state of the art, the trend seems clear.

Similar expansions of the hospitals and medical groups' responsibilities are also occurring, as was noted earlier.

At the same time that the scope of medical responsibilities is being widened, some indications reveal that society is at least willing to consider the idea that doctors may not have to do all of this and that other trained persons working with them can do some of it. Of course, in any individual case modifying traditional professional function remains a negotiable matter with the individual patient. However, the social understandings are important in regard to licensure and a broad operational definition of social roles. Social understanding is also important in determining how professionals will be educated and who will be paid for what services out of the pooled and quasipublic funds.

SUMMARY

Partly out of an abiding humanistic commitment to their patients' welfare, physicians have opposed trends in medical care organization and medical education which they perceive as diminishing the individual patient. They are concerned both with the orientation of reductionistic biology in medical schools and the depersonalization of medical care resulting from growing industrialization and institutionalization. The "doctor-patient relationship" has been the principal bulwark physicians have relied upon in opposing those trends, but that has been discredited, partly because it was not a precise enough delineation of the usages and issues involved and also because it was used to maintain a particular and exclusive professional status.

Clarifying the contract in the doctor-patient relationship and defining the evolving medical care system as a framework of complementary understandings or contracts will help retain the humanistic usages of clinical medicine while permitting more flexible accommodation to greater complexity in medical care.

Before, and certainly since the writings of Hippocrates, much of the altruism of medicine has for doctors been embodied in the concept of the doctor-patient relationship. We need to find ways in which that rather elite and exclusive professional altruism can be carried forward into changing arrangements in which physicians function as part of a system. Perhaps Tolstoy's admiring characterization of General Kutusov, who led the army which defeated Napoleon's, will help in this adaptation. "He will not introduce anything of his own . . . he will not stand in the way of anything expedient or permit what might be injurious. He knows that there is something stronger and more important than his own will—the inevitable march of events, and he has the brains to see them and grasp their significance, and seeing that significance, can abstain from meddling, from following his personal desires and aiming at something else."

FOOTNOTES

1 Note that when the patient pays directly, he is paying for something agreed upon in that private negotiation which was part of "diagnosis."

2 In New York (1957) and California (1958) similar court decisions had earlier affirmed essentially the same principle.

3 Of course, in a legal sense, such contracts now exist between any partnerships of physicians and individual patients of the partners. However, in that instance such contracts simply carry into a partnership way of doing business, the same kinds of obligations as exist between individual physician and patient. There is no implication that the collective group has a different responsibility to the patient than any one physician would have.

Chapter 16
Research:
The Promethean Dilemma
Joshua Lederberg, PhD, MD

It may be necessary to liberate technology and science and bring the institution of technology under more effective self-control, of the type exerted in medicine. Technology would then be collectively more responsible, while entrusting the detail of its work to the only community able to judge it well—itself.

PERSONAL PREFACE

As far back as I can recall, the ethical and intellectual precept that has guided my life-work has been the use of reason in the service of man. We have few other distinctions; integument, claws, and fangs have all atrophied in favor of the instruments that brain and hand could devise.

The most urgent and rewarding service to men surely is provided by the healing arts. My own career has been spent on the fringes of medicine, mainly in basic biological research, but along lines with an eye toward some eventual utility in protecting health or in the succor of medicine. My role in this volume is perhaps somewhat that of an outsider. Certainly I am bound to express some disagreement with some of my colleagues' admonitions against a commitment to research instead of clinical care.

Editor's Note: Dr. Lederberg, a Nobel Laureate, is one of the world's foremost geneticists. In recent years his career has been characterized by an increasing involvement in the social and philosophic implications of science and technology.

This was a choice I had to face 25 years ago: either to complete my medical studies (at Columbia College of Physicians and Surgeons) or further pursue my research in bacterial genetics. I am sure there are temperamental issues that each individual must answer to his own satisfaction. One personality may require the immediate rewards of benefaction to an individual patient whose life is trusted to his care and judgment. Others may be impatient with the complexities of individual behavior that seem to interfere with efficient solutions to a disease problem. But this is more a matter of taste than moral imperative.

One can argue, as I am sure I must have done during my own adolescence, that Louis Pasteur as a medical investigator did incomparably more good for man than he ever could have done as a personal physician. But today the Pasteurs are forgotten, and science is taxed with such morally complicated discoveries as dynamite and nuclear fission. Certainly, efficiency must not be deified as the cardinal principle in the choice of a life style. On the other hand, the existing art of medicine still

The existing art of medicine still fails in many tragic confrontations with disease and death; to condemn research is to perpetuate our blunders and our helplessness.

fails in many tragic confrontations with disease and death; to condemn research is to perpetuate our blunders and our helplessness.

Feelings against research that are expressed by certain practitioners of medicine and MD aspirants may be directed at the abstract and seemingly remote developments in contemporary science because these developments appear to be so removed from immediate human application. Some of these feelings are perhaps motivated by a fear of success, a fear that is promoted by the ambiguity of many large-scale ventures in recent times. Is the abolition of malaria or of smallpox an unmitigated good if it is merely followed by a population explosion and the perpetuation of poverty and exposure to famine? Will the discovery of a "cure for cancer" add more to the overall quality of human life than a few more years of senile decrepitude? Surely some of the rhetorical zeal that is often voiced about bringing medicine to the people, as if it were an alternative to the discovery of new scientific advances in medicine, is motivated by a desire to escape from these difficult questions of large-scale social influence. Providing care to specific, distressed individuals, in a one-to-one relationship, is surely free of some of the doubts that attend global interventions. However, there is no easy escape from these dilemmas. The ideology of diffidence about research may be as Promethean an intervention as any creation of the laboratory.

In this essay, I will deal with some broader aspects of the attack on science and technology. Many questions have been raised to which there are no simple answers, and to which no answers will be found if we rely on accusatory polemics or defensive dogmatism.

TECHNOLOGY AS DIABOLISM

In *The Myth of the Machine—the Pentagon of Power,* Lewis Mumford traces the philosophical roots of the contemporary techno-cultural-ecological crisis back to Galileo and Copernicus. He alleges that the enthronement of the "sun god" at the center of the solar system led eventually to an objective cosmology and demeaned the values inherent in earth-centered man. The intuition of some purpose outside of man could justify political absolutism, religious tyranny, and the destruction of the earlier ecological values which are implied by the numerous earthly gods of primitive cultures. We can argue in turn that Mumford's complaints are directed as much to monotheism as to heliocentrism; within the framework of his discussion, the sixteenth- and seventeenth-century conflict between church and science was a passing sectarian squabble. Monotheism's axial role was to liberate human thinking from polytheism, or animism—the interpretation of the world and every process in it as the work of spirits, demoniacal or beneficent, fabricated essentially in man's image.

Today we no longer deify the sun, the planets, the oceans, or the volcanoes. The One God of the Judeo-Christian tradition is inseparable from a universe ruled by law.

Animism is still a convenient metaphor and shortcut to detailed analysis. It is convenient, at times, to regard a computer *as if it were a* quasi-intelligent being, responding to instructions and replying to inquiries like a willful child. The scientist can better design certain experiments if he visualizes a molecule as a perceptive organism, and thinks how it can "be aware of" the physical and chemical details of its local environment. The most literal acceptance of the Darwinian theory does not hinder the experienced biologist from speculating about the "purpose" of an organ, as shorthand for a description of its evolution under the shaping influence of utility tested by natural selection. These are nevertheless metaphors, consciously preserved, which clearly can lead to error, folly, and disaster if they are misapplied outside the range of the appropriate analogy. We do not allow computers to vote, and we do not expect man to painlessly improve his genetic makeup merely by wishing for the good or needing to achieve it.

Many authors besides Mumford have tended to animize technology. Artful metaphors may be drawn, for example, the hypothesis that a technological society behaves as if technology were an autonomous malevolent force within it, that is, a devil. But this is a subject requiring careful definition and investigation and it is promptly obscured if the metaphor is taken for granted. The hypothesis can be made into a self-evident axiom by labeling the collective imperfections of society as "technology," as Theodore Roszak does in his book, *The Making of a Counter-Culture*. He attributes *Playboy*'s derogation of meaningful sexual relationship to technocracy. Such a definition does not help very much to discover who is a "technologist."

WHO IS A TECHNOLOGIST? Among engineers and scientists, technology means the concrete application of scientific knowledge to problems of human significance. It also means the organizational structure, the body of experience, the operational hardware, and the people who design and man it, and the end product. By further extension, technology may also be taken to mean science itself (knowledge about the natural world) and the community of scientists. The term technology conjures images of computers, suspension bridges, freeways, factories, nylon, jet planes, telephones, nuclear bombs, auto exhausts, pacemakers, television, penicillin, and DDT. These are products that are unique to the technology of the present century. It should also include the abundance of our crops for food and fiber, fire, and the domestication of dogs and horses. It also means cheap paperback books, a progressive relief of the burden of labor, and a standard of living whereby youth can spend 20 years getting an education, rather than go to the field or factory at 12. It is in fact the whole texture of modern life, based on the

> *Technology is in fact the whole texture of modern life, based on the level of industrial production that is possible only through the systematic application of scientific technology.*

level of industrial production that is possible only through the systematic application of scientific technology.

Insofar as technology is the indispensable instrument of social action, the most conspicuous faults in modern life are (by definition) the *misapplications* of technology. We have still to analyze the sources of that misdirection, for technology is a tool in the hands of men. This is neither to deny nor affirm the diabolical hypothesis that such a misdirection is inevitable, given the power of technology to amplify discrepancies of wealth and opportunity or the ideological impact of scientific skepticism on the shaping of human goals and aspirations. Nor can we give perfect marks to scientists and technologists for doing all that they might do to apply their special insights *about*, as well as *of*, science and technology for human welfare.

Do we, strictly speaking, live in a "technocratic society," if that implies that the major decisions are made by a scientifically trained elite?

There is much evidence to the contrary! It was one of our most respected Presidents who, against the advice and urging of many physicists, decided to end the war against Japan in 1945 by dropping the A-bombs on Hiroshima and Nagasaki (a complicated decision that is easy to criticize in hindsight). Indeed, it would be an intolerable arrogation of authority if scientists were to make such decisions against the informed conclusions of politically responsible leaders in a democracy. In recent months, scientists have been vehement in their denunciations of the SST and the ABM, and have been in the forefront of many other campaigns for restoring the quality of the environment. In the Soviet Union, they are the one irreducible focus of liberal thought, breaching national barriers to join the only effective world community functioning today.

The antitechnologist can, of course, find many texts to support his condemnations. The architect Albert Speer is much quoted for his remark that "some day the nations of the world may be dominated by technology—that nightmare was very nearly made a reality under Hitler's authoritarian system." But if we look more closely at this meaning, we find he refers above all to the radio and the telephone, systems by which a central authority could readily diffuse its commands without requiring the personal presence of the dictator. In fact, the Hitlerian regime did its utmost (and in many fields succeeded) to eradicate free scientific inquiry, and allowed only work judged relevant to the superiority of the German race to flourish. The technicians whom Speer describes as blindly following orders were simply bureaucrats. And, as Speer also documents, Hitler lost his bid for a millennial Reich in large measure because of the contradiction between objective scientific analysis and the central mystique of the German soil and race.

We could still profitably pursue parallel investigations that would help us to illuminate the sources of technopathy (the pathology of science and technology). Consider how many of the world's ills are attributable to language or to law out of control!

Language is, of course, the instrument of every deception and manipulation, as well as of man's utmost achievements. It is the means of reason and poetry alike, and confines them both. Should we not offer the same complaints against language that we do against technology? After all, language is the fundamental technique of the human species, which makes all others both possible and inevitable, through the process of culture. And could we not make a parallel argument about law—that it liberates and enslaves man at the same time?

These analogies have too much substance to be dismissed, but even apart from the obscene confusion of technician and technocrat, a valid indictment emerges not in spite of, but as a consequence of, the exoneration of technology. Technology, like law and language, is an institution whose realization depends on a particular community. Language comes closest to being a product of the whole community, and we share a collective burden for its advance and misuse; we do not confuse the linguists who merely study language with the whole culture that invents and enriches it. Law, at the other extreme, is shaped by a body of men—the legislators, lawyers, and judges—who are professedly responsible to the culture for its defects as well as its virtues. The law, like other organized professions, is also ruled by its own code. This is far from perfect, but it still serves as a specific nexus of confrontation with the culture's demands and an indispensable protection to the morale and efficacy of its individual members.

A definite though less tangible standard binds the behavior of the basic scientist who is dedicated to the exhibition of publicly verifiable discoveries. The technologist, however, sells his services to the highest bidder—producing whatever design a customer has the means to support. (The physician likewise does not judge the social virtues of his patient. Does this entail a moral copout?) He thereby transfers responsibility onto other shoulders, and in this particular sense the technologist (as distinct from a scientist) is a mere technician serving another master. This elusive irresponsibility of the technologist, in the face of the enormous amplification of power his work conveys, may be the ultimate exasperation that fuels the aquarian crusade. In one sense, technology is too ill-defined to be a legitimate target; in a deeper one, this is precisely the problem, given the disturbance it undeniably intrudes into the complacency and placidity of life. Science is somewhat better organized as a community, but suffers from the same vacuum of responsibility for the technical elaboration of discovery.

HOW TO CONTROL TECHNOLOGY It has been suggested that technology, and by extension science, should be brought under more explicit social control. The real need may be to liberate it, that is, to bring the institution of technology under more effective self-control, of the type exerted in medicine. Technology would then be collectively more responsible, while entrusting the detail of its work to the only community able to judge it well—itself.

Carried to a logical extreme, this would paralyze government and industry—if we mean that every technically trained employee in large organizations has the right and responsibility to judge every consequence of his efforts, and to sabotage whatever he deprecates. Furthermore, it goes beyond human reason to know the full outcome of any technological innovation. Shall we indict Alexander Graham Bell for the telephone that made Hitlerian totalitarianism possible? Shall we indict Mueller for DDT? And if so, should it be because of damage to wildlife, or rather because the effective control of malaria accelerated the population explosion? Would fewer lives have been ground up in war since August 1945 had the airplane or the atomic bomb not been developed? Or more? And what about the future?

There are, nevertheless, two major forms of socially useful control that a well-organized profession of technologists would advocate and could enforce.

First, major technological projects could be subject to disinterested review and licensure, to be certain that the intended profits in one area of the economy are not simply stolen, covertly, from another. This is the much discussed function of technological assessment. It deals with such questions as the true cost of the SST or of electric power, taking full account of the threatened impairment of the environment. It can equally be concerned with the full costs of technological displacement or monotonization of labor, invasion of privacy, or threats to any of the other cherished values of life. Almost all of the tangible grievances against technology can be covered by the extension of our economic system to take broader account of the values that make life worth-

while. It is furthermore within the power of a democratic society to insist on this—and scientists and technologists are just beginning to exercise their responsibility for systematic efforts to press public policy in this direction. The technology assessment need not all be delegated to a central authority, for regulatory agencies often ossify after their first flurry of reform. Alternatively, we should consider chartering pluralistic consumer and environmentalist organizations to allow them a standing in court as representatives of large groups with grievances that cannot be pursued on behalf of any one individual. There is already considerable momentum today by groups for conservation law and for consumer class actions to make equitable law in the courts. They would be greatly helped, however, if they had a firmer legal standing to match that of the corporations and the labor unions. If such groups could recover compensatory and penalty damages on behalf of their extended constituencies, entrepreneurship bolstering the interests of the consumer and inhabitant would be encouraged, balancing the entrepreneurship so effectively mobilized for the producer, distributor, and extractor.

Developing effective technology assessment would, furthermore, dilute any need to "control" technological innovation at its scientific roots, a step which is both impractical and tyrannical in its implications.

Second, since technology assessment can only be applied where the costs can be anticipated, much research is needed at earlier stages of development to look for unforeseen troubles and to develop antidotes. Technologists could insist that every project be taxed to support critical investigations of its consequences. (This need not imply any privilege in the specific control of the direction of technological changes, which is best left as a primary function of the market economy and of government support and regulation.) Without the same kind of expertise that produced DDT or high-energy fuels, we would not have known that DDT has deeper ecological effects than wiping out insect pests, or that Los Angeles smog is a consequence of unburned fuel in auto exhausts (rather than industrial pollution as would have been supposed by the naive observer). Technology has generated the environmental crisis, but science has discovered it, and is indispensable for planning the rational remedies. The closer some of this countertechnology can be placed in time, place, and motivation to the original sources of trouble, the more efficiently the latter can be neutralized.

To be sure, there are equally insidious social and economic roots to the environmental–technological crisis, and these may not be rectified without readjustments in the distribution of wealth and in our ideology about the meaning of human life and work. However, political solutions to these problems will be accelerated if we can expose and document the social costs of particular technologies. There is nothing in the ethic of science to oppose the reequilibration of values, and there is a great deal in its technique to help support it (and the technologists will work even more happily for consensual goals than for narrow ones). The trouble is that the consensual judgment does not always coincide with the most advanced insight—for example, on costs and pleasures of smoking cigarettes, allowing handguns to be freely available, investing in recreational lands versus strategic defenses, building freeways and dams, or making wars. The technologist is then caught in the middle, the most exposed target in the crossfire of social conflict. The university has been the chosen battleground partly as a by-product of its role as the seat of skeptical inquiry and to a lesser degree because of misconceptions about the potency of academic opinion on national policy. But this is the game of liberals. Radicalism sees the university as a place where bewildered and resentful youths, with unformed ideologies, can most efficiently be recruited as shock troops of revolution with expert assistance from indiscriminate doses of law and order.

As for the process of countertechnological inquiry, there are many kinds of incentives, taxes, and penalties that could encourage this kind of harmony, but none of them will be implemented if the technologists themselves do not respond to a crise-de-conscience and demand it. At the very least, professional groups could accredit and rate technological organizations in accordance with their acceptance of this responsibility, and government contracting and tax policy could take account of the ratings. Needless to say, the federal establishment itself requires the closest attention. It is idiocy that radiobiological research within the AEC should have been cut back, as it has been, at a time of increasing commitment to nuclear power development and militant, if highly controversial, complaints about the reliability of standards of public exposure to radiation.

What of the basic scientist, the investigator who seeks "the truth for its own sake," though sharing the well-placed confidence that it will fit somehow into the machinery of technological power?

Modern science was founded as a response to questions of everyday life—the motions of the stars, the forces of gravity and of magnetism, the continuity and evolution of life, the composition of familiar matter. It promptly dispelled the remaining relics of animism and did a great deal to shatter faith in revealed religion, insofar as these misguidedly justified themselves by assertions of a scientific nature. Well into the nineteenth century, science could be regarded as a liberating or counterreligion, wiping away many naive superstitions.

My own education, in the early 1930s, was still colored by this function of science as a general world outlook; but science was already hopelessly fragmented into innumerable specialties, in very poor communication with one another. By that time, a man who wished to understand nature could function far more efficiently by learning more of what was already known than by attempting to carve new facts and interpretations out of the unknown. The process today has reached the point where very few scientific reports tell of insights that can have any significance to the layman.

Apart from the jargon in which they are phrased, he would have to know more than he cares to about the background before he could understand why a particular fragment would interest the specialist.

The contemporary work of science is thus hard to justify in terms of individual man's "need to know." Yet the body of scientific knowledge would be a sterile scholasticism if it were not constantly challenged and restructured. Merely to resolve the many inconsistencies it still contains would require constant resort to new tests. No two men can learn quite the same material; except for rote parroting learning is thinking and questioning and speculating. Without the criterion of experimental verification, accumulated learning would again become dry rot (as has happened at times in the past). It is fortunate, then, that the thrill of *discovery,* as much as learning, motivates the researcher. Nor can we ignore the motives of competition for prestige and for material rewards that help label scientists as human.

It is still true that contemporary science, in its fragmentation, tends to become more remote from the basic questions about nature that were its original invigoration. The effective practice of a particular science requires an extraordinary narrowness of focus, and rare indeed is the man whose inherent abilities and training leave any room for broader education or philosophical and social wisdom commensurate with the pervasive impact of science on the human condition. The historical pattern for the use of talent has been too fruitful to warrant being disturbed, but everywhere the need is also seen for another kind of scholar: the contemporary humanist, who can understand science in its original terms without being engulfed by the detail of one speciality; the man who, to use a now banal phrase, can also bridge the two cultures. The social need for this kind of intercultural moderator has not carved out any evident niches in the prestige and career structure of the academy, perhaps because there is no easy way to measure the quality of his performance, to select the good from the bad, as we pretend to do in the established studies. We may then stumble along with the help of those stragglers who have dropped out of the race of strict science, especially elder scholars—although age is confused with wisdom at peril.

This gap does manifest harm to the understanding of science by scientists themselves, as well as by nonprofessionals and those in the corridors of political power. Even the methodology of science is impeded, for we still await a more rigorous formulation of the process of scientific thinking that is itself needed to do science scientifically; that is, in a way that would give us the full use of computer technology. With rare exceptions scientists are remarkably naive about the logical foundations of experiments and verification, and imprecise in their linguistics. The scientific specialist usually has rather naive ideas about the process of science in the large and is too enmeshed in detail to see it in a broad philosophical perspective. The challenge has been left to another discipline (the philosophy of science) which has remained so isolated from laboratory workers that, for example, few students majoring in a given science will have been exposed to it.

The prestige of the "scientific method," nevertheless, has peaked to the point where it is often invoked, almost mechanically, for areas whose complexity and inaccessibility to controlled experiment demand equal respect for other kinds of insight and analysis. Science itself is just such a process, and to speak of "a science of science" may be justifiable only insofar as one would define politics and history as science. The arrogance of occasional claims that the scientific method can be used to prove some particular value system, including the assignment of a value to the pursuit of science itself, has certainly added to the embarrassment of science as an institution. Science has also been criticized for being "value free." But it is only from men, not their instruments, that we can legitimately demand a commitment to values.

We still have a proletariat and we still have

poverty in the US, but they are shrinking rapidly in absolute terms. Science and technology can do little to furnish a sense of the purpose of life to accompany material affluence, except for the elite few who can find it in the actual processes of inquiry and invention. It is only by contrast with the possible future, not with historical reality, that technological culture also fails in terms of the objective quality of life.

Faced with the task of clearing the residue of superstitious rubble in the nineteenth century, science may have preempted the task of religious reconstruction. But it can function only as critic, and then mainly for the internal consistency of a rebuilt faith. I do not advocate science as a basis of religious commit-ment; but with all their faults, I know many scientists who are fulfilled. There is at least no inconsistency between the practice of science and leading the good life. Where scientists have rarely succeeded is in understanding themselves well enough to make their ethical and religious commitments a worthwhile source of leadership for many others, especially among the young. Many of their pronouncements and self-reports need insightful translation. What may have been left to isolated discovery by a pioneering generation must now somehow be built into the education of the next one—in order that the new generation be better equipped to make its own creative inventions.

Chapter 17
Feeling as Insight:
The Affective Dimension in Social Diagnosis
John J. McDermott, PhD

The sensitive diagnostician will not fit patients' complaints into an a priori context, but will strive to unearth their experienced roots so as to better follow the multiple hints and leads which yield genuine insight into the real and felt needs of the person.

MEDICINE AND PHILOSOPHY

The popular mind is deep, and means a thousand times more than it explicitly knows.[1]

As a teacher and student of philosophy, I welcome the opportunity to participate in a symposium with distinguished medical doctors devoted to rethinking the Hippocratic wisdom of antiquity and searching for new modes of inquiry in the art of healing. The history of philosophy has long been associated with medicine, as the careers of Aristotle and John Locke, among others, attest. Indeed, one of the most creative of nineteenth-century philosophers, William James, had but one earned degree, and that was in medicine. The comparative isolation of medicine as a discipline, particularly from the social sciences, is a phenomenon of our century and has done much to engender the unfortunate mystique which surrounds the practice of medicine and ensuing lack of social

Editor's Note: Professor McDermott has directed interdisciplinary studies at Queens College and has received the Harbison Award as national recognition for the quality of his teaching.

consciousness which too often affects public medical policy. And if similar charges can be placed against philosophy and other academic disciplines, the stakes in medical practice are far higher, for what more crucial ingredient of the human condition exists than physical and psychological well-being?

In the move to interdisciplinary studies, now characteristic of university curricula, little is accomplished if the important and powerful professions of law and medicine are left to pursue their professional paths unquestioned and unchallenged. The future of medicine is of secondary concern—it is the future

---

The future of medicine is of secondary concern—it is the future of man and the quality of his environment which are the primary issues.

---

of man and the quality of his environment which are the primary issues.

In this essay, I attempt to present in an interdisciplinary way some parameters relative to the problem of diagnosis as it applies to contemporary American man, especially in his urban setting. I make no claim to special medical knowledge other than the experience of my own body along with the complex and intense interactions of the medical history of my family. The significance of this limited experience is not, however, to be undersold, for it represents the empirical intimacy of everyone's experience with medicine.

Before turning to the problem of diagnosis, and speaking in general terms, the marvel of medicine is to be found in its achievement of an extraordinary correlation between knowledge and implementation. No other discipline has been so effective in obtaining concrete results from speculative and experimental probes. Catastrophic diseases have been wiped out and we have confidence that those remaining shall be eliminated. In recent years, dazzling reconstructions of essential bodily organs have given an aura of collective genius to medicine, accompanied by the capacity to outstrip human limitations long held to be inviolable. The existence of organ transplants, for example, connotes to the observer a bold transcendence of the boundaries of history and nature. In its intimacy and immediacy, the era of transplants is a more startling breakthrough than that of moonlanding the astronauts. The latter is an extension of man and continuous with nature, but the former is a rebirth, a bypassing of the heretofore inexorable laws of nature, as if man had transcended himself, albeit in single and isolated instances. At a minimum, the horizon of the possible has been immeasurably widened.

For those of us who are not in medicine, there is little question that the creative events of modern medicine are awe inspiring. Many achievements have an exotic ring to them and they seem to have elicited from even the reflective and informal observer a blank check for medicine to move forward as it wills. A closer look, however, at the activities of contemporary medicine and especially at the role and stance of the physician, yields a more complex evaluation. Without denying the achievement of modern medicine, we might ask the following questions:

Has the extraordnary success in dealing with highly specialized problems been at the expense of healing the entire community?[2] Said differently, has contemporary medicine, as so much of modern science, been guilty of dramatic linear breakthroughs while impervious to the highly negative implications they so often spawn?

Has contemporary medicine defined illness too narrowly, as if the human body has not undergone profound changes traceable not only to a new ecological setting but also to an entirely different social-psychological context?

The foregoing questions focus on human living as actually experienced in affective terms, rather than as speculatively projected. In a

In a word, we are calling for a cultural anthropology in which the affective dimension is at the center of our evaluation of the human condition, rather than peripheral to it.

word, we are calling for a cultural anthropology in which the affective dimension is at the center of our evaluation of the human condition, rather than peripheral to it. In doing so, relative to medicine, let us examine the diagnostic process, the new understanding of the nature of person, and finally some strands of an environmental aesthetic, significant for an amelioration of that form of pathology described variously as alienation, anomie, or cultural sadness.

PITFALLS OF DIAGNOSIS

Thus, our perceptions of, and our reactions to, other people and what they do or how they feel can be understood better if we consider the functional possibilities, the conditions and effects of their behavior, which are based on representation and openness to the environment.[3]

The euclidean point of view, with its emphasis on the measurable and its abhorrence of loose ends, still has influence. Despite the vast increase in the speculative versions of varieties of the human condition, our methodological approach to understanding others' experiences seems fixed both in point of origin and in the evaluation of implications. Even among those whose responsibility is to grasp the import of another's feelings, the assumptions about the nature of the human self are unrelievedly trite. Although the person who does not acknowledge the staggering change in environment, media, and pace of life in the last 50 years is rare, still more rare is the awareness of the profound transformation this development has worked upon human self-consciousness. The interiorizing, by the human self, of environmental changes has proceeded in an admittedly subtle but nonetheless significant way. It is not too much to say that the delicate fabric of self-consciousness, under the press of modern technology, has been altered in decisive ways, especially with regard to the experience of our bodies.

Despite these developments, social diseases —alienation, anomie, cultural deprivation, stimulant dependencies, and the afflictions of hard-core poverty—are still diagnosed relative to a classical image of human behavior. Erich Lindenmann, a psychiatrist, writes in his foreword to Herbert Gans's book on *The Urban Villagers*, an analysis of the relocation crises of the residents of the "urban-renewed" West End of Boston, that "The problems of medical care . . . and preventive services have been vastly complicated by our ignorance concerning basic attitudes and motivations of various types of people whom we are serving."[4,5]

If we look at this situation in methodological terms, we find most often that diagnosis proceeds from a fixed point of view, perhaps best resembling a self-fulfilling prophecy. The diagnostician assumes the contours of human behavior as known and deduces from those limits a set of symptom-question relationships, which follow step by lockstep to one of a number of familiar conclusions.[6] The person diagnosed has a sense of this ritual and he very much wants to receive a clarifying judgment as to the cause of his discomfort; therefore, he falls into the proscribed pattern. This can be described as an effort to avoid "being different." In analyzing our response to social pressures, Richard Sennett writes that "the enterprise involved is an attempt to build an image or identity that coheres, is unified, and filters out threats in social experience."[7] Sennett then proceeds to describe the burden we are under as we attempt to fit the model of expectancy.

The jarring elements in one's social life can be purified out as unreal because they don't fit that articulated object, that self-consciously spelled-out set of beliefs, likes and dislikes, and abilities that one takes to be oneself. In this way, the degree to which people feel urged to keep articulating who they are, what they want, and what they feel is almost an index of their fear about their inability of survival in social experience with other men.[7(pp 9, 10)]

In the process of diagnosis, as long as the questions asked are so structured as to elicit traditional responses, the judgments about their meaning are self-sustained. It is not that alternatives are ruled out but rather, not being sought, they never surface. This approach is a cardinal instance of what William James called "vicious intellectualism,"[8] wherein we define a situation such that all possibilities not included in the definition are thereby excluded, no matter the shifts in the overall context. From another vantage point, this methodological approach in diagnosis is the opposite of that encouraged by Martin Buber when he tells us that we should experience "from the standpoint of the other."[9] In this regard, focusing simply on the intake interview, we find countless instances of our insensitivity to the plight and standpoint of the "other."

As an evening counselor to an adult college program some years ago, I was struck by the disparity between the reasons for appointments, such as change of schedule and teacher complaints, and the extraordinary range of serious problems unearthed just in casual conversation. Under the guise of academic problems, many persons had a desperate need to discuss deep personal difficulties in their work and family life, and on a number of occasions they introduced into the conversation their recent suicide attempts.[10] The dramatic difference of the experience from the "other side" is caught in this text from Robert Sommer, as he describes reading 50 autobiographies of mental patients.

I found these books invaluable for understanding the ways in which being hospitalized affected a person's Weltanschauung. *Christmas and other holidays were times of loneliness and remorse. The admissions routine, which strips a patient of all personal belongings including his wedding ring (to protect his valuables) and his clothing (to send them to the laundry to be marked) and requires him to answer questions asked by people who do not bother to introduce themselves, lies somewhere between the tragic and the grotesque. Almost every case of visual hallucinations in these 50 autobiographies occurred under conditions of reduced visual stimulation, confirming the laboratory studies of sensory deprivation, in which people who are subjected to reduced sensory inputs are unable to focus their thoughts and frequently experience hallucinations.*[11]

In assuming that the person or persons under consideration proceed from the same basic understanding of experience as the one diagnosing, we find ourselves cut off from some of the most important factors in social diagnosis.

We may, for example, have profoundly different experiences yet develop the same symptoms, for as David Mechanic comments, "symptomatology and disability are very different aspects of illness and they must be studied independently."[12] As a case in point, a quest for drugs can be generated by an attempt to escape from the pressures of an outwardly successful life as well as from the horrors of a hopeless poverty condition. Surely the spread of heroin use among middle- and upper-class white youth disestablishes our previously held belief that the use of such drugs is a sign of economic and social deprivation. What about our tendency to trace listlessness and an anomic attitude to that classical social affliction, apathy? To the contrary, we now find that such disengagement proceeds frequently from the frustrations attendant upon an inability to convert intense moral concern into concrete forms of public amelioration, or, as we shall consider subsequently, traces to the antiseptic and bland character of much of our physical environment.

OTHER PROBLEMS IN DIAGNOSIS   Turning now to another serious oversight in traditional patterns of diagnosis, we focus on the common assumption that persons with deep afflictions of a personal and social kind have the necessary language to articulate these disturbances. Some years ago, Michael Harrington wrote a book entitled *The Other America*, in which he spoke about the invisibility of the poor, who "are increasingly slipping out of the very experience and consciousness of the nation."[13] One of the reasons for this invisibility is the drastic gap between the conventional understanding of poverty and the actual experiences of the poor. Harrington tried to show that the real malady of hard-core poverty was social-psychological. It was not so much the quantity of their food and clothing but rather the nutritional vacancy of their food, the difficulty in obtaining it, and the unkempt, styleless character of their clothing and furnishings which induced hopelessness and a loss of body tone. In turn, these characteristics generate environ-

mental conditions dangerous to health and ero-
sive of energy and mental stability, illustrat-
ing graphically what we now call the vicious
circle of poverty. The middle-class remark,
"How can they live that way," becomes a
telling instance of experiencing others' lives
only from the outside.

An anecdote told me by a poverty program
caseworker is indicative of how little we know
about the needs of others from their point of
view. In visiting an abjectly poor community

---

*In visiting an abjectly poor com-
munity in the Midwest, one literally without even substandard
housing or basic sanitation facilities, a social worker asked the
people what they wanted most
and first. Their answer was
startling but revealing: they
requested street signs.*

---

in the Midwest, one literally without even substandard housing or basic sanitation facilities,
a social worker asked the people what they
wanted most and first. Their answer was startling but revealing: they requested street signs.
Upon reflection this event teaches us much, for
the people in this community were not only
poor in traditional terms—lacking all the
fundamentals of living—but they had lost
their communal identity as well. Although
they may not have articulated it in this way,
apparently they felt that street signs would
give them a sense of place, a reference point
against which they could begin to evaluate
their wider needs.[14] It is difficult to judge
from the outside what will fulfill the needs of
another person's embattled recess of dignity.
Years ago, as a young man, I was a volunteer
worker at Bellevue Hospital in New York
City. My responsibility was to be of service
to the patients, all of them indigent, most of
them bereft of family and friends, many of
them terminal cases. One aged man had lost
his arms and legs and did not speak English.

Through gestures and halting translation, I
learned from him that he would like two cigars
of a certain Spanish make. No other type
would do. This man, faced with utter experiential deprivation, clung to a qualitative assessment of his world, while asserting an
irreducible pride in his taste.

In diagnosing and evaluating social affliction, the tendency is to proceed from a position of "knowing what is best" for those
involved and to scoff at the halting and
strange complaints that people have. Yet
every statement uttered out of the experience
of affliction is loaded with inferential meaning. The sensitive diagnostician will not fit
these articulations into an a priori context but
will strive to unearth their experienced roots
so as to better follow the multiple hints and
leads which yield genuine insight into the real
and felt needs of the person or community.

A still more difficult task for traditional
patterns of diagnosis is the ability to penetrate experiences that are difficult to articulate, that is, those experiences we undergo
which are vague in delineation or so profoundly different from the expected that we
feel awkward in describing them.[15,16]

Here we can think of the person for whom,
by all public accounts, "things are going
well," but who nonetheless is restless, on edge,
even hostile to his surroundings and his peers.
He may suffer from an interiorization of
heightened expectations, pressed subtly upon
him but not clear to his own consciousness.
Under the circumstances, for him to complain
seems "dopey" and "thankless," yet he suffers from deep disquiet and irritations, both
physical and mental. A pervasive presence of
this problem is found in the apparently per-
verse behavior of those people who are moved
from the ugliness of an urban slum to a clean
project. In many such situations, these residents proceed to deface their new environment in what seems to be a pathological effort
to duplicate the burdens of their original environment. Yet, consider the difficulty; how
does a community express its hostility against
a "clean" environment in terms that are sanc-

tioned publicly? What is it in their consciousness and their experience which engenders this hostility.[17-19] No doubt indicative of deepseated affective and communal needs, this distress defies expression to the larger community,[20] so often characterized by its clear-cut understanding of a hierarchy of social values.

Other experiences that are difficult to articulate abound. In what way, for example, does a person quantitatively rich in friends and family state his deep feeling of loneliness and anonymity? How awkward it has been for young people to justify their disinterest in perpetuating a society allegedly tuned to their every need. Also significant is the expansive role of shame or guilt in the patient's effort to mask his symptoms and throw the diagnostician off the trail, revealing a willingness to continue suffering rather than to admit to a "social" disease or an embarrassing event. How frequent it is that people retreat to a studied anonymity because the complex quality of their experience defies the recognized patterns of expression and explication.

Objective descriptions and evaluations of situations in which other persons find themselves, which fly in the face of the perceptions of those situations by the persons involved, result in a diagnostic charade. While it is true that we can doubt or deny the accuracy of a judgment about factual matters, we cannot deny the accuracy of another's feelings, however self-deceiving the cause. The vital center of diagnosis, then, is the ability to grasp the ongoing activity of the other person so that neither symptoms and complaints, nor their causes, are dealt with apart from the relational process of webbing and rejecting, which is what constitutes how one feels at any given time. It is important to realize that even agreement between the diagnostician and patient on a "cause" of the difficulty should not be interpreted as a clean-cut solution to the problem; people have an endless capacity and need to have answers, even if only to clear their minds. After all, we rarely have a one-to-one relationship between an event and a response. More likely, events bathe our con-

sciousness, churning up patterns of relationship, frequently novel, so that our deepest feelings are framed out of experiences far distant from what appeared to be the causal source. A richer sense of these dimensions should emerge if we sketch some characteristics of a different understanding of the nature of person than that assumed in most diagnoses.

THE PERSON AS RELATIONAL PROCESS

But don't you see that the whole trouble lies here. In words, words. Each one of us has within him a whole world of things, each man of us his own special world. And how can we ever come to an understanding if I put in the words I utter the sense and value of things as I see them; while you who listen to me must inevitably translate them according to the conception of things each one of you has within himself. We think we understand each other, but we never really do.[21]

Understanding another person is, indeed, difficult to achieve. Nonetheless, rich insights about the quality and direction of experiences shared with others is possible in sensitive interpersonal situations. The crucial factor in such a process is to cease treating the other person as an object; rather, we should make an effort to reach out beyond those accepted assumptions which often block us from grasping the distinctive versions of another's world view. This kind of sensibility has been steadily gaining ground on both a theoretical and a practical level. Beginning with William James, Henri Bergson, and the pioneering social psychology of Charles Horton Cooley and George Herbert Mead, our century has seen an extraordinary change in our approach to the nature of the person. More recent efforts in this direction include the work of Kurt Goldstein, Erik Erikson, Robert Jay Lifton, Erving Goffman, and the controversial philosophical psychiatry of Ronald Laing. Further, we have the imaginative efforts of Edward Hall, Kevin Lynch, and Robert Sommer, among others, in the comparatively new field of proxemics or person-space relationships.[22] Of a still more speculative cast is the work proceeding from existential and phenomenological sources, such as Jean Paul Sartre, Gabriel Marcel, and Maurice Merleau-Ponty. Utilizing the concepts of some of these thinkers, let us sketch some of those qualities in a person which, if taken seriously, would enable us to perform more fruitful diagnoses.

JAMES AND BERGSON   The initial breakthrough came in the thought of James and Bergson as they sought to overcome the traditional penchant for a dualistic interpretation of the person.[23] In so doing, they offered a radical reconsideration of the human body. Instead of claiming that the body is passive and merely receives external influences which are rendered meaningful by the active work of the mind, James and Bergson developed a position which delineates the body in more aggressive terms. In his book on *Matter and Memory*, Bergson points to the original quality of that image "which is distinct from all the others, in that I do not know it only from without by perceptions, but from within by affections: it is my body." [24] Further, he tells us that "my body, an object destined to move other objects, is then a centre of action; it cannot give birth to a representation." [24 (p 4)] In effect, we lead with our bodies, or better, our bodies are knowers in a primal way. The self, then, is not a privileged redoubt, not an archimedean point within our bodies, but is actually how and when the body acts. In a footnote to his essay on "The Experience of Activity," William James offers us an unusual text on the self as the activity of the body.

The individualized self, which I believe to be the only thing properly called self, is a part of the content of the world experienced. The world experienced (otherwise called the "field of consciousness") comes at all times with our body as its centre, centre of vision, centre of action, centre of interest. Where the body is is "here"; when the body acts is "now"; what the body touches is "this"; all other things are "there" and "then" and "that." These words of emphasized position imply a systematization of things with reference to a focus of action and interest which lies in the body; and the systematization is now so instinctive (was it ever not so?) that no developed or active experience exists for us at all except in that ordered form. So far as "thoughts" and "feelings" can be active, their activity terminates in the activity of the body, and only through first arousing its activities can they begin to change those of the rest of the world. The body is the storm centre, the origin of co-ordinates, the constant place of stress in all that experience-train. Everything circles round it, and is felt from its point of view. The word "I," then, is primarily a noun of position, just like "this" and "here." Activities attached to "this" position have prerogative emphasis, and, if activities have feelings, must be felt in a peculiar way. The word "my" designates the kind of emphasis.[25]

Speaking of Bergson, Ian Alexander claims that his "argument will consist in showing how the self inserts into the world and space through the body." [26] And John E. Smith, speaking of James's empiricism, holds it to be a "radically new account of how the self penetrates and is penetrated by the world." [27] It is important to realize that the role of the body, in the swarm of experiences which make up our world, is more than a neutral filter. We "intend" by virtue of our bodily activity. "Intentionality" is not limited to the processes of thinking, but is present in the selective character of our bodily responses. William James, in his *Principles of Psychology,* states that "out of what is in itself an undistinguishable, swarming *continuum,* devoid of distinction or emphasis, our senses make for us, by attending to this motion and ignoring that, a world full of contrasts, of sharp accents, of abrupt changes, of picturesque light and shade." [28]

In a similar vein, Bergson comments that "our representation of matter is the measure of possible action upon bodies: it results from the discarding of what has no interest for our needs, or more generally for our functions." [24(p 23)] The body, then, becomes a probe, an informing and selecting extension of our very being. We construct the focus of our experience by the activity of our bodies, for "the actuality of our perception thus lies in its *activity.*" [24(p 55)]

Writing closer to our time, Michael Polanyi, medical doctor and philosopher, comments on the bodily roots of man's thought and creative powers.

Our body is the ultimate instrument of all our external knowledge, whether intellectual or practical. In all our waking moments we are relying on our awareness of contacts of our body with things outside for attending to these things. Our own body is the only thing in the world which we normally never experience as an object, but experience always in terms of the world to which we are attending from our body. [29]

The most crucial difference in the post-Jamesian view of the self from that of traditional Western philosophy and psychology is the shift from spectator to constitutor as the delineating mark of self-consciousness. James had written that "*the pursuance of future ends and the choice of means for their attainment are thus the mark and criterion of the presence of mentality* in a phenomenon." [28(p 8)] The person constitutes a functional point of view and a series of interlocking goals, simultaneously forging relationships in order to sustain this anticipation. Some relationships are ultimately sterile, others obdurate when placed in a wider context. Adjustments and concessions must accompany the efforts of the person to constitute a world-frame compatible with needs, interests, and the ever-present facticity of the environment. It is, however, the perceiving activity of the person which is dominant, for the ordering of relations is in response to what we bring to the teeming continua of impressions. In effect, we each constitute a world whose perimeters are shared but whose center is distinctly personal and unrepeatable. One recent commentator, Robert Jay Lifton, refers to our time as the creation of "a new kind of man—a protean man."

For it is quite possible that even the image of personal identity, insofar as it suggests inner stability and sameness, is derived from a vision of a traditional culture in which man's relationships to his institutions and symbols are still relatively intact—which is hardly the case today. If we understand the self to be the person's symbol of his organism, then self-process refers to the continuous psychic recreation of that symbol. [30]

Protean man is an actualizer more than a recognizer, a formulator more than a spectator. Despite the accepted obviousness of the world, man, by virtue of distinctively personal emphasis, structures his own environment, whether by rejection or assimilation, whether by definition or by inference. A line from the lyrics of a contemporary rock group reads, "I see things I wish my eyes could see." [31] The reductionist character of our language often forces us to acknowledge similarities everywhere, thereby denying the novelty which lurks in all of our experiences. It was Soren Kierkegaard who said something to the effect that we live forward but understand backwards, as if upon retrospect the unique character of our experiences is flattened out so that others may understand them without having gone through them. In time this need for clarity becomes suffusive and we have our present experiences as already sanctioned by the canons of clarity and stripped a priori of their distinctively personal character. In his book on *Becoming*, Gordon Allport offers an ironic comment on this situation.

> *Striving, it is apparent, always has a future reference. As a matter of fact, a great many states of mind are adequately described only in terms of their futurity. Along with striving, we may mention interest, tendency, disposition, expectation, planning, problem solving, and intention. While not all future-directedness is phenomenally propriate, it all requires a type of psychology that transcends the prevalent tendency to explain mental states exclusively in terms of past occurrences.*
>
> *People, it seems, are busy leading their lives into the future, whereas psychology, for the most part, is busy tracing them into the past.*[32,33]

The point at issue is that contemporary man has access to a vast array of experiences and ways of experiencing, many of both becoming available only in the last half-century. He cannot fit into a framework of interpretation which assumes a one-to-one correspondence between the environment, as defined and clarified, and his affective experience of the environment. Recent commentators such as John Cage, Marshall McLuhan, and Edmund Carpenter have made much of the demise of Gutenberg or literate man, that is, he who experiences serially or linearly, with the major rubric the staccato of print. To this they contrast the emergence of the electronic medium, with its stress on instantaneity and the re-emphasizing of the senses, touch, taste, and smell, all of which are explicit body probes. The full ramifications of these judgments are complicated but, despite a flamboyance of style, they seem to characterize the more self-conscious and expressive aspects of our so-

ciety, particularly the young. The paradox, however, and this is a main thrust of the essay, is that "everyman" seems to be caught between the new experiencing and the contours of our old, desiccated environment. Thus, men learn by means of mass media about the incredible powers of contemporary man—they are placed in touch with global experiences representative of every land and every people. At the same time, especially in the great urban centers, the environment recedes in personal quality, while it takes a shape either hostile to human life or of a scope and function beyond a person's intimate reach. In a word, coupled with the majestic reach of global communication, with its concomitant increase on stress,[34] man's local environment, shrunken in affective dimensions, has become de-aesthetized. While not the only factor, this de-aesthetization is a major cause of the widespread anomie which affects contemporary man. It is a social disease and works a serious obstacle to the ameliorative goals of a truly social medicine.

DEAESTHETIZATION AS A SOCIAL DISEASE

Life is coexistent and coextensive with the external natural environment in which the body is submerged. The body's dependence upon this external environment is absolute—in the fullest sense of the word, uterine.[35]

Modern man is well aware of the obvious forms of repression and social affliction. Poverty, prejudice, and violence take their daily toll. We are less aware, however, of more subtle forms of dehumanization, namely, those brought on by the erosion of a genuinely human environment in aesthetic terms. John Dewey once wrote that "no experience of whatever sort is a unity unless it has aesthetic quality."[36] We refer here not to the world of art but to the drama of our doing, undergoing, celebrating, and suffering that comprises the rhythm of everyday ordinary living. Too often this rhythm is submerged in a bland environment, rendering us insensitive to differences, horizons, and crises. In time, we drift through life without variety or intimacy. Dewey writes:

> Things happen, but they are neither definitely included nor decisively excluded; we drift. We yield according to external pressure, or evade and compromise. There are beginnings and cessations, but no genuine initiations and concludings. One thing replaces another, but does not absorb it and carry it on. There is experience, but so slack and discursive that it is not an experience. Needless to say, such experiences are anaesthetic.[36]

How can this be a serious and pressing problem for contemporary man, especially urban man, living as we do in the midst of a technological explosion that has given us marvels of design, communication, and even extraterrestrial experience? We should keep in mind, however, that our analysis is from the perspective of the person rather than from the perspectives of a catalogue of wonders. A closer look at our environment and how we experience it will reveal some severe dislocations.

In the last 50 years we have witnessed a thoroughgoing movement from the affairs of nature to technological artifact as the context of our activity. The shifts from the horse to the automobile and from the stairs to elevator and escalator were aggressive symbols of a new sense of body, wherein we became packaged within a moving environment rather than physically continuous with it. The evolution of the automobile is characterized by an increasing discontinuity of our bodies with that environment, as we became simply steerers of a powerful and largely unintelligible container. The development of a host of appliances and the advent of packaging still further removed us from intimate contact with the fundamental affairs of our daily life. Even

our buildings are becoming containers, usually lacking the qualities that relate to the needs of the dwellers, and more often repressing the opportunity for affective participation. James Marston Fitch, Jr., writes:

> To a greater extent than perhaps any other nation, we Americans have become an "indoor" people. A large portion of our lives—working, sleeping, playing—is spent in buildings; buildings over whose design and construction we have little control: buildings whose physical and economic distribution are only remotely conditioned by our needs; buildings whose effects upon our health and happiness is only obscurely understood.[37]

A further source of the present alienation of our bodies from our immediate surroundings is the unfortunate fact that breakthroughs in technology were not accompanied by a rerouting of bodily interests into other areas of experience. I think that it can be said that we witnessed a steady loss in the role of our hands in the penetration and shaping of the world. Small children, as a case in point, are taught the intricacies of set theory and logic and the staggering speculative reach of modern science, but their bodies are still exercised exclusively under the traditional and time-honored ritual of sports and gymnastics. We rarely teach them to sculpt, to mime, or to experience technology tactilely through the spectrum of touch available to them, ranging over the variety of metals and plastics. Nor have we articulated adequately to ourselves a sense of taste and discrimination relative to our technological environment.

Traditionally, nature, which at one time occupied most of our lives, had an obviousness about it. Crops failed; they were not fecund, they had bugs crawling over and through them, or they simply died. Grass became parched, animals diseased, and water stagnant. On the other hand, our praise of nature responded to its colors, lushness, vitality, energy, texture, and its myriad of shapes and sounds, all deep aesthetic qualities. To the contrary, with regard to the world of artifacts, in our daily lives we seem to settle for "new" or "clean" or "convenient" as sufficient evidence of quality. This attitude has generated a sameness as witnessed by domestic housing, especially projects, roads, building façades, shopping centers, motels, and utensils. Consider also the dreariness of the institutional colors found in hospitals, schools, public housing projects, and, above all, prisons.

Our overall pattern seems to be developing subject to an attitude and a policy which we could describe as a systematic attempt to dilute or remove the sensuousness from our daily environment. Our buses and trains become more and more sterile without any visible recognition that they are to be occupied by human bodies. The seats in these vehicles are contoured as though for an indiscriminate lump and the hand straps have disappeared along with other personal amenities. The materials used in these vehicles are brittle or rigid and they neither take color well nor do they press back against our bodies as we touch them.[38] We have apparently lost our sense of tone and shape in the name of an unrelieved triteness, as if our culture were searching for the least common denominator. Mr. Allen Birnbach, a student of mine, is now preparing a photographic montage of New York City subway stations. His work vividly shows that in a systematic fashion we are replacing the extraordinary wall mosaics of those stations with strips of white tile, turning them into replicas of large public bathrooms.

Some may disagree with these judgments by pointing to the presence of exciting exceptions, as exemplified by isolated instances of monumental architecture found in great cities or cultural centers, or on university campuses.[39] It is instructive to realize that such achievements are experienced directly by only a small percentage of our society and serve frequently as a totally unreal horizon from which to evaluate our everyday experience.[40] Thus, Americans seem caught between amaz-

ing accomplishments which we admire from afar but do not experience in intimate terms, and an eroding aesthetic vitality in the rest of our environment. When those involved are also poverty stricken or otherwise socially trapped, this paradox becomes a cruel gap, rendering their environment still more tawdry and uninteresting.

Now what do these concerns have to do with diagnosis and the affairs of medicine? On one level, there is an obviousness to the problem recognized as such by modern medicine; namely, the disproportionate role of mental and psychological stress versus physical activity which characterizes contemporary man. Responses to this problem range from suggestions of periodic vacations to bicycle riding and jogging. While not opposed to these and similar remedies, our version of the problem cuts differently. The problem is not so much that contemporary man has insufficient physical activity, but rather that the environment in which we live is less and less receptive to our bodies and, further, that the nutrition which proceeds from affective stimulation brought on by aesthetic differentiation and rooted in the affective responses of our body has shrunk, especially in proportion to the range of experiences available to our intellect. My contention is that this situation has resulted in many persons experiencing a deep-seated listlessness, and experiential anomie, masked by using a jazzed-up contemporary idiom and the vicarious identification with the worlds portrayed by contemporary film and television, especially sports. This listlessness, not acknowledged as such, gives rise to a series of medical complaints, physical and/or psychological, which defy traditional modes of diagnosis. A pertinent remark on the medical implications of this development is offered by Serge Chermayeff and Christopher Alexander in a comment on the "Pathology of Boredom."

If man is restricted to one extreme, subjected exclusively to the excitement of the large scale, without the contrast of relief of the minuscule, it is easily con-

ceivable that the human organism might atrophy. Human sensibility, which may be seriously blunted by monotonous over-stimulation, may also be blunted if it is exercised exclusively in an environment of calculated and automatically controlled physical comfort. Our faculties function best and are best maintained at peak sharpness when effort is required of them. Monotony of any kind—dull or intense—is debilitating. Boredom is a word heard commonly today. It may be that the uniformity of the "air conditioned nightmare" fatigues both mind and body, that under such conditions the vital side of human life degenerates.

Possibly science will find that this balanced variety is not essential to man's physical well-being, but it seems unlikely. Equilibrium provided in nature for living organisms appears to be a compound of contrasts in a dynamic relationship. The man-made world must provide at least the same.

Today it is prevented from doing so because of two conspicuous invaders. The very instruments that have given man increased dynamic power—total mobility and instantaneous communication—are destroying the equilibrium in the human habitat.[37(pp 78–79)]

The use of the word pathology in the foregoing text is correct, for any situation which cripples or enervates the human organism, however unusual or vague its roots, is a pathological condition. The task of medicine conceived as a social science (which is not exclusive of medicine as a natural science) is to build into its diagnostic procedures a sensitivity to this dimension of contemporary human experience.

As a specific example of this approach consider the problem of drug use among the young and the increasing desire to be on the road, away from the formal structures of classrooms or conventional dress. Often accompanied by a backing away from tradi-

tional sanitary habits such as the use of shoes or patterns of hair grooming, the spectrum of these activities, ranging from a studied shabbiness up to the heavy use of hallucinogenic drugs, affirms a heightening of body sensibility. This development can also be read as an assault on the contemporary cosmetic masking of our bodies and an attempt to return to an explicit sense experience of the entire body, especially of a tactile kind.

Unfortunately, the causes of the attitudes among young people are often thought traceable to the classic explanatory scheme involving family conflict or the inherent social rebellion of youth. Environmental structures, however, play an important causal role in the disaffection of a younger generation. Over against the vast increase in mobility and the extraordinary heightening of sensory experiences by virtue of electronic media, contrast the average school building as an environment for adolescence. For the most part still an antique form, these buildings perform as rabbit warrens, with fixed space options and severe regimentation of movements. Even the occasional use of overhead projectors and other media aides only serves to intensify the enclosed and static experience presented by the classroom.[41] Spatial inflexibility generates an inflexibility about the processes of time, concretized by rigid scheduling, and contradicts a fundamental truth that "the same environment is not necessarily experienced in the same way by different individuals or, extending the argument, by different groups."[42]

Given a world wherein we can experience events instantaneously, we still cling to the belief that crucial processes such as education must occur as sanctioned in a fixed physical location. The fact that our private experiences evermore outstrip our public experiences in range, quality, and intensity causes considerable sensorial confusion and leads to skepticism about the worth of institutional life. Our point here is simply that environmental inadequacy is one of a series of factors in the emergence of a loss of energy and a need to escape, whether by studious withdrawal, as in the erosion of commitment, or more dramatically by the use of drugs or participation in the renascence of the occult and other counterculture fringe groups.

Certainly men of medicine should not function as the police department or as an extension of the clergy. On the other hand, they should leave no stone unturned in the effort to ameliorate human illness, whether it be of an explicit kind, as a result of epidemics, violence, or drugs, or of the more subtle type, brought on by a developing alienation from our work, our community, and even from ourselves. The local doctor has his hand on a barrage of symptoms and complaints. If he digs deep enough, he will find that environmental malaise plays a large role in developing and spreading social afflictions. In our society, the physician's role is extremely prestigious. Whether it should remain so is open to serious question, but so long as it does, this role should be put to better advantage. As diagnosticians of environmental sensibility, in concert with other socially sensitive agencies and individuals, the medical profession should lend its authority and wisdom to the urgent demand for creating environments which are continuous, supportive, and fertile for the very best of human living. In commenting on the relevance of the Hippocratic Oath, Rene Dubos makes the following point:

> *The well-being of man is influenced by all environmental factors: the quality of the air, water, and food; the winds and topography of the land; and the general living habits. Understanding the effects of environmental forces on man is thus the fundamental basis of the physician's art.*[43]

If the affective quality of an environment is a crucial factor in human well-being, and I believe that it is, then that aspect of medicine known as preventive medicine must attend to it, even if it is at the partial expense of those startling breakthroughs which affect the isolated few. American society is now in a bizarre situation where we have reached dizzying heights of scientific and technical achievement while we simultaneously experience an increase in violence, disaffections, and social disease. The call to education and government is to reorder priorities. Medicine should do likewise.

REFERENCES

1. Clendenning J (ed): *The Letters of Josiah Royce.* Chicago, The University of Chicago Press, 1970, p 586.

2. Cf Susser M: *Community Psychiatry: Epidemiologic and Social Themes.* New York, Random House, 1968, p 355. ''For instance, in New York City rates of perinatal, infant and maternal mortality that mortify conscientious health officials exist side by side with enormous medical virtuosity. The virtuoso performance of medicine is at the nub of the problem. In the great medical centers the effectiveness of care is likely to be measured, as we have noted, by its quality in an episode of illness at the point of delivery. In the twentieth century a more appropriate measure of acomplishment is the impact of a system of medical care on the health of a defined population.''

3. Heider F: Consciousness, the perceptual world, and communications with others, in Tagiuri R, Petrullo L (eds): *Person, Perception and Interpersonal Behavior.* Stanford, Stanford University Press, 1958, p 31.

4. Lindenmann E: Foreword, in Gans H: *The Urban Villagers.* Glencoe, The Free Press, 1962, p v.

5. For extensive support of Lindenmann's judgment, cf Fried M: Grieving for a lost home, in Duhl LJ (ed): *The Urban Condition.* New York, Basic Books, 1963, pp 151–171.

6. Laing RD: *The Divided Self.* Baltimore, Penguin Books Inc, 1965, pp 27–38; for penetrating remarks on the reduction of the patients' experiences to those proscribed by the doctor.

7. Sennett R: *The Uses of Disorder—Personal Identity and City Life.* New York, Alfred A Knopf, 1970, p 9.

8. Cf James W: *A Pluralistic Universe.* New York, Longmans Green & Co, 1909, p 60. ''The treating of a name as excluding from the fact named what the name's definition fails positively to include, is what I call 'vicious intellectualism.' ''

9. Buber M: Education, in *Between Man and Man.* London, Routledge & Kegan Paul, 1947, p 97.

10. McDermott JJ: Privacy and social therapy. *Soundings*, vol LI, no. 3, Fall 1968, pp 346–357; for a discussion and evaluation of some new approaches to ''interviews.''

11 Sommer R: *Personal Space—The Behavioral Basis of Design*. New York, Prentice-Hall, 1969, p 91.

12 Mechanic D: Community psychiatry: Some sociological perspectives and implications, in Roberts L et al (eds): *Community Psychiatry*. New York, Anchor Books, 1969, p 231.

13 Harrington M: *The Other America—Poverty in the United States*. New York, The Macmillan Co, 1963, p 4.

14 For a similar story, cf Ray G: An Anglo's barrio, in Cahill S, Cooper M (eds): *The Urban Reader*. New York, Prentice-Hall, 1971, p 34. A welfare mother chides a Vista volunteer. ''You kids come into our communities and are shocked by the garbage and rats. You want to start clean-up campaigns and get rid of the rats. I have lived with them for 40 years, and unless one bites my daughter, rats are the least of my problems. You find out what *I* am concerned about, even if it is a broken door hinge, and start to work on that.''

15 Cf James W: *Psychology—The Briefer Course*. New York, Henry Holt & Co, 1892, p 165. Long ago, William James wrote that ''it is, the reader will see, the reinstatement of the vague and inarticulate to its proper place in our mental life which I am so anxious to press on the attention.''

16 Cf Murphy G: *Human Potentialities*. New York, Basic Books, 1958, pp 302–329. For a discussion of novelty in human experience, especially in pp 312 313 where he considers the vast range of methods of articulation which differentiate cultures.

17 Witness the hatred of project living as expressed by Juan Gonzales in Mayerson CL: Two blocks apart, in Cahill and Cooper, ref. 14, pp 76–81.

18 Some discussion of the urgent reasons behind such hostility is to be found in Fried, reference 5, and McDermott JJ: Deprivation and celebration: Suggestions for an aesthetic ecology, in Edie JM (ed): *New Essays in Phenomenology*. Chicago, Quadrangle Books, 1969, pp 116–130. Also see reference 19.

19 McDermott JJ: Nature nostalgia and the city: An American dilemma. *Soundings*, vol LV, no. 1, spring 1972, pp 1–20.

20 Moore W Jr: *The Vertical Ghetto—Everyday Life in an Urban Project*. New York, Random House, 1969, pp 31–32n. A specific case of social-medical pathology caused by an absence of complaint is reported. ''In one case of acrophobia, a tenant and his family had been reassigned an eleventh-floor apartment from one that they had been assigned on the second floor. Although the man was a good tenant and appeared to be a good family man, he suddenly began to stay away from home for long periods of time, sometimes for days. Because his wife was concerned, she related the new behavior to a social worker, whom the husband agreed to see. After several discussions, it was revealed that the tenant was deathly afraid of height. Moreover, he could never ride the elevator. He would walk eleven floors.''

21 Pirandello L: Six characters in search of an author, in Bentley E (ed): *Naked Masks*. New York, EP Dutton & Co Inc, 1952, p 224.

22 Cf the extensive collection of materials by Proshansky, HM et al (eds): *Environmental Psychology—Man and His Physical Setting*. New York, Holt Rinehart & Winston, 1970. A number of these essays are directly pertinent to the problems of social medicine.

23 Cf Spicker SF (ed): *The Philosophy of the Body—Rejections of Cartesian Dualism*. Chicago, Quadrangle Books, 1970, for historical perspective on this problem.

24 Bergson H: *Matter and Memory*. New York, Doubleday & Co, 1959 (1896), p 1.

25 James W: The experience of activity, in McDermott JJ (ed): *The Writings of William James*. New York, Random House, 1967, p 284, n 180.

26 Alexander IW: *Bergson—Philosopher of Reflection*. New York, Hillary House, 1957, p 31.

27 Smith JE: Radical empiricism. *Proc Aristotelian Soc* **LXV**, March 1965, pp 205–218.

28 James W: *The Principles of Psychology*. New York, Henry Holt & Co, 1890, vol 1, pp 284–285.

29 Polanyi M: *The Tacit Dimension*. New York, Anchor Books, 1967, pp 15–16.

30 Lifton RJ: Protean man. *Partisan Review* 35:13, 1968.

31 From the vanilla fudge, cited in Carpenter E: *They Became What They Beheld*. New York, Ballantine Books, 1970.

32 Allport G: *Becoming*. New Haven, Yale University Press, 1955, p 51.

33 We should pay heed to the comment of the painter William de Kooning who remarked that ''The past does not influence me; I influence it.'' Cited in Cage J: *Silence*. Cambridge, The MIT Press, 1966, p 67.

34 Cf Meier RL: Living with the coming urban technology, in Geene et al (eds): *Man and the Modern City*. Pittsburgh, University of Pittsburgh Press, 1963, pp 59–70; for a discussion of the sensorial overload and the increase of harassment brought on by the expansion of mass media communications.

35 Fitch JM: Experiential bases for aesthetic decision, in Proshansky, reference 22, p 76.

36 Dewey J: *Art as Experience*. New York, Capricorn Books, 1958 (1934), p 40.

37 Cited in Chermayeff S, Alexander C: *Community and Privacy*. New York, Anchor Books, 1965, p 29.

38 Cf Berkley S, who makes urban play sculptures, in *New York*, 6 Sept 1971, p 52. She comments, ''Practically everything people touch in this city is rigid. With my things, they can feel, smell, pull, stretch, hit, punch and make noises. They are participants as well as viewers.'' A student in my seminar on ''Urban Aesthetics,'' Miss Jane Donenfeld, made a film of more than one hundred city signs. All but one said *No* or revealed some other form of prohibition. The one positive sign was a welcome to the city, which was followed by a series of prohibitions.

39 We should take notice that tedium has entered even monumental achievements. What could be more anesthetic than the simple jutting up of the formless twin towers of the World Trade Center in New York City, and what are we to make of the 747 airplane, which has removed from us the experience of flying?

40 Cf Jacobs J: *The Death and Life of Great American Cities*. New York, Vintage Books, 1961, p 13. Jane Jacobs, for one, criticizes the unreal character of city planning and design, comparing it at one point to the stage of ''bloodletting'' in medicine. She calls for an embarkation ''upon the adventure of probing the real world.''

41 Fitch JM: Experiential bases for aesthetic decision, in Proshansky, reference 22, p 79. He holds of ''good architecture'' that ''far from offering solid, impermeable barriers to the natural environment, its outer surfaces come more and more closely to resemble permeable membranes which can accept or reject any environmental force. Again the uterine analogy; and not accidentally, for with such convertibility in the container's walls, man can modulate the play of environmental forces upon himself and his processes, to guarantee their uninterrupted development, in very much the same way as the mother's body protects the embryo.'' A recent example of this approach is to be found in the retractable roofs and membrane dams of the German architect, Frei Otto.

42 Briggs A: The sense of place, in *The Fitness of Man's Environment*. Washington, Smithsonian Institution Press, 1968, p 79.

43 Dubos R: *Man, Medicine and Environment*. New York, Mentor Books, 1968, p 74.

Chapter 18
The Golden Rule and the Cycle of Life
Erik H. Erikson

The healer is committed to a highest good, preserving life and further-
ing well-being. He need not prove scientifically that these are, in fact,
the highest good; rather, he is precommitted to this basic proposition
while investigating what can be verified by scientific means. This, I
think, is the meaning of the Hippocratic Oath. It subordinates all
medical method to a humanist ethic.

As the Gay Lecturer of 1962, I take advantage of such leeway to offer a few insights coming from the study of life histories—a field of study first inspired by a series of physicians (from Sigmund Freud to William James and Henry Murray) who became psychologists and who created, out of the study of cases, the study of lives. The insights to be advanced will, it is hoped, prove to be relevant to "wise and proper conduct," even though the only kind of ethical investment to be recommended is that of one generation in the next.

THE GOLDEN RULE

My base line is the Golden Rule, which advocates that one should do (or not do) to another what one wishes to be (or not to be) done by. Systematic students of ethics often indicate a certain disdain for this all-too-

Editor's Note: The essay by Erik Erikson is reprinted from Erikson EH: The golden rule and the cycle of life. *Harvard Med Alumni Bull* **37** (2), Winter, 1963. Professor Erikson presented it on May 4, 1962, at the Harvard Medical School as the George W. Gay Lecture on Medical Ethics.

primitive ancestor of loftier and more logical principles. Yet this rule has marked a mysterious meeting ground between ancient peoples separated by oceans and eras, and is a theme hidden in the most memorable sayings of many thinkers.

I would like to take the *Talmudic* version of the Golden Rule for my opening: "What is hateful to yourself, do not to your fellow man." The Talmud adds, "That is the whole of the Torah and the rest is but commentary. Go and learn it." The Rule in this form, as critics have never tired of pointing out, is only the rockbottom of moral prudence. But then, it was so stated by Rabbi Hillel in answer to an unbeliever's challenge that he be told the whole of the Torah while he stood on one foot. Pressed for brevity, the great rabbi put basic things first. If he added that the rest was but commentary, nobody acquainted with the Jewish way of life would mistake *but* commentary for *merely* commentary, for surely sometimes the ongoing commentary is the very life of a rule.

The Golden Rule obviously concerns itself with one of the very basic paradoxes of human existence. Each man calls his own a separate body, a self-conscious individuality, and a personal awareness of the cosmos; and yet he shares this world as a *reality* also perceived and judged by others and as an *actuality* within which he must commit himself to ceaseless interaction. To identify self-interest and the interest of other selves, the Rule alternately employs the method of warning, "*Do* as you *would* be done by." For psychological appeal, some versions rely on the minimum of egotistic prudence, already quoted, while others demand a maximum of altruistic sympathy. It must be admitted that the formula, "Do not to others what if done to you would cause you pain," does not presuppose much more than the mental level of the small child who desists from pinching when it gets pinched in return; while mature insight and more is assumed in the saying, "No one is a believer until he loves for his brother what he loves for himself." Of all the versions, however, none commits us as unconditionally as, "Love thy neighbor as thyself." It even suggests a true love of ourselves.

I will not (I could not) involve us in comparative religion by tracing the versions of the Rule to various world religions; no doubt in translation all of them have become somewhat assimilated to our biblical versions. Yet the basic formula seems to be universal, and it reappears in an astonishing number of the most revered sayings of our civilization from St. Francis' prayer to Kant's moral imperative and to Lincoln's simple political creed: "As I would not be slave, I would not be master."

The variations of the Rule have, of course, provided material for many discussions on ethics weighing the soundness of the logic implied and measuring the degree of ethical nobility reached in each. My field of inquiry, the study of life histories, suggests that I desist from arguing relative logical merit or spiritual worth, and instead relate some variations in moral and ethical sensitivity to successive stages in the development of human conscience; in the framework of the life cycle, the most primitive rules and the most exalted may well prove to be necessary to each other.

MORALITY

This lecture [was originally] entitled "Upon Medical Ethics" and not "Upon Medical Mo-

---

This lecture [was originally] entitled "Upon Medical Ethics" and not "Upon Medical Morality." The implication is clear: he who knows what is legal or illegal and what is moral or immoral has not necessarily learned thereby what is ethical.

---

rality." The implication is clear: he who knows what is legal and what is moral or immoral has not necessarily learned thereby what is ethical. Highly moralistic people can do unethical things, while an ethical man's involvement in immoral doings becomes by inner necessity an occasion for tragedy. The dictionary, our first refuge from ambiguity, in this case only compounds it: morals and ethics are defined as synonyms and antonyms of each other. In other words, they are the same with a difference—a difference which I intend to emphasize.

I would propose that we consider *moral rules* of conduct to be based on a fear of threats to be forestalled—outer threats of abandonment, punishment, public exposure; or a threatening inner sense of guilt, shame, or isolation. In contrast, I would consider *ethical rules* to be based on a love of ideals to be striven for—ideals which hold up to us some highest good, some definition of perfection, and some promise of self-realization. This differentiation is, I think, substantiated by developmental observation, and the *developmental principle* is the first of those which will represent for us the kind of insight which we have gained by the study of life histories.

All that exists layer upon layer in an adult's mind has developed step by step in the growing child's, and the major steps in the comprehension of what is considered good behavior in one's cultural universe are related —for better and for worse—to different stages in individual maturation. The response to a moral tone of voice develops early. The small child, so limited to the intensity of the moment, somehow must learn the boundaries marked by *don'ts*. Here, cultures have a certain leeway in underscoring the goodness of one who does not transgress or the evilness of one who does. But the conclusion is unavoidable that children can be made to feel evil and that adults continue to project evil on one another and on their children far beyond the call of rational judgment.

Before discussing this early moral sense in more detail, let me mention the later steps which I will differentiate from it: they are the development of an *ideological sense* in adolescence, and an *ethical sense* in young adulthood. The imagery of steps, of course, is useful only where it is to be suggested that one item precedes another in such a way that the earlier one is necessary to the later ones, and that each later one is of a higher order. But development is more complex, especially since all manner of step formations take place simultaneously and in not-too-obvious synchronization.

CHILDHOOD To return to the moral sense, psychoanalytic observation first established in a systematic fashion what certain Eastern thinkers have always known, namely, that radical division into good and bad can be a sickness of the mind. It has traced the moral scruples and excesses of the adult to the childhood stages in which guilt and shame are ready to be aroused and are easily exploited. It has named and studied the superego which hovers over the ego as the inner perpetuation of the child's subordination to the restraining will of his elders. The voice of the superego is not always cruel and derisive, but it is ever ready to become so whenever the precarious balance which we call a good conscience is upset, at which times the secret weapons of this inner governor are revealed: the brand of shame and the bite of conscience. Are these "caused" or merely accentuated by the pressure of parental and communal methods, by the threat of loss of affection, corporal punishment, public shaming? Or are they by now a proclivity for self-alienation which has become a part—and to some extent a necessary part—of man's evolutionary heritage?

All we know for sure is that the moral proclivity in man does not develop without the establishment of some chronic self-doubt and some truly terrible—even if mostly submerged —rage against anybody and anything that reinforces such doubt. The "lowest" in man is thus apt to reappear in the guise of the "highest": irrational and prerational combinations of goodness, doubt, and rage can reemerge in the adult in those malignant forms of righteousness and prejudice which we may call *moralism*. In the name of high moral principles we can employ all the vindictiveness of derision, torture, and mass extinction. One surely must come to the conclusion that the Golden Rule was meant to protect man not only against his enemies' open attacks, but also against his friends' righteous encroachments.

EVOLUTION

Lest this view, in spite of the evidence of history, seem too "clinical," we turn to the science of evolution which in the last few decades has joined psychoanalysis in recognizing the superego as an evolutionary fact— and danger. The *developmental* principle is thus joined by an *evolutionary* one. Waddington even goes so far as to say that superego rigidity may be an overspecialization in the human race, like the excessive body armor of the late dinosaurs. In a less grandiose comparison he likens the superego to "the finicky adaptation of certain parasites which fits them to live only on one host or animal." In recommending his book, *The Ethical Animal* (in addition to the works of J. Huxley and G. G. Simpson), I must admit that his terminology contradicts mine. He calls the awakening of morality in childhood a proclivity for "ethicizing," whereas I would prefer to call it moralizing. As do many animal psychologists, he dwells on analogies between the very young child and the young animal instead of comparing, as I think we must, the young animal with the preadult human, including the adolescent.

I cannot dwell here on the new insights regarding the cognitive and emotional gains of adolescence which enable the young, often only after a severe bout with moralistic regression, to envisage more universal principles of a highest human good. The adolescent learns to grasp the flux of time, to anticipate the future in a coherent way, to perceive ideas and to assent to ideals—to take, in short, an *ideological* position for which the younger child is cognitively not prepared. In adolescence, then, an ethical view is approximated, but it remains susceptible to an alternation of impulsive judgment and odd rationalization. It is, then, as true for adolescence as it is for childhood that man's way stations to maturity can become fixed, can become premature and stations for future regression—in the individual person and in masses of individuals.

The moral sense, in its perfections and its perversions, has been an intrinsic part of man's *evolution,* while the sense of ideological rejuvenation has pervaded his *revolutions,* both with prophetic idealism and with destructive fanaticism. Adolescent man, in all his sensitivity to the ideal, is easily taken in by the promise of a new and arrogantly exclusive identity.

The true *ethical sense* of the *young adult* at its best encompasses moral restraint and ideal vision, while insisting on concrete commitments to those intimate relationships and work associations by which man can hope to share a lifetime of productivity and competence. But young adulthood engenders its own

dangers. It adds to the moralist's righteousness—and to the ideologist's repudiation of all otherness—the territorial defensiveness of one who has appropriated and staked out his earthly claim and who seeks eternal security in the superidentity of organizations. Thus, what the Golden Rule at its highest has attempted to make all-inclusive, tribes and nations, castes and classes, moralities and ideologies have consistently made exclusive again —proudly, superstitiously, and viciously denying the status of reciprocal ethics to those "outside."

If I have so far underscored the malignant potentials of man's slow maturation, I have done so not in order to dwell on a kind of dogmatic pessimism which can emerge all too easily from clinical preoccupation and often leads only to anxious avoidances. I know that man's moral, ideological, and ethical propensities can find, and have found on occasion, a sublime integration, in individuals and in groups who were both tolerant and firm, flexible and strong, wise and obedient. Above all, men have always shown a dim knowledge of their better potentialities by paying homage to those purest leaders who taught the simplest and most inclusive rules for an undivided mankind. But men have also persistently betrayed them, on what passed for moral or ideological grounds, even as they are now preparing a potential betrayal of all human heritage on scientific and technological grounds in the name of that which is considered good merely because it *can* be made to work—no matter where it leads.

We begin to see where it may lead. But only in our time, and in our very generation, have we come to view with a historical start the obvious fact that in all of previous history the Rule, in whatever form, has comfortably coexisted with warfare. A warrior, all armored and spiked and set to do to another what he fully expected the other to be ready to do to him, saw no ethical contradiction between the Rule and his military ideology; he could, in fact, grant to his adversary a respect which he hoped to earn in return. This tenuous co-existence of ethics and warfare may outlive itself in our time. The military mind may well come to fear for its historical identity when technical mass annihilation replaces tactical warfare. The Golden Rule of the nuclear age, which is, "Do not unto others unless you are sure you can do them in as totally as they can do you in," creates not only an international deadlock, but a profoundly ethical one as well.

One wonders, however, whether this deadlock can be broken by even the most courageous protest, the most incisive interpretation, or the most prophetic warning—a warning of catastrophe of such immensity that most men will ignore it, as they ignore certain death and have learned to ignore the monotonous prediction of hell. It seems instead that only an ethical orientation, a direction for vigorous cooperation, can free today's energies from their bondage in armed defensiveness. We live at a time in which, for all the species-wide destruction possible, we can think for the first time of a species-wide identity, of truly universal ethics, such as have been prepared in the world religions, in humanism, and by some philosophers. Ethics cannot be fabricated; they can only emerge from an informed and inspired search for a more inclusive human identity which a new technology and a new world image make possible as well as mandatory.

Man's sociogenetic evolution is about to reach a crisis in the full sense of the word: a crossroads offering one path to fatality, and one to recovery and further growth. Artful perverter of joy and keen exploiter of strength, man has learned to survive "in a fashion," to multiply without food for the multitudes, to grow up healthy without reaching personal maturity, to live well but without purpose, to invent ingeniously without aim, and to kill grandiosely without need. But the processes of sociogenetic evolution also seem to promise a new humanism: the acceptance by man—as an evolved product as well as a producer, and a self-conscious tool of further evolution of the obligation to be guided

in his planned actions and his chosen self-restraints by his knowledge and his insights. In this endeavor, then, it may be of a certain importance to learn to understand and to master the differences between infantile morality, adolescent ideology, and adult ethics. Each is necessary to the next, but each effective only if they eventually combine in that wisdom which, as Waddington puts it, "fulfills sufficiently the function of mediating evolutionary advance."

At the point when one is about to end an argument with a global injunction of what we must do, it is good to remember Blake's admonition that the common good readily becomes the topic of "the scoundrel, the hypocrite, and the flatterer"; and that he who would do some good must do so in "minute particulars." And indeed, I have so far spoken only of development and the evolutionary principle, according to which the propensity for ethics grows in the individual as part of an adaptation roughly laid down by evolution. Yet, to grow in the individual, ethics must be generated and regenerated in and by the sequence of generations. This generational principle we must now make more explicit.

SCIENTIFIC MAN

Let me make an altogether new start here; let us look at scientific man in his dealings with animals. Harry Harlow's studies on the development of affection in monkeys are well known. He did some exquisite experimental and photographic work attempting, in the life of laboratory monkeys, to "control the mother variable." He took monkeys from mothers within a few hours after birth, isolated them and left them with "mothers" made out of wire, metal, wood, and terry cloth. A rubber nipple somewhere in their middles emitted piped-in milk, and the whole contraption was wired for body warmth. All the "variables" of this mother situation were controlled: the amount of rocking, the degree of "body warmth," and the exact incline of the maternal body necessary to make a scared monkey feel safe and comfortable. Years ago, when this method was presented as a study of the development of affection in monkeys, the clinician could not help wondering whether this was *monkey* affection or a fetishist addiction to inanimate objects. And, indeed, while these laboratory-reared monkeys became healthier and healthier, and much more trainable in technical know-how than the inferior monkeys brought up by mere monkey mothers, they became at the end what Harlow calls "psychotics." They sat passively, they stared vacantly, and some did something terrifying: when poked they bit themselves and tore at their own flesh until the blood flowed. They had not learned to experience "the other," whether as mother, a mate, a child—or enemy. Only a tiny minority of the females produced offspring, and only one of them made an attempt to nurse hers. But science remains a wonderful thing. Now that we have succeeded in producing "psychotic" monkeys experimentally, we can convince ourselves that we have at last given scientific support to severely disturbed mother-child relationships as causative factors in human psychosis.

It speaks for Harry Harlow's methods that what they demonstrate is unforgettable. At the same time, they lead us to that borderline where we recognize that the scientific approach toward living beings must be with concepts and methods adequate to the study of ongoing life, not of selective extinction. I

One can study the nature of things by doing something to them, but one can only learn about the essential nature of beings by doing something with them or for *them.*

---

have put it this way: one can study the nature of things by doing something to them, but one can only learn about the essential nature of beings by doing something with

them or *for* them. This, of course, is the principle of clinical science. It does not deny that one can learn by dissecting the dead, or that an animal or a man can be motivated to lend circumscribed parts of their being to an experimental procedure. But for the study of those central transactions which are the carriers of sociogenetic evolution, and for which we must take responsibility in the future, the chosen unit of observation must be the generation, not the individual. Whether an individual animal or human being partook of the stuff of life can only be tested by the kind of observation which discerns his ability to transmit life—in some essential form—to the next generation.

One remembers here the work of Konrad Lorenz, and the kind of "interliving" research which he and others have developed, making, in principle, the life cycle of certain selected animals part of the same environment in which the observer lives his own life cycle, and studying his role as well as theirs, taking his chances with what his ingenuity can discern in a setting of sophisticated naturalist inquiry. One remembers also Elsa the lioness, a foundling who was brought up in the Adamson household in Kenya. There, the mother variable was not controlled, it was in control. Mrs. Adamson and her husband even felt responsible for putting grown-up Elsa back among the lions and succeeded in sending her back to the bush, where she mated and had cubs, and yet came back from time to time (accompanied by her cubs) to visit her human foster parents. In our context, we cannot fail to wonder about the built-in "moral" sense that made Elsa respond—and to respond in very critical situations, indeed—to the words, "No, Elsa, no," if the words came from human beings she trusted. Yet even with this built-in "moral" response, and with a lasting trust in her foster parents (which she transmitted to her wild cubs), she was able to live as wild lions do. Her mate, however, never appeared; he apparently was not too curious about her folks.

The point of this and similar stories is that

our habitual relationship to what we call beasts in nature and "instinctive" or "instinctual" beastliness in ourselves may be highly distorted by thousands of years of superstition; there may be resources for peace even in our "animal nature" if we will only learn to nurture nature, as well as to master her. Today, we can teach a monkey, in the very words of the Bible, to "eat the flesh of his own arm," even as we can permit "erring leaders" to make of all mankind the "fuel of the fire." Yet it seems equally plausible that we can let our children grow up to lead "the calf and the young lion and the fatling together"—in nature and in their own nature.

MUTUALITY AND TRUST

To recognize one of man's prime resources, however, we must trace back his individual development to his premoral days, his infancy, which are marked by basic trust—an overall attitude integrating what in the newborn organism reaches out to the caretakers and establishes with them what we will now

---

The failure of basic trust and of mutuality has been recognized in psychiatry as the most far-reaching development failure, undercutting all development.

---

discuss as mutuality. The failure of basic trust and of mutuality has been recognized in psychiatry as the most far-reaching development failure, undercutting all development.

MUTUALITY I would call mutuality a relationship in which partners depend on each other for the development of their respective strengths. A baby's first responses can be seen as part of an actuality consisting of many details of mutual arousal and response. While the baby initially smiles at a mere configuration resembling the human face, the adult cannot help smiling back, filled with expecta-

tions of a "recognition" which he needs to secure from the new being as surely as it needs him. The fact is that the mutuality of adult and baby is the original source of the basic ingredient of all effective as well as ethical human action: *hope*. As far back as 1895, Freud, in his first outline of a "Psychology for Neurologists," counterpoints to the "helpless" newborn a "help-rich" ("hilfreich") adult and postulates that their mutual understanding is "the primal source of all moral motives." Should we, then, equip the Golden Rule with a principle of mutuality, replacing the reciprocity of both prudence and sympathy?

A parent dealing with a child will be strengthened in his vitality, in his sense of identity, and in his readiness for ethical action, by the very ministrations by means of which he secures to the child his vitality, his future sense of identity, and his eventual readiness for ethical action. On this mutuality, then, all ethical potentialities are built—and we know how tragic and deeply pathogenic its absence can be in children and parents who cannot arouse and cannot respond.

But we should avoid making a new utopia out of the "mother-child relationship." The paradise of early childhood must be abandoned—a fact which man has not yet learned to accept. The earliest mutuality is only a beginning and leads to more complicated encounters as both the child and his interaction with a widening cast of persons grow more complicated. I need only point out that the second basic set of vital strengths in childhood (following trust and hope) is autonomy and will, and it must be clear that a situation in which the child's willfulness faces the adult's will is a different proposition from that of the mutuality of instilling hope. Yet any adult who has managed to train a child's will must admit—for better or for worse—that he has learned much about himself and about will that he never knew before, something which cannot be learned in any other way. Thus each growing individual's developing strength "dovetails" with the strengths of an increasing number of persons arranged about him in the social orders of family, school, community, and society. These orders, in turn, safeguard themselves by formalizing the Golden Rule in a hierarchy of institutions. But all orders and rules are kept alive by those "virtues" of which Shakespeare (in what appears to me to be *his* passionate version of the Rule) says that "shining upon others [they] heat them and they retort that heat again to the first giver."

AMENDING THE GOLDEN RULE

With such high encouragement I will try to formulate my amendment to the Golden Rule. I have been reluctant to come to this point; it has taken thousands of years and much linguistic acrobatics to translate the Rule from one era to another and from one language into another, and at best one can only confound it again in a somewhat different way.

It would, at any rate, seem irrelevant to formulate any new or better *do's* or *don't's* than the Rule already implies in its classical forms. Rather, I would advocate a general orientation not too narrowly hemmed in by scruples and avoidances and not too exclusively guided by high promises and rewards. This orientation has its center in whatever activity or activities give man the feeling, as William James put it, of being "most deeply and intensely active and alive." In this, James promises, each will find his "real me"; but, I would now add, he will also acquire a conviction that truly ethical acts enhance a mutuality between the doer and the other—a mutuality which strengthens the doer even as it strengthens the other. Thus, the "doer unto" and "the other" are one deed. Developmentally, this means that the doer is activated in whatever strength is appropriate to his age, stage, and condition, even as he activates in the other the strength appropriate to his age, stage, and condition.

Our next step is to demonstrate that the inequality of parent and child, or better, the uniqueness of their respective positions which has served as our model so far, has significant analogies in other situations in which uniqueness depends on a divided function. Here, eventually, we may come closer to an application of our amendment of the Rule to medical ethics as well.

ACTIVE CHOICE   But there is one more principle which must be added to the developmental one, to mutuality, and to the generational principle. I already implied it in the term "activate," and I would call it the principle of active choice. It is, I think, most venerably expressed in St. Francis' prayer: "Grant that I may not so much seek to be consoled as to console; to be understood, as to understand; to be loved as to love; for it is in giving that we receive." Such commitment to a decisive initiative in love is, of course, contained in the admonition to "love thy neighbor." It is not in our domain, however, to discuss that religious frontier of existence where man expects to derive his most decisive ethical initiative from a highest grace. Yet I think that we can recognize in these exalted words a psychological verity which determines that only he who approaches an encounter in an active and giving attitude (consciously and unconsciously), rather than in a demanding and dependent one, will be able to make of that encounter what it can become.

SEXUALITY   To return to particulars, I will attempt to apply my amendment to the diversity of function in the two sexes. I have not dwelt so far on this most usual subject of a psychoanalytic discourse, sexuality. So much of this otherwise absorbing part of life has in recent years become stereotyped, and not the least among the terminological culprits to be blamed for this sorry fact is the psychoanalytic term "love object." For the word "object" in Freud's theory has been taken too literally by many of his friends and by most of his enemies. (Moralistic critics do delight in misrepresenting a man's transitory findings as his ultimate "values.") The fact is that

Freud, on purely conceptual grounds, and on the basis of his scientific training, pointed out that drives have objects; but he never said, and he certainly never advocated, that men or women should treat one another as objects on which to live out their sexual desires.

Instead, his central theory of a mutuality of orgasm which combines strivings of sexuality and of love points, in fact, to one of those basic mutualities in which a partner's potency and potentialities are activated even as he activates the other's potency and potentialities. Freud's theory implies that a man will be more a man to the extent to which he makes a woman more a woman—and vice versa—because only two uniquely different beings can enhance their respective uniqueness for one another. A "genital" person in Freud's sense is thus more apt to act in accordance with Kant's version of the Golden Rule, namely, that one should so act as to treat humanity (whether in his person or in another) "always as an end, and never as only a means." What Freud added, however, was a methodology which opens to our inquiry and to our influence the powerhouse of inner forces which provide the shining heat for our strength—and the smoldering smoke of our weaknesses.

THE UNIQUENESS OF WOMEN I cannot leave the subject of the two sexes without a word on the uniqueness of women. One may well question whether the oldest versions of the Rule meant to acknowledge women as partners in the golden deal; and today's study of lives still leaves quite obscure the place of women in what is most relevant to men. True, women are being granted equality of political rights and the recognition of a certain sameness in mental and moral equipment. But

---

What women have not begun to earn, partially because they have not cared to ask for it, is the equal right to be effectively unique.

---

what they have not begun to earn, partially because they have not cared to ask for it, is the equal right to be effectively unique, and to use hard-won rights in the service of what they uniquely represent in human evolution.

One senses today the emergence of a new feminism as part of a more inclusive humanism. This coincides with a growing conviction —highly ambivalent, to be sure—that the future of mankind cannot depend on men alone and may well depend on the fate of a mother variable uncontrolled by technological man. The resistance to such a consideration always comes from men and women who are mortally afraid that by emphasizing what is unique one may tend to reemphasize what is unequal. The study of life histories certainly confirms a far-reaching sameness in men and women insofar as they express the mathematical architecture of the universe, the organization of logical thought, and the structure of language. But such study also suggests that while boys and girls can think and act and talk alike, they naturally do not experience their bodies (and thus the world) alike: one could illustrate this by pointing to sex differences in the structuralization of space in the play of children. But I assume here that a uniqueness of either sex will be granted without proof, and that the "difference" acclaimed by the much-quoted Frenchman is not considered a mere matter of anatomical appointments for mutual sexual enjoyment, but a psychological difference central to two great modes of life, the *paternal* and the *maternal* modes.

The study of creative men reveals that only a vital struggle makes it possible for them to reconcile in themselves the paternal and the maternal dimensions of all mental productivity. It may well be that there is something in woman's specific creativity which has only waited for a clarification of her relationship to masculinity (including her own) in order to assume her share of leadership in those fateful human affairs which so far have been left entirely in the hands of gifted and driven men, and often of men whose creativity eventually has yielded to ruthless self-aggrandizement. Mankind now obviously depends on new kinds of social inventions and on institutions which guard and cultivate that which nurses and nourishes, cares and tolerates, includes and preserves. Mere conquest and invention alone, and more expansion and organization, will make life more exciting but not more livable. And if my amendment to the Rule suggests that one sex enhances the uniqueness of the other, it also implies that each, to be really unique, depends on a mutuality with an equally unique partner: only when women dare to assume the motherhood of man, may men be emboldened to overcome the boyhood of history.

MEDICAL ETHICS

By now, one may well have reached the conclusion that my discursiveness was intended to leave me little time for the problem of medical ethics. However, medical ethics can only be a variation of a universal theme, and it was necessary to establish the general context within which I could hope to give a slightly different emphasis to a subject so rich in tradition.

There is a very real and specific inequality in the relationship of doctor and patient in their roles of knower and known, helper and sufferer, practitioner of life and victim of disease and death; for which reason, medical people have their own and unique professional oath and strive to live up to a universal ideal of "the doctor." Yet the practice of the healing arts permits extreme types of practitioners: from the absolute authoritarian over homes and clinics to the harassed servant of demanding mankind; from the sadist of mere proficiency to the effusive lover of all (well, almost all) his patients.

Here, too, Freud has thrown intimate and original light on the workings of a unique relationship. His letters to his friend and mentor Fliess illustrate the singular experience which made him recognize in his patients

what he called "transference"—that is, the patient's wish to exploit sickness and treatment for infantile and regressive ends. But more, Freud recognized a "countertransference" in the healer's motivation to exploit the patient's transference and to dominate or serve, possess or love him to the disadvantage of his true function. He made systematic insight into transference and countertransference part of the training of the psychoanalytic practitioner. I would think that all of the motivations necessarily entering so vast and intricate a field could be reconciled in a Golden Rule amended to include a mutuality of divided function. Each specialty and each technique in its own way permits the medical man to develop as a practitioner and as a person, even as the patient is cured as a patient and as a person. A real cure transcends the transitory state of patienthood; it is an

---

A real cure transcends the transitory state of patienthood; it is an experience which enables the cured patient to develop and to transmit to home and neighbor an attitude toward health which is one of the most essential ingredients of an ethical outlook.

---

experience which enables the cured patient to develop and to transmit to home and neighbor an attitude toward health which is one of the most essential ingredients of an ethical outlook. This variation on the overall theme of an amended rule is all I can offer in the framework of this lecture; intensive discussion will, I hope, lead to more detailed and more concrete matter vital to medical practice.

A NEW ETHICAL OUTLOOK? Beyond this, can the healing arts and sciences contribute to a new ethical outlook? This question always recurs in psychoanalysis and is usually disposed of with Freud's answer that the psychoanalyst represents the ethics of scientific truth only, and is committed to studying ethics (or morality) in a scientific way. Beyond this, he leaves "Weltanschaungen" (ethical world views) to others.

It seems to me, however, that the clinical arts and sciences, while employing the scientific method, are not defined by it or limited by it. The healer is committed to a highest good, preserving life and furthering well-being. He need not prove scientifically that these are, in fact, the highest good; rather, he is precommitted to this basic proposition while investigating what can be verified by scientific means. This, I think, is the meaning of the Hippocratic Oath, which subordinates all medical method to a humanist ethic. True, a man can separate his personal, his professional, and his scientific ethics, seeking fulfillment of needs in personal life, the welfare of others in his profession, and, in his research, truths independent of personal preference or service. However, there are psychological limits to the multiplicity of values a man can live by; and, in the end, not only the practitioner, but also his patient and his research, depend on a certain unification in him of temperament, intellect, and ethics; this unification clearly characterizes great doctors.

While it is true, then, that as scientists we must study ethics objectively, we are, as professional individuals, committed to unifying personality, training, and conviction which alone will help us to do our work adequately. At the same time, as transient members of the human race, we must record the truest meaning of which the fallible methods of our era and the accidental circumstances of our existence have made us aware. In this sense, there is (and always has been) not only an ethic governing clinical work, and a clinical approach to the study of ethics, but also a contribution to the ethics of the healing orientation. The healer, in addition, has now committed himself to prevention on a large scale, and he cannot evade the question of how to assure ethical vitality to all lives saved from morbidity and early mortality.

THE INTERNATIONAL SITUATION

And now a final word on what is, and will be for a long time to come, the sinister horizon of the world in which we all study and work: the international situation. Here, too, we cannot afford to live for long with a division of personal, professional, and political ethics—a division endangering the very life which our professions have vowed to keep intact, and thus cutting through the very fiber of our personal existence. But again, I can offer you only another variation of the theme, and propose, in all brevity, that what has been said here about the relationships of parent and child, of man and woman, and of doctor and patient, may have some application to the relationships of nations to each other, nations which by definition are units at different stages of political, technological, and economic transformation. I know that it is all too easy for us to believe that nations thus engaged should treat one another (or at least that we should treat others) with a superior educative or clinical attitude. This is not what I mean. The point is, again, not one of underscored inequality, but one of respected uniqueness within historical differences. Insofar as a nation thinks of itself as a collective individual, it may well learn to visualize its task as that of maintaining international relations of mutuality. For the only alternative to armed competition seems to be the effort to activate in the historical partner what will strengthen him in his historical development even as it strengthens the actor in his own development—toward a common future identity. Only thus can we find a common denominator in the rapid change of technology and history and transcend the dangerous imagery of victory and defeat, of subjugation and exploitation, which is the heritage of a fragmented past.

Does this sound utopian? I think, on the

The only alternative to armed competition seems to be the effort to activate in the historical partner what will strengthen him in his historical development even as it strengthens the actor in his own development—toward a common future identity.

contrary, that all of what I have said is already known in many ways, is being expressed in many languages, and is practiced on many levels. At our historical moment it becomes clear in a most practical way that the doer of the Golden Rule, and he who is done by, is the same man, *is* man.

Men of clinical background, however, must not lose sight of a dimension which I have taken for granted in what I have said. While the Golden Rule in its classical versions prods man to strive consciously for a highest good and to avoid mutual harm with a sharpened awareness, our insights assume an *unconscious* substratum of ethical strength and, at the same time, unconscious arsenals of destructive irrationality. The last century has traumatically expanded man's awareness of the existence of motivations stemming from his animal ancestry, from his economic history, and from his inner dividedness; but it has also created methods of productive self-scrutiny. It will be the task of the next generation to begin to integrate such new awareness with the minute particulars not only of advancing proficiency but also of ongoing mutuality by which alone man's ready rage is neutralized.

It does not seem easy to speak of ethical subjects without indulging in some moralizing and ideologizing. As an antidote I will repeat the final words of the quotation from the *Talmud* with which I began. It does not say: "Here is the rule; go, and act accordingly." It says: "Go, and learn it." Here lies our challenge.

Chapter 19
Autoexperimentation:
An Unappreciated Tradition in Medical Science
Lawrence K. Altman, MD

Some physicians consider autoexperimentation a late nineteenth-century fad—a methodology of the past—but it is indeed a rather common means of contemporary investigation.

AUTOEXPERIMENTATION

Throughout medical history, the ethics of medical practice have concerned physicians. Traditionally, responsibility was for the patient and his naturally acquired disease; later, when deliberate investigation was introduced, concern expanded to the ethics of human experimentation.

In centuries past, only a few conducted medical investigations. As apprentices, often these investigators remained in the same laboratory for years, absorbing much of the character of their tutors, who instilled in them the principles and ethics of experimentation. One of the guiding principles through these years was that of autoexperimentation—serving as the subject of one's own experiment—a tradition which continues, although largely unappreciated, today.

In recent decades medical science's major advances have been associated with significantly larger budgets for research, thus creating the opportunity for more physicians and scientists to carry out clinical investigations.

A BRIEF HISTORY Since World War II, over a wider geographic area of this country, there has been a dramatic increase in the number of clinical investigators as well as academic institutions. Despite this crescendo, rarely do new investigators receive a background course concerning ethics, selection of the human subject, or the history of medical experimentation as medical students, house officers, fellows, or subsequently as medical researchers. Indeed, on his first day, a doctor may begin his clinical investigations on patients. Because this phase of the investigator's education is often omitted, perhaps less thought has been devoted to the selection of the human subject and the validity of the particular experiment than has been given to the technical method-

Editor's Note: Dr. Altman is now in his thirties. For more than a decade he has been pursuing the philosophy and nature of self-experimentation. The philosophic implications of this subject have broad application to clinical medicine. Portions of his article first appeared in Altman LK: Auto-experimentation: An unappreciated tradition in medical science. *New Eng J Med* 286:346–352, 1972.

ology and the number of subjects required for a statistically valid study. These factors, as well as public criticism of some experimental procedures during the past decade, have raised questions concerning possible neglect of the traditions in clinical research and have created a climate of furthered interest in the ethics of human experimentation. Consequently, this has resulted in more discussion of these issues in the medical literature.[1,2]

Surprisingly, these and previous articles have mentioned only briefly, if at all, one of the most common and perhaps most fundamental methodologies of clinical investigation —autoexperimentation. Those few articles which have discussed autoexperimentation have presented only a handful of examples. Few writers (Ebstein,[3] Ivy,[4] Beecher,[5] and Pappworth[6]) along with one editorial[7] and one leading article,[8] discuss and provide examples of autoexperimentation.

Ebstein's 1931 article[3] did not contain a list of true autoexperimenters; several of his examples were physicians whose morbidity and mortality resulted from occupational or environmental exposure, not from deliberate experimentation. Ivy[4] listed about ten autoexperimenters, none more recent than a half century before his 1948 paper; all were unreferenced. Ivy[4] cited them critically, as random experiments on man. "While these experiments may be a tribute to the enthusiasm and the bravery of these early medical scientists, they clearly show the limitations and dangers of uncontrolled self-experimentation," he concluded.

Beecher[5] in 1959 commented, "experimentation on other men requires a willingness to experiment on oneself as evidence of good faith, although in a given case self-experiments may be wholly impractical." Beecher, however, added no new autoexperimenters to Ivy's small list and Beecher's discussion of autoexperimentation paraphrases Ivy's critical attitude.

Pappworth[6] cites only four examples, all of which have been included in Ivy's paper. Pappworth's conclusion ("all these experi-

---

1820, Boston, Massachusetts Enoch Hale, Jr.,* age 29, injected 1/2 cc cold pressed castor oil intravenously into himself over a 25-minute period to determine whether the cathartic effect would result from this route of administration. "Having been persuaded from my own observations and those of others, that some of the milder medicines may be injected into the veins with safety, I resolved to make the experiment on myself." †

A nervous assistant fumbled his attempts to introduce the silver tube into Hale's vein, so, "I took the tube myself, and after several ineffectual trials, which gave considerable pain, I succeeded in introducing it. . . . The injection of the oil was a slow operation . . . the princi-pal obstruction arose from the difficulty of carrying the oil forward into the circulation, after it had entered the vein . . . it was necessary to press it forward gently by the fingers upon the arm, until it disappeared." ‡

Hale experienced an oily taste in his mouth, "copious eructations of wind, and slight nausea" § and a mild cathartic effect. His dissertation won the 1821 Boylston Medical Prize.

* Hale E Jr: Dissertation on the Propriety of Administering Medicine by Injection into the Veins. Boylston Medical Prize Dissertations for the Years 1819 and 1821, unpublished. Boston, Everett & Ingraham, 1821, pp 70–135.
† Ibid, p 111.
‡ Ibid, pp 112–113.
§ Ibid, p 115.

1874, Odessa, Russia Gregor Munch, age 38, injected blood from a patient with relapsing fever into himself, refusing medical treatment, to observe the natural course of the disease. He suffered four relapses, the last of which proved nearly fatal. He did not publish his experiment, and thus forfeited to Motschutkoffsky the claim of being the first to transmit relapsing fever. Many years later, Munch's nephew, **Dr. Podjapolsky**, discovered Munch's protocol preserved between old newspapers.*

* Podjapolsky P: Zwei Worte uber den Ruckfalltyphus und den Flecktyphus und 3 Memuaren des Prof GN Munch. *Rev Microbiol Epidemiol* Saratow T IN 2, 1922. Cited in: Podjapolsky P: GN Munch. *Arch Geschichte Med* **18**:361–368, 1926. Zeiss H: Otto Hugo Franz Obermeier (1843–1873). *Arch Geschichte Med* **15**:161–164, 1923.

---

ments could justifiably be described as foolhardy'') echoes the attitude presented by Ivy and Beecher.

Superficially, these experiments, performed more than a century and a quarter earlier, may seem unwise today. But viewed in historical perspective, they may not have been as foolhardy as Ivy, Beecher, and Pappworth considered.

For example, Ivy, Beecher, and Pappworth cite Enoch Hale's intravenous self-injection of castor oil as an unwise experiment. Ironically, Hale's essay was awarded the Boylston Prize for 1821. As the *New England Journal of Medicine and Surgery*'s review of Hale's prize dissertation noted, "Although the injection of foreign substances into the veins of animals in various physiological investigations has been a frequent experiment among philosophers . . . these inquiries have not been made with any particular view to the improvement of practical medicine, or to the safety or expediency of extending the same operations to the human subject. . . . This is, we believe, the only well authenticated one upon record, in which any medical substance has been introduced into the veins of any individual of our own species. . . ."[9] Thus, Hale's contemporaries considered his experiment to have significant merit.

If the medical literature neglects autoexperimentation as a subject, so too do the various codes of ethics concerning human experimentation. Interestingly, the Nuremberg Code[10] mentions autoexperimentation, and then in ambiguous terms. Article 5 states, "No experiment should be conducted where there is an *a priori* reason to believe that death or disabling injury will occur; except, perhaps, in those experiments where the experimental physicians also serve as subjects."

Autoexperimentation appears to have been neglected and inaccurately portrayed in the medical literature. The purpose of this chapter is, therefore, to call attention to the rich tradition of this particular type of human experimentation and to document a number of the contributions that this method has made to medicine.

THE EXPERIMENTS The boxed extracts located throughout the chapter give examples of a number of physicians and medical scientists who, to demonstrate an hypothesis about an etiologic agent, drug, diagnostic method, or physiologic response, purposely performed their experiments upon themselves. The examples cited have been selected from a much longer list, collected from the medical literature over the past 14 years. Since no index, reference book, or catalog classifies experiments according to the subjects used, these examples merely reflect my reading. Accordingly, the complete list of 137 experiments involving more than 185 investigators cannot be construed as an encyclopedia of autoexperi-

Ca 1600, Padua, Italy Santorio Santorio, age 39, was the first to understand the necessity of evaluating "insensible perspiration." To quantify it, he invented a steelyard, or balance. "He placed his work table, his bed and even all his other necessities needed for existence, upon suitable balances constructed by himself, and began experimenting to see to what alteration the bodily weight is subject, deducting solid and liquid secretions in their various physiological and pathological states; he conducted these experiments . . . for more than thirty years. . . . It was the first time and the first case in which a physician thought of verifying theoretical statements, by testing, retesting and with experiments. . . . There is a picture of Sanctorius, seated in a chair, facing a prepared table which rests upon balances, partly hidden in the ceiling of his room. . . . The chair was at a finger's height from the floor so that it could be displaced laterally. When the experimenter took nourishment, the chair lowered itself somewhat, and he was easily able to establish when he had taken the right quantity of food and drink. The elevation of the chair indicated the quantity of perspiration, since the sum of the excretions was deducted from the total amount of the loss of weight. Assuming that the healthy adult body generally retains the same weight for twenty-four hours, the experimenter indicated with his balance the absorbed substances, the secretions and excretions, noting the rest of the loss until he obtained the actual weight effective on the next day." *

Instead of describing the exact technique and results of each experiment, Santorio summarized his deductions in hundreds of aphorisms which comprise his *De Statica Medicina*. But Garrison and others† acknowledge that Santorio did these experiments on himself although Sontorio does not specifically so state in his aphorisms.

* Santorio S: *Ars de statica medicina*. J Quincy (trans), London, W & J Newton, 1972, sec 1, pp 43–122.
† Garrison, FH: *An Introduction to the History of Medicine*, ed 3. Philadelphia, WB Saunders Company, 1924, pp 258–259. Castiglioni A: Life and work of Sanctorius. *Medical Life* 38:729–785. Foster M: *Lectures on the History of Physiology During the Sixteenth, Seventeenth, and Eighteenth Centuries.* Cambridge University Press, 1901, pp 145–147.

mentation in medical science. Probably, they reflect no more than a small fraction of the experiments so performed.

These references span four centuries, from the seventeenth century through the present, and four continents, Asia, Europe, and North and South America. The documentation of more than 137 such experiments performed in diverse geographic areas and cultures during this period certainly would establish this methodology as a tradition.

The criteria for selection were:
Publication of the experiment in the medical literature

Documentation of the autoexperimental approach in the original report (by narrative description or by matching the subject's and the author's initials) and/or in a reliable secondary source

Whenever ambiguities arose, I solicited verification or clarification from the autoexperimenter. The element of risk, the degree of difficulty or sophistication, the suspected motivation, or the significance of its contribution to medical science were *not* used as criteria for inclusion. Papers in which medical students and other physicians served as subjects of the experiments are not listed if these subjects were not included among the authors of that publication.

A critical factor in compiling such examples is the definition of an experiment. What is an experiment to one, may not be to another; one labels an experiment what another considers merely an observation. Where to draw the line can be a difficult decision. Mc-Cance's definition is the broadest and perhaps the most realistic.[11] "Let us start with the word experiment, which most biologists use very loosely to cover any investigation, however trifling, made to advance knowledge. The term generally implies some deliberate change of conditions without foreknowledge of the results but with subsequent observation of them. It may be used, however, even when the conditions are not being deliberately changed, when the term observation would be more correct. . . . We should, I think, for present purposes, regard anything done to a patient, which is not generally accepted as being for his direct therapeutic benefit or as contributing to the diagnosis of his disease as constituting an experiment, and falling, there-fore, within the scope of the term experimental medicine.'' McCance's definition formed the background for my selections.

Although the boxed extracts contain a brief narrative of some of these examples, a few are repeated in the following discussion to demonstrate some general points about this methodology.

EARLY AUTOEXPERIMENTS

The earliest recorded example of autoexperimentation appears to be that of Santorio Santorio (Sanctorius, 1561–1636) of Padua, the father of metabolism. He constructed scales (a steelyard) on which he weighed himself before and after meals—as many as four times a day—over a period of several decades. He attributed differences in weight of food ingested and the body's excretions to "insensible perspiration." These experiments, seemingly, were riskless. Yet, two decades later, Stark found his autodietary studies risky. He died.

The first known deliberate experiment in-

1769, London, England   William Stark,[*] age 29, lived on bread and water augmented with an item such as sugar, egg, olive oil, salt, fig, or various meats, in a series of dietary experiments. "If possibly it could be pointed out to mankind that some articles used as food were hurtful, whilst others were in their nature innocent, and that the latter were numerous, various and pleasant they might, perhaps, from a regard to their health, be induced to forego those which were hurtful, and confine themselves to those which were innocent. To establish such a distinction as this, from experiment and observation, is the chief object of my enquiry: and I confess it will afford me a singular pleasure if I can prove, by experiment that a pleasant and varied diet is equally conducive to health, with a more strict and simple one; at the same time I shall endeavour to keep my mind unbiassed in my search after truth, and, if a simple diet seems the most healthy, I shall not hesitate to declare it.'' [†]

Stark's death in 1770 was attributed to these experiments and to "the imprudent zeal with which he prosecuted them." [‡]

[*] Stark W: *The Works of the Late William Stark, MD, Consisting of Clinical and Anatomical Observations with Experiments, Dietical and Statical.* Revised by James Carmichael Smyth, London, J Johnson, 1788.
[†] Ibid, p 90.
[‡] Ibid, p xi.

1760, Vienna, Austria Anton Storck,* age 19, encouraged by the therapeutic success of the external application of hemlock to the skin, investigated its use by the oral route. After a dog survived a test of hemlock's safety, Storck ingested increasingly larger amounts twice daily for more than a week. He experienced no unusual symptoms. "I was, therefore, now justified, in reason and conscience, to try this on others" † for the treatment of cancers, tumors, ulcers, and cataracts.

* Storck A: *An Essay on the Medical Nature of Hemlock*. London, J Nourse, 1760.
† Ibid, p 8.

---

volving significant risk to the investigator was Anton Storck's studies on the medicinal values of hemlock. This 19-year-old Viennese physician, encouraged by the therapeutic success he had had with the external application of hemlock to the skin, ingested increasingly larger quantities of hemlock solution. Having demonstrated its safety, he justified further investigational studies of its systemic use on others.

John Hunter's 1767 venereal study ranks among the most famous of the autoexperiments. At age 39 Hunter inoculated himself with matter obtained from the penis of one of his patients, whom Hunter thought to have gonorrhea only. Unfortunately for Hunter, the patient probably had a dual infection—syphilis in addition to gonorrhea. When Hunter developed signs and symptoms of both diseases, he drew the erroneous but, retrospectively, understandable conclusion that the two diseases were one and the same.

Although some physicians consider autoexperimentation a late nineteenth-century fad and a methodology of the past,[12] it is indeed a rather common means of contemporary investigation. I have found 12 examples during the past decade; personal discussions with a number of investigators indicate that the practice continues to be common—so common that these men were unaware that it has not been the subject of a medical experimentation monograph.

Despite autoexperimentation's limited application to human investigation, the examples cited in the boxed extracts cover a spectrum of medicine's subspecialties. Perhaps the large number of examples from research in infectious disease may reflect my special interest, yet it may represent a more accepted and applicable tradition in that field.

OTHER AUTOEXPERIMENTS Pharmacologists often use themselves as experimental subjects. Indeed, one leading contemporary pharmacologist, Dr. Chauncey Leake, has stated: "Those of us who were interested in the drugs in the laboratory were the first to administer them to ourselves. It was only after we ourselves were convinced of their relative safety that we would undertake their use in human subjects. . . . I think pharmacologists have a

---

1967, Seattle, Washington Ralph E. Cutler, age 39, became thyrotoxic in order to study the renal physiology of this metabolic disease state.*

* Cutler RE, Glatte H, Dowling JT: Effects of hyperthyroidism on the renal concentration mechanism in humans. *J Clin Endocr* 27:435–460, 1967. Cutler RE: Personal communication.

moral obligation to try such drugs on themselves after appropriate clearance with experimental animals before using them experimentally on any other human being." [13]

Similarly, physiologists often have used themselves as their experimental subjects, not only when studying the "normal" but also when studying a specific disease process. Cutler's deliberately self-induced hyperthyroid state is one such example; his aim was to study the renal physiology of hyperthyroidism.

One of the most famous—certainly one of the most dramatic—examples of autoexperimentation led to a new dimension of cardiology. Werner Forssmann, a surgical house officer in Germany, was dismayed at the dangers resulting from the external approaches to intracardiac injections at times of cardiac emergencies. In 1929, he wrote:

These experiences have induced me to seek new ways in which one can enter the heart, without danger, and thus I investigated the catheterization of the right heart from the venous system. I have tested out these considerations in experiments upon cadavers. . . . After the experimentation on the cadavers had succeeded, I undertook the first experiments on the living human in auto-experimentation. First of all, I permitted a colleague, who cooperated in the experiment, to puncture my right antecubital vein with a thick needle. I then introduced, as in the experiments on the cadavers, a well oiled uretal catheter of a thickness of four on the Charriere scale, through the canule into the vein. The catheter was easily introduced, 35 cm. upwards. As it seemed too dangerous to the colleague to go further, we stopped the experiment, although I felt completely well. One week later, I repeated the experiment, alone. Because venipuncture with a thick needle is technically too difficult to perform upon one's own body, I performed, under local anesthesia, a venisection in my left

elbow and introduced the catheter, without resistance, its entire length, 65 cm. This distance appeared to me, according to a measurement on the body surface, to be equivalent to the catheter. I had only a slight feeling of warmth, similar to that which we feel upon the intravenous injection of calcium chloride. Upon jerky movements, the catheter rubbed against the upper and lower walls of the clavicular vein, and I noticed a particularly intense heat below the clavicle . . . and a mild urge to cough. I checked the position of the catheter in the x-ray picture, and, indeed, I observed the forward progression of the catheter itself in a mirror held up by a nurse before the fluoroscopy screen. . . . Even the rather long trip in our Institute from the operating room to the x-ray department, during which I had to climb stairs, traveling on foot with the catheter located in the heart, was not associated with any annoyances. The insertion and removal of the catheter was completely painless, accompanied only by the above described sensations. Later, I could not establish anything detrimental to myself except a mild phlebitis at the site of venisection; this occurred apparently because of an imperfect asepsis at the site of operation.[14]

Two years later, Forssmann wrote about the need to develop angiographic studies of the heart.

Thus it is the intention and purpose of the procedure described here to make it possible to study the anatomy and physiology of a living chamber of the heart and . . . to work out as in the case of the digestive tract, the functional patterns and functional types of the various heart diseases.[15]

Again, Forssmann autoexperimented with radio-opaque substances.

Hunter and Forssmann represent the pitfalls and benefits, respectively, of conclusions

1767–1770, London, England John Hunter, age 39, inoculated himself with venereal matter, contracting both syphilis and gonorrhea. He punctured his penis "with a lancet dipped in venereal matter from a gonorrhea; one puncture was on the glans, the other on the prepuce. This was on a Friday; on the Sunday following there was a teasing itching in those parts, which lasted till the Tuesday following" when "the parts of the prepuce where the puncture had been made were redder, thickened, and had formed a speck. . . . On Saturday morning the slough came off. . . . On the Wednesday the sore on the prepuce was yellow, and therefore was again touched with a caustic. . . . Four months afterwards the chancre on the prepuce broke out again. . . ."* He treated himself with mercury. "The time the experiments took up, from the first insertion to the complete cure, was about three years. The above case is only uncommon in the mode of contracting the disease. . . . It proves, first that matter from a gonorrhea will produce chancres."† Subsequently, this conclusion was proven incorrect.

Hunter did not state specifically that he was the subject of his experiment, but the above provides the distinct impression that the subject could have been none other than Hunter.

George Babington's editorial note to the 1841 edition of Hunter's *Treatise* states clearly, "The author Hunter inoculated himself with the matter of gonorrhea. . . ."†

Corroborating evidence can be found in Paget's biography of Hunter. In a letter about a new surgical technique, Hunter wrote, "I go no further in theory than I would perform in practice . . . nor do I go further than I now think I would have performed on myself were I in the same situation. . . . I would have no one perform an operation that he is not clear about the propriety of himself."‡

---

* Hunter J: *The Works of John Hunter: A Treatise on the Venereal Disease.* JF Palmer (ed), London, Longman, 1837, vol 11.
† Hunter J: *A Treatise on the Venereal Disease.* George C. Babington (notes), Philadelphia, Haswell Barrington & Haswell, 1841, p 27.
‡ Paget S: *John Hunter, Man of Science and Surgeon.* London, T Fisher, 1897, p 172.

---

inferred from the results of autoexperimentation. Forssmann, after appropriate cadaver trials, performed what then were daring experiments. Although made on only one subject, they proved the important point. Cardiac catheterization was ridiculed in spite of the clearly stated potential benefits of Forssmann's successful experiments. Forssmann was "subjected to criticism of such exaggerated severity that it robbed him of any inclination to continue."[16] He became a transoceanic spectator as Cournand and Richards, a decade later, developed further that technique for which the trio shared the 1956 Nobel Prize in Physiology and Medicine. Hunter drew conclusions on the basis of only one case; even today, gonorrhea and syphilis coexist in about 3% of cases.[17] The results might have been equally erroneous had his experiment been performed on any one human volunteer other than himself.

Several individuals used themselves for more than one series of experiments. A few, in fact, made it an established lifetime practice. Indeed, it even became a family tradition; two generations of one of the most famous medical science families—the Haldanes—devoted much of their lives to investigations

1873, Berlin, Germany Otto Obermeier, age 30, after discovering spirochetes in the blood of relapsing fever patients, injected these organisms into animals, but did not succeed in reproducing the disease in them. "The failure of infecting animals spurred Obermeier to perform a crucial experiment on himself. Without any bluster or announcement of his intention, he injected himself intramuscularly with 5 ml of blood removed from a relapsing fever patient. Again he failed to reproduce the disease. This led him to believe that a special relapsing fever diathesis was essential to contract the disease. This erroneous conclusion could possibly have been averted had he only ascertained beforehand if spirochetes were present in the relapsing fever blood with which he inoculated himself in the left forearm." *

A few weeks later, when a cholera epidemic hit Berlin, Obermeier turned his research efforts toward this disease, injected blood from a cholera patient into himself, and died. Obermeier's professor, Virchow, delivering the funeral oration, stated: "Desirous of investigating the nature of cholera and doubtlessly with the purpose of evolving new curative methods for this devastating disease, he injected himself with blood from a cholera patient. During one of his clear moments he confided this fact in his nurse. Unfortunately, it is too late to ponder on whether Dr. Obermeier took ill following the self-inoculation or whether the disease would have occurred without it. The fact remains that Dr. Obermeier was anxious to have the opportunity to make an exact study of the disease on himself, perhaps to discover its cause." *

* Obermeier OHF: *A Symposium on Relapsing Fever in the Americas.* K. Birkhaug (ed), Ass Advancement of Science Monograph 18, 1942, pp 7–14.

involving themselves as subjects. The Finch cousins have served as subjects in their hematology experiments.

Surprisingly, these studies resulted in apparently relatively few catastrophes, although such reports may be understandably incomplete. Of course, outsiders and even associates might never learn about the ultimate catastrophe, death, in association with an autoexperiment. Indeed, facts might be changed to protect the investigator and his family. Hench's[18] version of Lazear's yellow fever autoexperiment documents one such instance. Luck must have favored some of the early random experimenters. Most of the more recent autoexperiments were conducted with appropriate medical precautions.

Stark, Obermeier, Lazear, and Carrion are the only four fatalities known, although Scott[19] attributes Carroll's death from myo-carditis, years after his mosquito experiment, to his yellow fever infection. Hunter's angina may have been a late manifestation of the lues he induced in himself; thus, conceivably, the experiment could have caused death. Sertuner, Perkinje, Fraser, Munch, and Wright survived the complications their experiments wrought. Halsted, however, had to interrupt his surgical career to recuperate from the addiction resulting from his enthusiasm for cocaine anesthesia. Harrington, Smith, and several of the catheterized cardiologists required the close medical supervision available to them. Brown-Sequard continually tasted the sequella of his autodigestion studies; he had a persistent rumination, forced to chew a second time what he had swallowed earlier.

Seldom did these investigators indicate motivation for their autoexperiment. Only the experimenter, however, can answer why he

---

1825, Breslau Germany Jan Purkinje, age 38, performed at least thirty-five experiments on himself. Purkinje overdosed himself with digitalis to study its effects on vision. Among other experiments he studied the actions of camphor, belladonna, stramonium, and turpentine on himself.*

*Kruta V (ed): Jan Evangelista Purkyne, 1787–1869, Centenary Symposium held at the Carolinum, Prague, 8–10 September 1969. Universita Jana, Evangelisty Purkyne, Brno, 1971.

---

chose himself instead of a volunteer as his subject. Even the investigator may not know his reason(s); or the true reason may have become clouded in the course of time. His version, when provided in the original paper or in later accounts, must be accepted; others, including myself, may only speculate about their impressions regarding the motivations of the autoexperimenter.

WHY CHOOSE YOURSELF? On the basis of the overall impressions I have gained from my interviews with a limited number of these autoexperimenters, and from reading the literature, both practical and ethical considerations were apparent in the choice of oneself. Of course, reliability, dependability, convenience, curiosity, a spirit of adventure, and an ethical code were strong influences. Sometimes one category predominated over the other, but usually factors in both were mentioned. Often, a combination of practical factors governed.

Whether practical or ethical, they raise pertinent questions about clinical investigation. The practical considerations included a number of points.

CONVENIENCE Many investigators, including those who have not published results of some autoexperiments, have cited factors of convenience: simplified schedules, time-saving, eliminating the need of explanation ("informed consent"), and so forth. Most referred to experiments involving simple procedures or measurements; that is, blood drawing, insertion of tubes into the gastro-intestinal tract, or ventilation measurements. Many investigators use their own blood when they need repeated samples or other tissues for calibration of their techniques and for controls. Thus, they can maintain a reliable standard conveniently. "I think the bureaucratic paperwork has led to a lot more auto-experimentation because it makes safe experiments simpler. We don't bother with the forms," one investigator explained frankly.

RELIABILITY The need for reliability in clinical investigation is obvious. For example, in an experiment which extends over a long period of time, a minor lapse of memory or "slip-up" could devastate the study's results. Consider a long-term dietary study in which one essential ingredient has been omitted purposely, and which requires the ingestion of items specially prepared by the research unit. If a volunteer, momentarily fed up with the monotony of the study, decided to eat a forbidden item, and then was too embarrassed to tell the investigator that he had done so, or if the volunteer honestly forgot that he ate a forbidden item, an erroneous conclusion might be reached.

Martin and Robinson called attention to this problem in 1922.[20] "This is inconvenient but advantageous, for the experiments are exacting and necessitate constant supervision of one's actions if sources of error are to be avoided. The partial abandonment of the joys of life is to some extent compensated by interest in the results."

Reliability was the prime practical factor

1962–1965, Boston, Massachusetts Victor Herbert, age 35, proved that pure folic acid deficiency (on a nutritional basis) could be produced in man by maintaining himself on a folate-free diet for four and one-half months.[*]

After Herbert proved that folate deficiency could cause megaloblastic anemia, three of his laboratory assistants, Nancy Cunneen, Louise Jaskiel, and Carola Kapff, ages 24, 24, and 25 respectively, ate a diet containing approximately 5 μg daily of folate activity, supplemented with oral tablets of pteroylglutamic acid. The studies, lasting five to seven weeks, sought the minimal daily adult folate requirement. An additional incentive was the subjects' desire "to lose weight during the course of the study."[†]

In 1962 and 1963, Herbert and Louis Sullivan, age 30, each ate one pound of raw beef spleen daily for a week and followed their platelet counts to determine whether spleen contains an agent affecting platelet production. Herbert experienced "headache, polyuria, some increase in stool and, he, in fact, for his second and third trials ate two pounds daily. As part of the study we each did a sternal marrow aspirate on the other." Thrombocytopenia resulted then and again when the experiment was repeated a week later. A third trial led to no change in their platelet counts. The study is unpublished.[‡]

[*] Herbert V: Experimental nutritional folate deficiency in man. Trans Ass Amer Phys 75:307–320, 1962.
[†] Herbert V, Cunneen N, Jaskiel L et al: Minimal daily adult folate requirement. Arch Intern Med 110:649–652, 1962.
[‡] Herbert V: Personal communication.

governing Victor Herbert's selection of himself as the subject of his folate deficiency diet studies. "I lived on a diet of prewater extracted food for the period necessary to produce megaloblastic anemia, which turned out to be four and a half months.

"Whenever I went out to eat, I carried along my plastic bag of prewater extracted food. I would not have trusted a patient to do it, but I trusted myself. I understood the factors involved. For example, some candies (chocolate) contain lots of folate but others (gum drops) contain none. I chewed gum drops because I knew they were safe. But a patient, misunderstanding the difference in candies, may have eaten a chocolate," Herbert explained.[21]

Had a "normal volunteer" been the subject, and had he inadvertently eaten such a folate-containing item, Herbert's study might have been ruined. Instead of establishing, for the first time, that folate deficiency could produce megaloblastic anemia, Herbert's experiment instead might have corroborated the two previous studies which established the opposite conclusion.

CURIOSITY Satisfying one's own curiosity might have been a factor in many, if not in each of the examples cited. Several items in the boxed extracts indicate that an accidental event led to an observation, experience, or deduction by the investigator, who then, after correctly interpreting the facts, chose purposely to repeat on himself, as an experiment, the event which had happened accidentally.

A pruritic, erythematous skin reaction developed where Looss (in 1898) had spilled a drop of water containing hookworm larvae on his hand. He associated the two events, and suspected that they were cause and effect. To satisfy himself on this point, he tried it again. Eventually this purposeful experiment led to the recognition of a hitherto unappreciated mode of hookworm infection, a finding of great epidemiologic significance.

Hofmann's laboratory notes describe his unintentional LSD poisoning. "I was forced to stop my laboratory work in the middle of the afternoon and to go home, as I was overcome by a peculiar restlessness associated with mild dizziness. Having reached home, I lay down and sank into a kind of delirium which was not unpleasant and which was characterized by extreme activity of the imagination. As I lay in a dazed condition with my eyes closed (I experienced daylight as disagreeably bright), there surged in upon me an uninterrupted stream of fantastic images of extraordinary vividness and accompanied by an intense, kaleidoscope-like play of colors. The condition gradually passed off after about two hours." [22]

As a result, Hofmann purposely autoexperimented with the compound and described other psychomimetic reactions. The results of his discovery are well known.

A peculiar sensation aroused Hald et al's interest in a compound, disulfiram, so they autoexperimented for its use as an antihelmintic. Unusual symptoms resulted "after an occasional intake of relatively small doses of alcohol." Their curiosity aroused, they continued to autoexperiment. Eventually, this compound was introduced into therapeutics as Antabuse, the antialcoholic drug.

Also, curiosity may represent a certain spirit of adventure. Where explorers invade the unknown of the physical world, the autoexperimenter may seek the unknown reactions of the human body and mind. This spirit of adventure includes the self-satisfaction of being *the* first to have experienced something new, not just experiencing for oneself that which already has been experienced by others.

CONTROLS   When the experiment involves subjects with a specific disease state, frequently the experimenter performs the studies on himself, a "normal," for control purposes, even when the results do not affect the study's conclusion. His main objective is to determine whether the changes are specific for the diseased patient, or occur in others free of that disease. He shares the test of safety with these patients, and he assumes the same risks as his diseased subjects, albeit that a given risk may be less to a "normal" than to an ill patient. The other factors mentioned herein may apply also to the investigator's selection of himself as a control.

PREPARED ANTICIPATION   The autoexperimenter, with the expertise of his specialty, is better able to comprehend and to solve un-

---

1948, Copenhagen, Denmark   Jens Hald, Erik Jacobsen, and Valdemar Larsen, ages 43, 45, and 46 respectively. During pharmacologic autoexperiments with disulfiram (tetraethylthiuram disulfide) as an antihelminthic, Hald and Jacobsen experienced unusual symptoms "after an occasional intake of relatively small doses of alcohol. . . . The effect was further examined in a series of self-experiments by Hald and Jacobsen who eventually found that a formation of acetaldehyde from the ingested alcohol caused the observed hypersensity to alcohol after the ingestion of disulfiram." *

Further studies led to disulfiram's use in the treatment of alcoholism under the trade name Antabuse.

* Hald J, Jacobsen E: A drug sensitizing the organism to ethyl alcohol. *Lancet* 2:1001–1004, 1948. Jacobsen E: Personal communication.

1947, Boston, Massachusetts, and Seattle, Washington   Clement Finch, age 32, received 0.5 gm of sodium nitrite intravenously to rapidly produce methemoglobin to compare that compound's fate in himself, "a normal control," with that in a patient with congenital methemoglobinemia. One-half the methemoglobin Finch formed disappeared after three hours; the patient's level showed no tendency to fall even after seven hours.*

* Eder HA, Finch C, McKee RW: Congenital methemoglobinemia. A clinical and biochemical study of a case. *J Clin Invest* 28:265–272, 1949. Finch C: Personal communication.

expected complications in the course of the study. Herbert relates the following:[21]

The only person who knows all the variables of the study is the subject. If a physician, he has the capacity to understand the unpredictable.

On Christmas morning when I got out of bed, I collapsed. I could not walk. I returned to bed and thought about what could cause lower extremity paralysis. I knew folic acid deficiency couldn't—or at least it had never been reported. Suddenly it occurred to me that potassium depletion could cause muscle weakness. My diet was water extracted. I had not replaced potassium. I had some samples of Tedral and Potassium Iodide. I took them. I managed to get to the lab where the resident on duty happened to be interested in potassium metabolism. He measured my potassium that morning— it was 2.77—and my EKG showed the typical changes of potassium depletion. We made the diagnosis.

I wonder how long it would have taken [someone else] to understand the problem—particularly on Christmas day. I suspect that if it had been a patient describing these symptoms, I would have thought it was psychiatric and put him off a day or two on a holiday.[21]

AVAILABILITY   An investigator who wishes to study a particular disease state may find that suitable cases are admitted to his institution only infrequently. Furthermore, this admission may occur when the investigator is absent, committed to another ongoing project, or simply at a time inconvenient to the investigator's schedule, thus depriving him of the opportunity to take full advantage of the situation. Accordingly, it may be easier to deliberately create the reversible pathologic process in oneself at a convenient time and place, with provision for adequate medical supervision.

SELF-INTEREST   At least one infectious disease investigator was prompted to develop an immunization technique not just for the benefit of society, but also as a means of protecting himself against a potentially dangerous agent with which he and his colleagues were working. With reference to the development of the Rocky Mountain spotted fever vaccine, De-Kruif quotes Spencer, "I was scared of this spotted fever. Look at all that hot virus we were breeding, with all those ticks around here. Why shouldn't I have grabbed at *any* way to protect myself?"[23]

"I think there's a certain pleasurable facet which encourages autoexperimentation. We are not supposed to think in those terms, but we tend to look upon autoexperimentation as something admirable," one autoexperimenter admitted.

LEGAL   Nonphysician scientists have used themselves as experimental subjects, perhaps

1924, Hamilton, Montana Roscoe R. Spencer, age 36, performed the first human test of the Spencer-Parker Rocky Mountain spotted fever vaccine on himself.*

* Aikawa JK: *Rocky Mountain Spotted Fever.* Springfield, Thomas, 1966, pp 51–52. DeKruif P: *Men Against Death*, New York, Harcourt Brace & Co, 1932, pp 140–145.

---

as the obvious consequence of their curiosity or a combination of the other factors mentioned here.

One additional reason must be considered. Had the nonphysicians performed the very same experiment on volunteer subjects other than themselves, could legal issues be raised against these investigators? Conceivably, would they be guilty of practicing medicine without a license?

For example, from 1942 to 1951, a group of University of Illinois biochemists studied the dietary role of the essential amino acids in humans, themselves. They wrote that "For the most part, these young men have been graduate students in biochemistry, or students in related fields who have had sufficient experience in biochemistry courses to appreciate the significance of the findings. Thus, they had a personal interest in the outcome of the studies."[24]

More than 25 years after these experiments began, one of the investigators, Haines, reflected, "Isn't it interesting that we were able to accomplish so much in days gone by without the 'benefit' of present-day Investigational New Drug (IND) procedures of the FDA? In fact, the 'investigators' in our studies would never have been qualified so as to be allowed to treat the 'subjects'."[25] Haines' comment deserves attention with respect to the newer federal regulations governing clinical research. Properly trained nonphysician scientists have conducted significant autoexperimental research in the past. Will they be able to continue to do so? Should they not be allowed to do so?

Haines' comment raises the issue of whether nonphysicians as well as physicians should

---

Properly trained nonphysician scientists have conducted significant autoexperimental research in the past.

---

subject their proposed autoexperiments to the institution's clinical investigation committee.

Are physicians violating their institution's clinical investigation committee if they fail to gain clearance in advance for the autoexperiment? Must they wait for such a decision if the subjects are themselves?

If the investigator disagrees with the committee's decision, may he still proceed? Consider the would-be autoexperimenter, his proposal rejected, who, convinced the committee's decision is wrong, has the strength of conviction to defy its authority. What penalties would ensue? Would such defiance jeopardize his future research career even if the experiment were successful? Could the Nobel Committee, aware of such defiance against an authoritative body, still award him a Prize in Medicine if he qualified otherwise?

These are interesting questions for which the federal and other ethics codes provide no basis for an answer.

SUICIDE Evidence exists for only one autoexperiment as a means of an attempted suicide. Olga Metchnikoff wrote in her biography of her husband that he had chosen to experiment with relapsing fever on himself, so as

---

1881, Odessa, Russia Elie Metchnikoff, age 36, "to spare his family the sorrow of an obvious suicide . . . inoculated himself with relapsing fever, choosing this disease in order to ascertain at the same time whether it could be inoculated through the blood. The answer was the affirmative; he became very seriously ill," his wife wrote.*

Later in France, in 1892, he swallowed a culture of cholera vibrios to demonstrate his doubts of the specificity of cholera vibrios; he escaped clinical illness.†

* Metchnikoff O: *Life of Elie Metchnikoff.* London, Constable & Co Ltd, 1921, p 104.
† Ibid, pp 154–156.

---

to benefit society and in preference to a more conventional and obvious means of suicide.[26] Metchnikoff recuperated from his attack of relapsing fever, and his experience provided further documentation of the hematologic transmissibility of this disease.

Others, however, may have succeeded not only in their suicide goal, but also in concealing this motivation from their family and/or the public.

ETHICAL CODE Application of the Golden Rule ("and as ye would that men should do to you, do ye also to them likewise")[27] to medical research seems to have been a major factor in the decision of many to have used themselves as subjects. Many of the essays on human experimentation have emphasized the fact that the investigator must be willing to perform the experiment on himself, but the crucial issue seems to be in the actual performance of the experiment on oneself, not the mere willingness to do so.

Welt's queries to 66 university departments of medicine provided a similar response: "Some recommend the Golden Rule at least as a minimal requirement. They recognize the special interests and motivations of the investigator and hence do not imply that because the investigator is willing to be a subject it is permissible to impose this on others; but, rather, that he has no right to subject others to an experiment in which he himself would not be willing to serve. The ultimate proof of this willingness to serve is, of course, serving," he wrote.[28]

Evaluating risk is unfeasible, if not impossible. Risk represents a different value or magnitude to each person. Withdrawing a mere 10 cc of blood could represent a greater psychological risk to some nonanemic individuals than the physiologic risk of bleeding an anemic person several liters. Others may agree on the risk involved, but each may differ on the degree he would accept. It is easier to state, "I would be willing to take the same risk as the volunteer," than act, "I will actually take this same risk."

"While I had never thought about the specifics until you asked," one investigator commented to me, "I certainly would never consider not doing the experiment on myself if I were to ask someone else to volunteer; no matter how minimal or great the anticipated risk."

"Nothing we do in medicine is without risk, and I could never tell a volunteer that the experiment was without risk. But I could tell him that I had actually taken the same risk. Somehow that creates a better feeling and understanding for both the investigator and the subject," another said.

"I always believe in taking twice as much as the next person in any of the vaccine or ingestion studies undertaken in our laboratory," an immunologist asserted.

"I always operate on the Golden Rule concept in all my research whenever it involves anything unknown," Herbert stated.[21] Reflecting on his folic acid autoexperiment, he remarked, "It hadn't occurred to me, as it should have, that water extraction would have led to potassium depletion. It would have scared the hell out of a patient, as it did to me."

Obviously, willingness to experiment on oneself is difficult to define. An investigator can state that he would be willing to do the experiment on himself. But does that statement have any meaning unless he actually does the experiment on himself? Proving intent in medical research may be as impossible as proving intent in judicial matters. It may be meaningless. To carry the analogy in human experimentation ad absurdum, Hitler could have justified the Nazi atrocities, in these terms, by stating that as a medical investigator he would have been willing to do the same experiments on himself!

Equally obvious is the fact that the mere act of doing the experiment on oneself neither justifies a poorly designed experiment nor justifies doing the same, well-designed experiment on someone else. But one wonders if it is justifiable to do the experiment on a willing, properly informed volunteer unless one had done the experiment on himself. Sir George Pickering addressed himself to the same problem: "The experimenter has one golden rule to guide him as to whether the experiment is justifiable. Is he prepared to submit himself to the procedure? If he is, and if the experiment is actually carried out on himself, then it is probably justifiable. If he is not, then the experiment should not be done."[29]

Autoexperimentation is criticized on the grounds of the overenthusiasm of the investigator, his bias and lack of ability to critically evaluate his results. Whether that is true or not, participation in one's own study cannot bias the result any more than can an enthusiastic investigator's subconscious interpretation of the results of a study in which he is an objective observer. It is the rare study which can provide valid results on the basis of an experiment on only one subject. Most studies are based on many cases, the number determined by the particular study at hand. In such instances, when the investigator is among the subjects, it is hard to see how his participation could bias the interpretation of the overall study. As the boxed extracts indicate, many of the important experiments in medicine have been performed by the autoexperimental method, and criticism of these studies has not been made because of the methodology. If the criticism of autoexperimentation centers on the investigator's weakness to defend a bias, the same can be said for studies in which, as an objective observer, he has conscious or subconscious biases also.

Overt practical factors may also involve additional, complex, ethical reasons. Studies on disease states raise frequent ward conver-

---

1885, Lima, Peru Daniel A. Carrion, age 26, inoculated himself with verruga peruana to learn the nature and incubation period of the disease and then succumbed to "Oroya fever" (bartonello- sis). As an unintended consequence of his experiment, Carrion demonstrated that these were two manifestations of the same disease.*

* Medina C, et al: *La Verruga Peruana y Daniel A. Carrion.* Lima, Imprenta del Estado, 1886. Schultz MG: Daniel Carrion's experiment. *New Eng Med* **278**:1323–1326, 1958.

Schultz MG: A history of Bartonellosis (Carrion's disease). *Am J Trop Med* **17**:530–515, 1968.

sational questions such as, "Is it fair to the patient to protract his disease state—not to curtail it as soon as possible?" This raises the conflict between the physician and the investigator, often the same person.

Such discussions often elicit the justification that the investigator indicated he would be willing to have the experiment done on himself if he were in the same situation. But would he? It is a question easier to answer as a bystander than as a patient. At least one of the investigators in the boxed extracts answered the question by making himself the patient with the particular disease state. But this was a study in which the practical factors mentioned earlier were important. Might not this technique be applied to other treatable, reversible disease states?

Obviously there are limitations to autoexperimentation, for it is not applicable to all clinical research. That experimentation which offers potential benefit to the patient himself, such as a heart transplant to an individual with apparent terminal cardiac disease, differs markedly from experiments which are done, not to directly benefit the patient himself, but to possibly benefit others.

In cardiac transplants, the deceased donor, presumably "normal," receives no direct benefit from the transplant. Indeed, many are concerned about the liability to him of a premature declaration of his death. If the Golden Rule applies, should not the surgeon investigator will his heart for a transplant, accepting application of the same criteria of death to himself at the appropriate moment? At least one cardiac transplanter has made such provision.

Scientific research and war hardly seem related subjects. Yet the principle of enlightened responsibility over the affairs, health, and lives of others is shared by the clinical investigator as well as the political leader.

Might not HG Wells, commenting on the responsibility of the political leaders who willfully made war and promoted international dissension, have been discussing human experimentation when he wrote, "It is not reasonable that those who gamble with men's lives should not stake their own"? [30]

REFERENCES

1　Ladimer I, Newman RW (eds): *Clinical Investigation in Medicine: Legal, Ethical and Moral Aspects.* Boston, Law-Medicine Research Institute, 1963.

2　Ethical aspects of experimentation with human subjects. *Daedalus* 98 (no. 2): Spring, 1969.

3　Ebstein E: Medical men who experimented upon themselves—A contribution to the causes of death in physicians. *Medical Life* 38:216–218, 1931.

4　Ivy AC: The history and ethics of the use of human subjects in medical experiments. *Science* 108:1–5, 1948.

5　Beecher, HK: Experimentation in man. *JAMA* 169:461–478, 1959.

6　Pappworth MH: *Human Guinea Pigs.* London, Routledge & Kegan Paul, 1967, pp. 78–80.

7　Martyrs of medicine. *JAMA* 90:1712–1713, 1928.

8　The doctor as the guinea pig. *Med J Aust* 2:65–66, 1969.

9　Review. Boylston Medical Prize Dissertations for the years 1819 and 1821. *New Eng J Med Surg* 11:163–175, 1822.

10　US Adjutant General's Department. *Trials of War Criminals Before Nuremberg Military Tribunals Under Control Council Law No. 10 (October 1946–April 1949); The Medical Case,* Washington, US Gov Printing Office, 1949, vol 11, 181–183. Reprinted in reference 1, p 117.

11　McCance EA: The practice of experimental medicine. *Proc Royal Soc Med* 44:189–194, 1951.

12　Schultz MG: Daniel Carrion's Experiment. *New Eng J Med* 278:1323–1326, 1968.

13　Leake CD: Discussion of technical triumphs and moral muddles. The changing mores of biomedical research. A colloquium on ethical dilemmas from medical advances. *Ann Int Med* 67 (suppl 7): 43–56, 1967.

14　Forssmann W: Die Sondierung des rechten Herzens. *Klin Wchnschr* 8:2085–2087, 1929, addendum 2287, 1929.

15　Forssmann W: Ueber Kontrastdarstellung der Hohlen des lebenden rechten Herzens und der Lungenschlagader. Munchen. *Med Wchnschr* 78: 489–492, 1931.

16   Liljestrand G: Presentation Speech 1956 Nobel Prize: *Physiology or Medicine.* Amsterdam, Elsevier, 1964, vol 3, p 502.

17   Beaty HN, Petersdorf RG: Gonococcal infections, in Harrison JR et al (eds): *Principles of Internal Medicine,* ed 6. New York, McGraw-Hill, 1970, pp 798–801.

18   Hench PS: Conquerors of yellow fever. *Proceedings of the Staff Meetings of the Mayo Clinic* 16:785–792, 1941.

19   Scott HH: *A History of Tropical Medicine.* Baltimore, Williams & Wilkins, 1939, vol 11, pp 1022–1023.

20   Martin CJ, Robison R: The minimum nitrogen expenditure of man and the biological value of various proteins for human nutrition. *Biochem J* 16:407–447, 1922.

21   Herbert V: Personal communication.

22   The history of LSD 25 (lysergic acid diethylamide). *Triangle* 2:117–124, 1955.

23   DeKruif P: *Men Against Death.* New York, Harcourt Brace & Co, 1932, pp 140–145.

24   Rose WC, Johnson JE, Haines WJ: The amino acid requirements of man: I. The role of valine and methionine. *J Biol Chem* 182:541–556, 1950.

25   Haines WJ: Personal communication.

26   Metchnikoff O: *Life of Elie Metchnikoff.* London, Constable, 1921, p 104.

27   St. Luke 6:31.

28   Welt LG: Reflections on the problems of human experimentation. *Connecticut Med* 25:75–78, 1961.

29   Pickering GW: The place of experimental method in medicine. *Proc Roy Soc Med* 42:229–234, 1949.

30   Wells HG: *The Salvaging of Civilization: The Probable Future of Mankind.* New York, Macmillan, 1922, p 42.

Part V
On Passing the Torch

Chapter 20
Concerning Teachees
Leonard K. Nash, PhD

Teachers promote learning less by the answers they give than by the questions they raise, less by their explicit instruction and profound erudition than by their example and commitment, less by concern to gloss over the difficulties of their subject than by their respect for the students' capacity to penetrate those difficulties.

TEACHING

Good students are what make teachers look (and feel) good, but students must somehow learn what their instructors cannot teach them. Nobody learns to ride a bicycle because he has been instructed to steer in "a curve with radius proportional to the square of his velocity divided by the angle of his imbalance"—though this is actually the way in which the competent cyclist, all unknowingly, maintains his balance.

At a higher level of abstraction, anybody who has taught a subject like ionic equilibrium or thermodynamics must be painfully aware that no encapsulated mathematical or verbal formula suffices to impart his own competence to those who do not have it. About all the teacher can do is point to the problems and tools for their solution—guiding the students' endeavors by his own example, and stimulating their efforts by demonstrations that the problems are not only soluble but

Editor's Note: Dr. Nash delivered these remarks in 1966 on receipt of an award for outstanding teaching at the 94th Annual Meeting of the Manufacturing Chemists' Association.

worth solving. If he succeeds in this the teacher is able to place his students in a learning situation. More than this he cannot do, but if he does less he is doomed to fail

ASKING QUESTIONS   To put his students in a learning situation, the teacher must somehow get them engaged in *inquiry*. For this purpose good questions are far more effective than good answers. A profound insight is contained in Weizsacker's comment, "Even if someone came today who knew the answers to all unsolved problems, we should not understand him if our own need had not already driven us to put the questions which he answers." Demonstrably sound where scientific discovery is concerned, this view surely is equally applicable in pedagogy. Everybody who has sought to master a new subject finds that he begins to grasp the subject only at that instant when he first apprehends the thrust of the inquiry: the sense of what is being sought, and how. As teachers our task is not simply to give answers; our primary responsibility is to ask questions. Answers become meaningful only if students have seen the force of our

> *Everybody who has sought to master a new subject finds that he begins to grasp the subject only at that instant when he first apprehends the thrust of the inquiry: the sense of what is being sought, and how.*

questions, only if we have been able to make the questions live issues students can regard as significant enough to justify their efforts to grasp our answers.

MAKING PROBLEMS INTERESTING How can we make problems come alive for students? We seek to relate chemistry to their lives by stressing, for example, its vast economic importance, but most often this seems too remote for students to feel it is their concern. We try to convey, both in lecture and in laboratory, the challenge of science as an open frontier, but we first have to convince students they want to explore this domain. We confront them with lecture experiments that pose arresting problems, rather than with the more usual lecture demonstrations that merely enforce trite answers. Yet even this may be insufficient. It seems to me that students become engaged with the problems of a subject only after they have chosen for themselves a certain life image. The most effective thing the teacher can do, then, is to act out for them what it means to be a chemist, seeking to evoke their commitment by his own.

The teacher asks questions; he encourages students' participation by answering theirs. My own experience is that one can do this in a limited way even in a class with as many as 300 students. Answering students' questions offers the teacher a magnificent opportunity to be seen thinking things through on his feet —filling the role for which he destines his students. There's no harm in being a little slow, or even occasionally confused; this dissolves the sense of magic and one's performance encourages students to feel they too could

fill this role. The same priceless opportunity can arise from lecture experiments. I deplore the current decay of the art of lecture experimentation. Filmed or televised experiments, though tremendously useful as supplements, fail to express the teacher's active personal involvement. Even more notable, they fail to offer the prime virtue of the live, on-the-spot experiment: it can, and often does, go wrong. Nature, not the students, then poses a sharp question which the teacher must try to solve in their presence. My students seem to remember best, and to get the most from, just those experiments that nominally have failed.

If a teacher wants his students to respect a subject, he must show his respect for them; respect is a two-way relationship. Laboratory

> *There's no harm in being a little slow, or even occasionally confused; this dissolves the sense of magic.*

work, homework assignments, and examinations must appear to students not as sterile police measures, but as still further extensions of the kind of inquiry in which he wishes to involve them. A searching question rather than a demand for pat answers is the best way of conveying to students his respect for their potential competence as inquirers. Students are capable of such inquiry. Indeed, recent experiments in secondary-school (and even elementary-school) education convince me that our students are far more capable than we have supposed. There is then every reason to offer them the opportunity to wrestle with modern subjects—living inquiries in which they can imagine themselves taking part. They can get surprisingly far with advanced subjects if the teacher is content to do a few things in depth rather than many things superficially, and if he deals as honestly as he can with all that he teaches.

By honesty I mean the conscientious effort to distinguish fact from theory, and even to distinguish the element of theory in fact and the element of fact in theory. By honesty I mean the frank admission that theories can never be proven beyond all doubt, thus preparing students themselves to make discoveries. Honesty also means rejecting reasoning more notable for its plausibility than for its integrity, and spurning facile pseudoexplanations (using such words as "tend" and "tendency," for example), which make a mockery of the critical inquiry we seek to promote. In my opinion, honesty calls for greater emphasis on how we know rather than on what we know, never seeking to conceal ignorance or doubt by invoking dogma or a smokescreen of specious (though technical) verbalisms. The concealment is in any case illusory. Students are astonishingly acute in detecting all such lapses from honesty. We can earn students'

respect for our subjects only by treating both subject and student with respect.

Teachers don't teach; at most they stir students to learn.

My message very simply is this. Teachers don't teach; at most they stir students to learn. Teachers promote learning less by the answers they give than by the questions they raise, less by their explicit instruction and profound erudition than by their example and commitment, less by concern to gloss over the difficulties of their subject than by their respect for the students' capacity to penetrate those difficulties. The most active role in education belongs not to the teacher but to the student.

Chapter 21
Two Views of Present Trends
in the Teaching of Clinical Medicine
Tinsley R. Harrison, MD

Imagine that a time machine apparatus has moved Cassandra some 3,000 years into our own era, where she encounters Pollyanna. They discuss modern education in internal medicine in the United States. The result?

In one of his many fantasy tales of science fiction, HG Wells, who out-Verned even Jules Verne in terms of imagination, wrote of the "time machine." With it one could move backward into the past or forward into the future. Let us imagine that such an apparatus has moved Cassandra some 3,000 years into our own era. She encounters Pollyanna. They meet in a large auditorium, and their audience consists entirely of full-time clinical teachers. They discuss modern education in internal medicine in the United States.

MODERN EDUCATION IN INTERNAL MEDICINE

Pollyanna
   One of the great things is that our full-time faculties are bigger than ever before.

Editor's Note: Dr. Harrison's essay is reprinted from Harrison TR: Two views of present trends in the teaching of internal medicine. *Ann Intern Med* 73: 475–478, 1970. It was presented on April 15, 1970 as the American College of Physicians Distinguished Teacher Award Lecture. For many years Dr. Harrison has been one of the most influential teachers of clinical medicine in America.

Cassandra
   Bigness and greatness are not the same thing. Indeed, they are sometimes antithetical. Besides, the amount of teaching which our volunteer teachers do is steadily diminishing in most schools. Often these are the best teachers. I need cite only the names of James B. Herrick, Louis Hamman, and Samuel A. Levine to prove my point.
Pollyanna
   But when our young people are exposed to so many dedicated investigators, each an expert in his own field, they are literally compelled to learn.
Cassandra
   That's the trouble with you moderns. You never read the classics. Don't you know what Plato said: "Knowledge that is acquired under compulsion obtains no hold on the mind." At least you must have read the relatively recent works of Chaucer, who wrote: "The gretteste clerkes been noght the wysest men."
Pollyanna
   But . . .

Cassandra

(Interrupting) I do not know the full-time teachers personally. But I manage to read the journals. There are a few excellent papers that are not only true and new but important. However, there are many more that are true but rarely new and relatively unimportant. Are those who write such trivialities the best-qualified persons to teach our students?

Pollyanna

You overlook the multitude of new and valuable techniques. It is our full-time teachers who apply them best because they have had the most experience with them.

Cassandra

Some of the newer techniques such as radio scans of various organs have great value in patient care. Others such as cinecardiography are mainly of research value.

Pollyanna

But almost all new techniques are initially used for research only. After a time they tend to be used for patient care.

Cassandra

It is true that the full-timers are likely to be more experienced and skillful with these new techniques. But here we encounter a difficulty that stems from a defect in human nature. Those who begin by using new methods for research only tend subconsciously to exaggerate the importance of these techniques in the practical care of patients. As a consequence we have much overuse, a large increase in medical costs, and sometimes—fortunately very rarely—an unnecessary death.

Pollyanna

But frequently we obtain practical information that cannot be obtained in any other way.

Cassandra

Not frequently but sometimes. The less

a man knows about history-taking the more he relies on objective methods. But I must confess that I do not blame our younger colleagues for their abysmal shortcomings in history-taking. Their teachers have not taught them how to secure a good story of the present illness. The reason is that many of the teachers do not themselves know how to do so. Every physician and especially every teacher of clinical medicine should have these words engraved on his left frontal lobe, "They look upon the instrument as all-sufficient . . . they neglect or disdain to make those careful and minute inquiries that no sound and sensible physician ever fails to do and thereby convert an invaluable auxiliary into what, in their hands at least, proves but an imperfect and treacherous substitute." This remark was not made, as you may suspect, concerning the cardiac catheter, the x-ray, or the electrocardiograph.

Pollyanna

Unless I am mistaken, the man who described pernicious anemia and also Addison's disease said it in 1846, about the stethoscope.

Cassandra

In any case, the remark indicates that the degradation of the history had already begun a century and a quarter ago. The rate of the process seems to be accelerating. Our Greek physicians on the island of Cos made no such error.

Pollyanna

I am truly amazed. You seem totally unimpressed by an obvious fact. Patients are now being studied more carefully than ever before.

Cassandra

Insofar as this leads to new and important knowledge, obtained without hazard to the patient and without an outrageous and unnecessary expense, I am all for such studies. But more thorough study does not invariably lead to better treatment. It may have the reverse effect when the senior staff sets the bad example of greater concern with the disease than with the patient.

Pollyanna

You cannot deny that our students and house officers are more familiar with scientific principles than ever before. And you surely approve of this.

Cassandra

Of course I do. But that doesn't excuse the scandalous neglect of symptoms which pervades the profession and is especially harmful to internal medicine, that branch of practice in which the history is more important than in any other. A knowledge of scientific principles is fundamental to good patient care. However, such knowledge should be, as so ably expressed by Thomas Addison, in addition to rather than in place of "those careful and minute inquiries which no sound and sensible physician ever fails to do." It is probable that such inquiries, if universally used, would reduce the number of laboratory tests requested by 50% to 80%. The expense of these tests, many of them unnecessary and ordered only because of the physician's sub-conscious feeling of insecurity in bedside medicine, is one of the major causes of the rapid increase in the cost of medical care. You perhaps have forgotten the curse placed on me long ago by Apollo. Because I refused him my favors he, having previously conferred on me the gift of prophecy, ordained that my prophecies would never be believed. I therefore am unwilling to prophesy about the future of medicine.

Pollyanna

But surely you are glad to see that we have so many more internships and residencies than ever before. Are you not?

Cassandra

Let me ask you a question. Do you believe that our house staffs are receiving better training than previously?

Pollyanna

Of course. Like Candide, I believe that we live in the best of all possible worlds. Everything always gets better and better.

Cassandra

It all depends on the type of training these young men and women are receiving. Subspecialty rotations teach them techniques but are not likely to make them better doctors. If they stay on a nose-to-the-grindstone general medical ward during the entire period, which they almost never do, then I will agree that the training is better than ever before. But actually it is often worse than 30 or 40 years ago. The proof is the high number of failures on the practical or oral examinations of the Board of Internal Medicine. We are training good written-examination-passers but poor bedside doctors. Our house officers are made so dizzy by rotating from cardi-ology to hematology to endocrinology to what-have-you that their vertigo makes them stagger and even fall when they come up against a really rough problem in internal medicine. By this I mean an elderly patient with multiple diseases involving multiple organ systems.

Pollyanna

But what about teaching them the new techniques?

Cassandra

That's easy. They should learn the techniques by actually performing them —under proper supervision, of course— on their own patients on a general medical ward. In my view a man learns

---

In my view a man learns more by reading 100 electrocardiograms on patients for whom he has responsibility than from reading 1,000 when he has no such responsibility.

more by reading 100 electrocardiograms on patients for whom he has responsibility than from reading 1,000 when he has no such responsibility. The same goes for many techniques. In other techniques the essential thing is to learn the indications (or contraindications) for a given procedure, but learning to perform it is unnecessary for most of our house officers. Cardiac catheterization is an example. The principle involved in learning techniques is that it is responsibility for a patient that makes the mind retain knowledge. Without such responsibility most men will soon forget much of what has been temporarily learned.

Pollyanna

You seem to me to be biased and against everything new. Surely you will agree that patients are receiving better care than ever before.

Cassandra

That depends on what you mean by care. If you mean only preventing death and alleviating physical suffering, then care is far better than a few decades ago.

My definition of care is much broader than that. I believe that the medical tree has three roots. The youngest but thickest is the scientific root; this root is much stronger than in the past. Then there is the intermediate root, the skills or, if you wish, art of medicine. I use the term art to signify not bedside manner but bedside skill. This began with Hippocrates, the first to secure thorough histories. It was strengthened by Auenbrugger and much more so by Laennec and many others including surgeons who led the way not only in operative skills but also in the art of palpation. Insofar as physical diagnosis is concerned, today's young physician is often superior to his forebears. But I strongly suspect that we have been deteriorating in the art of eliciting information concerning the subjective manifestations of disease.

The third root, which is much older and deeper than the others, is the priesthood of medicine. The latter goes back to the temples of Egypt and thousands of years before that to the medicine men of primitive tribes. They were often good psychiatrists and probably helped many of their patients. When one reads the works of William Osler, Weir Mitchell, and Francis Peabody, one wonders whether we are not losing ground during the present century in our obligations to medicine as a priesthood. Are we not falling behind in the care of those patients, once the majority and still a large minority, for whom, as Alan Gregg expressed it, "the physician himself is the treatment"?

Pollyanna

In terms of the potential treatment of structural disease medical care is much better than two decades ago. The major credit for this goes to research, which is, in the main, conducted by the teachers of medicine.

Cassandra

Regarding the actual treatment patients receive, there are three aspects of medical care. These are quality, availability, and cost. If the investigators and teachers are to receive their deserved credit for the present potential higher quality, should they not also assume a major share of the blame for the diminished availability to a large segment of our population and for the skyrocketing costs? Regardless of the method of payment, whether direct, through insurance, or from tax funds, this huge expense comes from the pocket of society. At least some of it might be prevented by better medical education.

Pollyanna

I don't agree with . . . What's this?

The dialogue is abruptly terminated by the sudden appearance of a dense, white cloud enveloping the figures of five persons. At first their visages are masked by the cloud. Soon the fog lifts, and the audience can discern the faces of Hippocrates, Sydenham, Boerhaave, Osler, and Peabody. Hippocrates steps forward and says:

"Greetings. My friends have journeyed with me from the Great Beyond on our time machines. We are self-appointed judges of your debate. They have asked me, as the oldest among us, to tell you our decision. It is unanimous. We believe that each of you being partly wrong has received some intellectual blows. But each being partly right has scored points. The question is who has scored the most."

As Hippocrates steps toward Pollyanna and shakes her hand a thunderous roar of applause comes from the enchanted audience of full-time clinical teachers. The Father of Medicine continues, now addressing Pollyanna:

"My kindly daughter, we too believe that the teaching of internal medicine is better than before."

The applause is now deafening.

"But," resumes Hippocrates, "we deem it only slightly better." He now moves to Cassandra's side, shakes her right hand, and says, "Old friend, the great Apollo has, at the urging of his son Aesculapius, granted me the honor of removing his curse placed on you so long ago. Henceforth your prophecies will not only be true. They will be believed."

Slowly Hippocrates raises the right hand of Cassandra above her head. "You, my dear, have scored the most points. We timeless ones are not content with improvement, only slight, over the past."

The silence in the auditorium is now absolute. One can hear a pin drop. But there is not a pin in the place. Pins are used for testing sensation as part of bedside medicine.

There is no rattle of a stethoscope because there are no stethoscopes. Nor is there the sound of the scrape of a pencil because pencils are used to take histories, which are often inadequate. Each member of the audience remains rigid, his hands clasping his briefcase, the now recognized symbol of a professor of medicine.

Again addressing Cassandra, Hippocrates proceeds. "We all," glancing at his four colleagues, "believe that if we take the absolute view and compare the present teaching of internal medicine with what it should and could be, it is decidedly mediocre."

Cassandra replies, "And I prophesy that it will become worse before it becomes better. Thank you. I shall soon see you again on Mount Olympus."

Cassandra then turns and, mounting her time machine, rides back into the past. The five Giants of Medicine do likewise.

At once the members of the audience rush for the exits. Each one remembers that he has an appointment for a committee meeting.

Soon Pollyanna is left standing alone. There is no one with whom she can talk. Furthermore, she has nothing to say.

As Cassandra is being wafted back through time and space, she muses, "How nice of Apollo. And after all these years. He asked for nothing in return. So unlike a man. He is still very handsome despite his age. But then I am not so young myself. Perhaps I should change my mind about my favors. At least it is a pleasant thought."

Cassandra did change her mind. Soon she and Apollo were spending much time discussing their forthcoming child. They hoped it would be a boy who could again do for medicine what Apollo's older son, Aesculapius, had done so long ago.

Their hopes were partially fulfilled. The new infant was indeed a boy. But alas, alas! He was born with a tiny briefcase clutched in his hand.

Chapter 22
The Humanities and Medical Education
Roger J. Bulger, MD

It seems embarrassingly self-evident to me that physicians in training should be continually exposed to the type of analysis and thinking that the humanities offer; if they are not, they will be painfully inadequate as they try to understand the world in which they live.

THE HUMANITIES IN MEDICINE

In April 1971 an interdisciplinary conference sponsored by the Society for Health and Human Values was held at Arden House in Harriman, New York, to explore the desirability and implications of formal attempts to bring scholars and teachers of the humanities into the structure of medical education in a significant way. Philosophers, theologians, historians, and physicians at the conference generally accepted the distinction between the disciplined studies that make up the humanities and the process of being humanized; everyone was acquainted with people who excelled in the humanities but were unappealing as human beings. Despite this, and although a minority concern was expressed that an overt attempt to hire teachers of the humanities by medical schools might only be an administrative sham to counteract the growing public disillusionment with what some people regard as an increasingly inhumane profession, the general feeling of the group was that the humanities should occupy a more prominent place in medical education and that subsequent consideration should be given as to how this should be accomplished.

Certainly, for whatever reasons, there has been minimal use of the humanities in examining and resolving health-related ethical problems of all sorts. Technical advances, from organ transplantation to eugenics, force ethical matters into the laps of physicians, who will often take moral decisions upon themselves, however unsophisticated and uninformed they may be particularly if the rest of society chooses to ignore the issues. There are broad moral and ethical issues to be considered, such as:

Under what conditions, if any, can we allow transplantation of an unpaired organ?

What should be society's position on euthanasia and abortion?

What proportion of our health budget will go to increasing the availability of expensive, life-saving procedures and devices and what proportion will be directed toward preventive medicine?

In the future, scholars of the humanities and social sciences must be more involved in discussing issues at these broad levels.

In addition, there are problems about individual patients which arise every day in the hospital wards and clinics; often the young doctor or student is forced to take a stance which may have more far-reaching ethical or philosophic implications than he or she imagines. It is particularly at this level that experience in participation and interaction with the humanities is needed; up until now it has been minimal. At a few medical schools, ward rounds often include nonphysician faculty members with training in philosophy, sociology, and theology and thus far these activities apparently have proved to be fruitful. Most of the recent dialogue between the humanists and medical educators has focused on issues at these two levels (that is, the broad philosophic and ward consultation levels) and, appropriately, the dialogue has emphasized the moral and ethical implications of medical science and medical practice.

There is another potentially fruitful and as yet largely unexplored area of mutual interest between the humanities and medicine; it is with this third area, which involves the personal development of the physician, that this essay is primarily concerned.

The thrust in medical education is to turn out more practitioners and, once a person has gone into practice, medical education should provide him or her with a sufficiently satisfying life so that he or she will not want to leave the patient-care situation. What satisfies the physician in family or general practice? What gets him or her up at odd hours? What thread can make such a person happy, when he or she must face birth and death, sickness, anxiety and grief, tremendous character weaknesses and strengths? I suggest that this thread has little to do with science directly, but is a cultivated interest in human nature, an interest that may sometimes equal that of the artist.

Hemingway chased all over the world to find his apocalypse in the bullring; others went to Montmartre or Greenwich Village to engage real life. But the aware and sensitive physician can find it all in his practice. If his sensitivities have been sharpened in chasing symbols through *Moby Dick*,[1] *A Light in August*,[2] or *The Hollow Men*[3] and *The Waste Land*,[4] he may be able to find that much more enrichment in his day-to-day life. Instead of escaping from death and suffering in a cold or cynical denial, he may learn about them from those people he calls "patients." I believe the complete physician must at some point contemplate such things as the confrontation with horror; the relationship between comedy and tragedy; the role of suffering in human development; the history of the work ethic and what it may mean to be deprived of the capacity to work; the concept that emotional maturity is related to the acceptance of one's own death, that death is a part of life; the role of "indifference" in the professional bearing of the physician; the beauty intrinsic to a well-established personal or professional relationship; the idea of a profession; the rights of patients. No one has a greater opportunity to be closer to human nature than does the physician. The man or woman who sees this and enjoys that close-

> *The humanities can help broaden a physician's sensitivities and deepen his insights.*

ness will stay in clinical medicine. The humanities can help broaden his sensitivities and deepen his insights.

THE HUMANITIES' FUNCTION

A primary function of the humanities could be to focus upon the individual physician and his personal growth, emphasizing the need to work around the central issue of motivation and the nature of the satisfactions of a service-oriented life. As the medical student becomes more deeply enmeshed in his career, a wide variety of personal questions will present themselves. The appropriately sensitized teacher of the humanities can help the student recognize that the questions exist and can help him develop his own answers.

QUESTIONS At the risk of confusing the reader by introducing a bewildering array of subjects, it might be useful to illustrate the kinds of questions which have been raised in my mind during my own medical education, which officially began in 1956. In raising these questions, I have sometimes proposed my own answers or have described pertinent educational experiences for the reader's consideration. Where this is done, my aim has been only to illustrate more clearly the potential value of an interaction with scholars of the humanities. My goal is not to convince the reader that my current views on these matters should be his.

Some of the questions that have crossed my mind follow. What is the role of the physician regarding his patients? Can he simply be himself or should he at times play a role for his patient's benefit? How much authority should he claim? When the physician is confronted with a sick patient who views the physician as a superhuman being riding a white charger, should the physician force his humanity and the imperfections and ambiguities of his skills and knowledge upon the patient, or should the physician gracefully accept the role in which the patient has cast him?

Most mature physicians are more aware of the magnitude of their ignorance as compared with the depth of their own knowledge; is it wise, then, not to manifest an air of confidence for the patient's sake? Confidence is not synonymous with certainty and is not incompatible with humility.

What are the "rights" of patients? What kinds of psychologic roles can we sometimes force upon them and what roles do some of them take regardless? We frequently hear of the person who when hospitalized is treated like an infant by the health care team; laymen seldom realize that many aggressively

independent individuals literally regress and become like little children when they get sick or think they are sick. The sensitive doctor needs to be able to make these distinctions.

How does a physician learn how to deal compassionately with suffering and anxiety of all sorts? It is necessary to have the capacity in every instance, almost intuitively, to ask "How would I feel in such a setting"? This alone, however, is not sufficient. The physician must indeed understand himself well enough to know how he would feel—and that means *all* the feelings he would feel—in situations in which his patients find themselves; but he must also have enough humility to realize that he cannot react blindly according to his knowledge of his own feelings and should appreciate that others might react differently.

Has the physician the right to make moral judgments about his patients, especially those with different life styles? Has he a right to be a doctor to just certain kinds of people, or should he be constantly attempting to understand and become empathetic with different styles and groups? On what legitimate grounds may a physician decline to take care of a person who seeks his help?

What role does "indifference" play in the bearing of the physician? T.S. Eliot, in his play *The Confidential Clerk*,[5] seems to make this quality of indifference an essential ingredient in the personal growth of his major character; to my reading, this quality is the opposite of emotional involvement. What is the difference between empathy and sympathy? How can one be empathetic and indifferent at the same time, and what good do such reflections do for the individual attempting to be a useful physician?

What are the significant elements of the doctor-patient relationship? Medical faculty and students frequently discuss a well-worked-up diagnostic problem or the careful unraveling of a fascinating epidemiologic puzzle and wide appreciation is given in a variety of ways to the exquisite surgical procedure. It is difficult for me to recall in my own education any development of the concept of the beauty and importance of the successfully established doctor-patient relationship. This relationship is a difficult matter indeed for a patient and a physician living in an ever more transient America, bereft of home towns and a sense of permanency. There is a knack to establishing this working relationship and it must be defined and developed if more effective humane delivery of health care is to occur.

Once I have become proficient at my trade and primarily involved in dispensing the fruits of my expertise, what can I learn and where is my chance for growth? With the apparent decline of orthodox religions, people these days seldom talk about spiritual development; and personality development seems to be something one should worry about only in the so-called formative years. Most of us somehow have come to accept the idea that everything important about our psyche was settled before our second birthday, so why bother? Some students may fail to see various possibilities if the process of medical education does not emphasize and capitalize upon the almost unique opportunity the physician has to work on his own development through his daily interaction with the gravest

It is appalling to reflect upon the number of people, including physicians, who do not recognize that the basis for the modern restlessness, ennui, and dissatisfaction is a deep and almost universal quest for individual meaning.

human personal problems. It is appalling to reflect upon the number of people, including physicians, who do not recognize that the basis for the modern restlessness, ennui, and dissatisfaction is a deep and almost universal quest for individual meaning.

The physician, like everyone else, needs periodic refreshment and redirection, a refixing of his eyes upon his goals. As a pro-

fession, perhaps we have been a little embarrassed to speak of these things. The quality that separates the best physicians from the others is the degree of their motivation and their job satisfaction; and that in turn means they have to find meaning in what they do, to enjoy working with people and their problems, their strengths, their weaknesses, and their responses to crises.

DEATH How do I deal with dying patients and those who feel they have no hope? It is commonplace now, but nonetheless true, to point out that one of the greatest American taboos is the subject of death. In my own mind, maturity implies a realistic personal confrontation and handling of the idea of one's own death. As Americans become more aware of this taboo and attempt to counteract it in their individual lives, we are also experiencing the dissolution of the national gestalt of perpetual progress towards an attainable, perfect, just, and bountiful society. Thus, as a nation and a culture we are dealing with emptiness and potential meaninglessness while increasing numbers of us are attempting to deal with the concept of our individual deaths. I think these are two dimensions of the same subject. Recent literature on these two subjects illustrates how the humanities can offer much to the understanding of the physician, who, after all, will need to deal with patients wrestling with the prospect of death, dread, or great suffering on the one hand or with the implications of a meaningless existence on the other.

Elisabeth Kubler-Ross' book *On Death and Dying, What the Dying Have to Teach Doctors, Nurses, Clergy and Their Own Families*[6] has passages in it which seem analogous to ideas expressed by Michael Novak, the American philosopher and theologian, in his recent book *The Experience of Nothingness*,[7] which deals with the apparent meaninglessness of twentieth-century existence.

Kubler-Ross makes a strong case for the prospect of personal growth through an effective confrontation with the concept of death rather than perpetuating the denial of death and suffering. Similarly, Michael Novak speaks about recognizing and dealing with the "experience of nothingness" and contends that by refusing to run away from it or deny its existence, the individual personality may be taking the first step to a creative synthesis of individual personality and meaningful existence in the modern world. Mr. Novak says, "The experience of nothingness is an incomparably fruitful starting place for ethical inquiry. It is a vaccine against the lies upon which every civilization, the American civilization in particular, is built."

What is this experience of which Novak speaks and which he feels we Americans tend to deny as readily as we have denied death? He says it is a personal experience closely akin to the experiences of feelings about the meaninglessness of existence brought to the world's attention by people like Camus, Kierkegaard, Sartre, and illustrated most recently by the Theater of the Absurd. A recent quote from the interesting TV personality Dick Cavett describes at least a portion of the experience.

I'm at my worst when I come out of a nap, and I can see with some kind of crystal clarity the existential absurdity of life. You can never do one-millionth of what's available. There's a sense of lassitude and emptiness about it all. And there's a clarity about it, which doesn't last very long, when I think, oh God, it isn't worth it. It's almost like seeing life from a photograph in the planetarium, where the earth is a small thing in all that space.

Perhaps part of Mr. Cavett's appeal is that his viewing audience recognizes this perspective in him and more and more Americans are finding it in themselves.

Kubler-Ross classifies the experience of dealing with death as she has recognized it among her patients roughly as follows (and it is of interest to substitute Novak's "experience of nothingness" for "death"): Step one —the abyss of death (or the experience of nothingness); step two—despair or depression; step three—there is no disintegration of the psyche and the issue has been faced; step four—the individual realizes he has faced it and that it hasn't ruined him and his own courage gives him a sense of dignity and achievement. The latter must be akin to what I saw in my little daughter's eyes the other day when she was so proud at having come down a big slide she had never previously had the courage to negotiate. In a very real sense, people who face death (or the experience of nothingness) accept it and have the courage to proceed with whatever else remains to them —have conquered it. They develop a dignity others recognize. They have done what the astronauts appear to have done; they have dealt with the prospect of being blasted into infinity and have accepted that fate as a real possibility. Although it may in fact be true that some astronauts are fearless because they are among the world's best at denying death (it can't happen to me!), it is possible that in large measure they are such popular heroes because most of us transfer our own fears to them and assume that these men have dealt with death and have in fact conquered its fear.

Whether or not one shares Dr. Kubler-Ross's or Mr. Novak's ideas, it should be clear that the perceptions of people like them can be significant and stimulating elements in the continuing education of the developing physician.

COMMUNICATION AND UNDERSTANDING

What is nonverbal communication and which of its modalities are most likely to be useful to a health care worker? As the physician matures, he can learn more and more about this interesting area and can develop competence and pride in his abilities to communicate in a meaningful way with an increasingly greater variety of people. The white Anglo-Saxon Protestant presents a different problem in communication for the physician than does the hippie, the American Indian, the black, the aged Irish Catholic, the Gypsy, the Orthodox Jew, the paranoid individual, the stray or maverick, or the tracheotomized quadriplegic. There is much to be learned from artists and writers in this difficult matter of making a personal connection and I believe my own attempts at understanding some of the elements of novels by writers like Henry James, Virginia Woolf, and Dostoevsky have been helpful in later years as a physician. Patients have been helpful, too!

I can recall an experience with a severely psychotic hospitalized patient whom I saw as a fourth-year medical student over a two-month period. We met for an hour, three times a week, during that time and I still frequently reflect on some of the lessons she taught me. The patient was a gigantic black lady in her mid-thirties who had gained her PhD at a leading university and possessed an extraordinary intellect. On top of her massive six-foot frame, she had trained her hair so that it rose upward from her head somewhat grotesquely an additional 10 to 12 inches. Her speech was apparently unintelligible, her language symbolic, and people thought her to be hallucinating. Her eyes sought out direct contact and I felt her to be challenging me to figure out what she was saying; she seemed to be rejoicing at the perplexity and confusion of those of us who tried ever so intently and compulsively to interpret her ramblings. She seemed to enjoy these victories over smaller intellects.

After each session, I would review what had happened with the teaching psychiatrist whose practice and major interest was primarily with schizophrenics. As the weeks wore on, he got more excited about the fact that I was making unusual progress with her and that she was telling me more and more about what was bothering her most deeply. Intermingled with unintelligible babbling, one could piece together a story she was telling about a great ancestral princess, from some wondrous primordial tribe, who got lost as an infant among a wild bunch of lesser beings and who was forced to grow up amongst these sometimes well-meaning but clearly inferior

beasts. One day, the princess' true father, a great king and possibly god, came amongst the barbarians, identified his daughter, anointed her in some way, and placed a tremendous crown upon her head. None of the lesser creatures were aware of the meaning of all this or of the princess' greatness, and they continued to think of her as an ugly stranger. All this came out over two or three sessions amidst babblings and ramblings delivered at the wall and ceiling, but not at me. Suddenly she stopped and looked directly at me and asked, "Do you understand?"; and for the first time she waited for an answer. For some reason I said, "Yes, you are that princess; your hair is your crown; the rest of us are the barbarians. But I want you to know that I respect you." And I did respect her! I must have been right, because from that turning point, she seemed to speak more directly and honestly and formed the beginnings of some kind of human relationship. It is even possible that all of this did her some good.

Not all patients are so cryptic, but in order for the primary therapeutic physician-patient relationship to become established, the patient must learn, in some way or other, that the physician accepts the patient in a nonjudgmental way and accords that patient a necessary and basic human respect. Once this has been achieved, I believe there are then at least three important messages to get across to the patient. To the extent that I can convey these points successfully to the patient and to the extent that I live up to them is the measure (aside from the crucial matter of the quality of the technical medical ability and knowledge brought to bear on the case) of my success in achieving an effective therapeutic relationship with that particular patient. These three important messages which may or may not be delivered by explicit oral statements follow:

"I, as a physician, accept personal responsibility for you as a patient. I will do all I can to find out what is wrong with you and get you the best available treatment.

If I can't find out or am confused in any way, I will seek consultation and help from others. If you develop a fatal disease, I will stand by you and do all that is possible to minimize suffering and pain.'' Once the physician understands the reality of this basic underpinning of the most creative kind of doctor-patient relationship, then he can begin to explore at a conscious level whether he is well-suited to deal with all patients, or whether some patients will be more difficult or impossible for him. If he can't look a badly burned or disfigured or quadriplegic or dying patient in the eye and make this kind of commitment, then he shouldn't attempt to be that patient's primary physician.

"I, as a physician, wouldn't recommend anything for you as a patient that I wouldn't do for myself or my immediate family under the same circumstances.'' Implicit in this message is the principle that the patient shapes or participates in the critical decisions involving his care. The patient may elect to delegate these decisions entirely to the physician or he may need to participate more actively in the decision-making process. For better or for worse (and I think it's for the better), physicians are having to deal more and more frequently with patients who demand full participation in the crucial elements of their care.

"I, as the physician, am not emotionally involved with you as the patient.'' Implicit here is a guarantee of scientific objectivity, a steady hand in surgery, a clear mind in diagnosis.

As an intern, I cared for an extraordinary man who came into our hospital for cardiac catheterization studies and evaluation for possible cardiac surgery. He was over 60 years of age, lean, muscular, hard-working, honest, kind, and tough. He had come to Montana many years before with nothing and had worked up to ownership of a huge and productive farm. He was very proud of his children, all of whom had received magnificent educations. His respect for education seemed to me to be not that of the average hard-working fellow who had missed the college experience, but rather came from a rather deep, intuitive philosophic love for knowledge.

Five years before coming to us, his heart failed so that he couldn't work any more, a condition completely unacceptable to him. When doctors at several medical centers refused to recommend surgery and in essence told him to learn to live with it, he went to the East Coast where he went through a dangerous heart operation successfully. He had won the gamble and had returned to work. Now his heart was failing badly again, but incredibly he had worked for ten hours on his tractor the day before coming to our hospital for evaluation. I lived through the tests with him and helped him interpret the findings and their implications. In essence, they were as follows: no operation, little chance of improvement, and a probable gradual downhill course with a sedentary existence—versus dramatic open-heart surgery with a 50% operative mortality but a reasonable chance of significant improvement if he survived the hospital stay. Without batting an eyelash, he chose surgery and returned to Montana to get a few things in order. I admired him immensely.

Some days later when he returned to the hospital under the care of other physicians,

---

When I walked into the room, he suddenly began to cry; I barely made it from the room without breaking down similarly. Outside I did cry openly and I knew then that I could never again be of any use to him as a physician.

I went to the surgery ward to wish him well with the operation the following morning. When I walked into the room, he suddenly began to cry; I barely made it from the room without breaking down similarly. Outside I did cry openly and I knew then that I could never again be of any use to him as a physician. I learned from this experience about the quality of "indifference," something I couldn't quite learn from reading T.S. Eliot's *The Confidential Clerk*. The trick is to care, but to be "indifferent," that is, not emotionally involved. It is not always possible.

Although my tears were inappropriate because they were really for me and I didn't die, the man had cried appropriately, for he never regained consciousness after surgery.

I am not suggesting that my positions on these proposed elements of the doctor-patient relationship are the right ones or the only ones, but I am suggesting that the concerned physician must come to grips with these questions, and that humanities teachers may be helpful in aiding each maturing physician in developing his own particular answers.

It seems embarrassingly self-evident to me that physicians in training should be continually exposed to this type of analysis and thinking or else they will be painfully inadequate as they try to understand the world in which they live. I believe that one of the challenges to medical education in the immediate future is to learn how best to implement this proposed interaction of the humanities and medicine so that the students are engaged on their own grounds. It will not be an easy challenge to meet.

REFERENCES

1 Melville H: *Moby-Dick; or The Whale*. Chicago, Encyclopedia Britannica, 1952.
2 Faulkner W: *Light in August*. New York, Random House, 1932.
3 Eliot TS: "The Hollow Men—1925," in *Collected Poems* 1909–1962. New York, Harcourt Brace & World, 1963, pp 51–76.
4 Eliot TS: "The Waste Land—1923," in *Collected Poems* 1909–1962. New York, Harcourt Brace & World, 1963, pp 79–82.
5 Eliot TS: "The Confidential Clerk," in *The Complete Plays of T.S. Eliot*. New York, Harcourt Brace & World, 1963, pp 217–291.
6 Kubler-Ross E: *On Death and Dying*. New York, The Macmillan Co, 1969.
7 Novak M: *The Experience of Nothingness*. New York, Harper & Row, 1970.

Chapter 23
Can One Teach Medical Ethics?
Louis Lasagna, MD

The question is not can *we teach medical ethics—since we must—but rather how can we* best *teach it?*

MEDICAL ETHICS

The last quarter century has seen a remarkable burgeoning in our societal concern with problem areas in medicine with special implication for ethics. There are good reasons for the increased emphasis on medical ethics—the shocking Nazi medical experiments, several well-publicized scandals connected with medical research in this country, the concern with definitions of life and death prompted by advances in transplantation techniques, to name a few. It is also a time when one hears an ever-growing chorus of voices (often, but not exclusively, young ones) proclaiming the overriding importance (and dangerous neglect) of "humanism," "sensitivity," and so forth in medicine.

Editor's Note: Louis Lasagna, MD, is Professor and Chairman, Department of Pharmacology and Toxicology, University of Rochester School of Medicine and Dentistry. Dr. Lasagna is well known for his effective and provocative attempts to educate the profession and the public concerning vital issues in medicine.

THE CLASSROOM

This essay will describe my experiences in teaching a course entitled "The Doctor and Society." While many students referred to the course as "Medical Ethics," its purview was larger than the latter title would suggest. It was really concerned with the mutual impact of several important cultural forces. Medicine was the central focus, but the interacting forces included religion, philosophy, law, history, the communications media, and politics. One thing was clear: the course was not "Introductory Empathy 104" or "Intermediate Social Consciousness 203," or "Advanced Compassion 301." The sessions were not intended to create sensitive, compassionate people (is that a realistic goal for any course?) but to deal as rigorously as possible with complex issues, hoping to educate bright young men and women about problems and to suggest an approach for handling them.

The students were a mixed lot: most were premedical or medical students; a few "nonmedical'' undergraduates and graduate students were also enrolled. The format was the Socratic discussion and was most easily applied the first year (when there were a dozen students or so) and least effective the last year (when the class attendance averaged 30). Sessions lasted approximately two hours. Each week, packets of reading material were handed out, to be read before the next session. This posed a small fiscal problem: there are no adequate texts that can be used for a course such as this, and the readings used were culled from all sorts of obscure places. Library references seemed out of the question, if one expected (and demanded) reading by everyone before each session.

The point was made, however, that I was uninterested in off-the-cuff pontifications by anyone about something about which he knew nothing. The readings were not intended to make "instant experts" out of anyone, but they did provide a common meeting ground and a starting point. So, too, did the questions provided with each reading assignment. The questions were not always taken up in class, but they forced the student to think out specific issues, so as to facilitate the discussion in class and help those shyer students who might tend to panic if asked to supply answers on the spur of the moment.

MY FUNCTION   My own function was a mixed one. I asked questions, "pushed" students a little on their opinions (to show more fully the implications of a position), played the devil's advocate, and tried to keep the discussion from being too one-sided. I attempted (apparently with success) to hide my own feelings and preferences, an approach that was frustrating to those students who preferred an "answer," and who believed my opinion to be more valid than their own or that of their classmates.

The general approach was simple in concept, if not so in application. As already indicated, the first step was to acquire the relevant data that would allow choices to be made. The "facts" were not always readily at hand,

especially since the pertinent data were often nonmedical in character. If one is considering a matter such as the population explosion, the important information is about equally split between the medical and the nonmedical. Religious, economic, and political factors, for example, are of major significance. The same is true for the field of heart transplantation. For some questions, like the approach to nonpsychotic "disturbed behavior" or to abortion, the entire discussion can be readily oriented to nonmedical considerations. (It doesn't have to, and it isn't necessarily best to do so, but it can.)

The material and the discussions were made as specific as possible, with real or theoretical "case histories" almost always utilized because of my bias that vague discussion about medical ethics is usually both boring and sterile.

Alternative courses of action or proposed solutions were then weighed in regard to the "cost" of each. It was also necessary to discuss the goal or goals. If the class could agree on goals, there was at least the possibility that we might agree on the best path. If we could not achieve consensus on the goals, it was at least helpful to know that, and to realize that we were unlikely as a group to agree on the best solution.

SESSIONS   The first session, since it preceded any opportunity for reading assignments, was given over to a lecture on factors that affect the social functioning of the doctor. I discussed, for example, the pressures and background characteristics that push many physicians in the direction of conservatism, authoritarianism, and entrepreneurism. Next I would point out the conflict between the doctor *qua* physician and *qua* researcher or student. The problem of "man versus men" or "statistical morality" was also taken up, using such examples as what the doctor and society should do with typhoid carriers or alcoholic drivers.

It was also helpful, I found, to group together in pairs other opposing pressures: the need for the doctor to be (or at least seem) omniscient, and the importance of his maintaining a fallibilistic humility; the conflict between contemplation and decisive action in making medical decisions; the need to maintain both critique and credulity; the importance of influencing public opinion versus the safety of the cloistered office practice or university life; the contrast between the drama of person-to-person medical confrontation and the low-key, nondrama of most public health or preventive medicine measures; and so forth.

Finally, I would stress the fact that individual action, with significant social impact, was still possible, even in our complicated modern world. A few dramatic instances, such as the influential "citizen witnesses" at congressional hearings, or the victory of John Francis Banzhaff III, the young lawyer who singlehandedly managed to get "equal time" for antismoking commercials on TV, usually sufficed in this regard.

After the first year it seemed worthwhile to begin a Socratic discussion even during the opening session, despite the students' lack of preparation for it. So, after a preliminary talk along the lines described above, we would begin to argue about a given real-life problem. One year it was the question of who should be immunized against rubella, and why. Another year we argued over who should be immunized first against influenza if vaccine were scarce and priorities had to be set (health workers, such as hospital doctors and nurses? the critically ill?).

EXAMPLES   Perhaps some examples of individual sessions would best convey the flavor of our discussions. The one on "Human Heart Transplantation," for instance, used a collection of references that included the script for Dr. Barnard's "Face the Nation" TV appearance. Some questions given out with the readings were:

Was the first (Washkansky) operation "premature"? Were the donor and recipient treated ethically?

Were the other transplants done soon after the first Cape Town procedures just "an international race"? What would you want to know about the scientific credentials of Drs. Shumway and Kantrowitz, for example, to help render a judgment on this point? If not a race for glory, how do you explain the small "epidemic" of heart transplants?

Comment on these words of the sixth scheduled case, JW Van Huyssteen: "I want to see what chance I have to live longer than two months."

Who should make the decision as to whether an institution should perform heart transplants? Which surgeons? Who should determine the criteria for picking the recipient? The donor? Who should explain the risks and possible benefits? The surgeon? Another doctor? How much should the recipient be told?

Should our laws be changed to facilitate heart (and other) transplants? Who "owns" a dead person's heart?

Some scientists have suggested a moratorium on further heart transplants to allow "reassessment and taking stock of where we are." Do you agree?

Does the success of a heart transplant operation make the procedure "ethical"? Do the ends justify the means?

How would you have handled the publicity regarding Washkansky if you were director of the Groote Schuur Hospital? What do you think of the $50,000 contract between NBC and Dr. Blaiberg for exclusive story and picture rights to his operation?

Suppose that you are a *New York Times* reporter in Cape Town and have just heard of the Washkansky story. Dr. Barnard asks you not to file a story because the operation is to be kept secret for a month. What would you do? Discuss the harm caused by "raising false hopes."

If you were the producer of "Face the Nation," would you have handled it any differently? Should they have placed some critic of heart transplantation on the panel?

- Discuss the shortage of hearts for transplantation. Suppose you had only one heart available and four persons equally in need (medically speaking) of a new heart. How would you choose among the potential recipients? Suppose one were President Kennedy, dying of an assassin's wound through the heart (instead of the brain), one a 25-year-old housewife with three children, one a 53-year-old alcoholic vagrant, and one a 14-year-old child with congenital heart disease and an IQ of 190. On whom would you operate, if you knew the graft would be successful?

- How important are the economic aspects of heart transplants? Should people be allowed to bid for the few available hearts, high price winning? Discuss the following quote from the *Manchester Guardian*: "If you have a rare disease, it can be cured, and if you have a common one it is too expensive." Could the funds, manpower, operating rooms, and so forth used for heart transplants be put to better use? Can our society afford 500,000 U.S. heart transplants? Should money and effort be directed primarily to developing artificial hearts? To preventing heart disease? Is there really a national "pot" of resources that is finite in size, or can a society afford "what is necessary for the health of the people"?

The question about the shortage of hearts and the four potential recipients served almost as a Socratic Rorschach test. One medical student protested that a choice couldn't be made, "it's too painful." Another medical student picked the housewife, saying that "three children depend on her." One student selected President Kennedy, because "the welfare of the world hinges on his life." Still another found it possible to make the choice "easily" by considering "only medical grounds." Thus he ruled out Kennedy because of the

unsterile nature of the operative field, the alcoholic because of his concomitant disease, the young child because of the extra risk entailed by his polycythemia.

ETHICAL CODES   Our session on "Codes, Consent, and Captive Groups" utilized a broad range of reading material, from the various oaths formulated during Hippocrates' time to Pappworth's inflammatory book, *Human Guinea Pigs*. Here are some of the questions for that session:

- Is the ethical code an effective way of moulding moral behavior? (Reflect on the Ten Commandments.) In what ways can ethical codes do harm? Should one rely, instead, on punishments and rewards of a more specific kind, such as via the legal system? Does the law inhibit unethical behavior? Could it? Are there other systems or techniques that you believe more desirable than presently available ones? What of the NIH regulations?

- What are the main arguments against using prisoners as experimental volunteers? What are the arguments in favor? What two main types of motivations characterize those who would prohibit all use of prisoner volunteers?

- Should prisoners be "paid" for participating in research? How much? What types of payment (money, cigarettes, parole credits)? Should the nature and extent of payment be discussed before a prisoner consents to be a subject, or after? Could one satisfy those who object to parole credits as an "unfair" inducement by eliminating such credits or even by "subtracting" from credit achieved by "good behavior"?

- Is parole credit for volunteering to be a subject fundamentally different from parole credit for working in the prison laundry? Should a man sentenced to death be allowed to risk his life in an experiment in return for eliminating the death sentence? If a prisoner is deprived of his right to volunteer, is this a further abuse of his freedom? Could it affect his rehabilitation?

New York State Senator S.J. Thaler introduced a bill in 1967 that would in essence have banned all experimentation with children unless supported by a court order. What effect might such an edict—if nationally applicable—have had on the national polio field trials?

Should children only be subjected to an experimental drug if they stand a chance of obtaining therapeutic benefit from it in the near future? Can a healthy minor volunteer for an experiment? Should consent for experimenting on minors involve only the parents, or the child himself? At what age should a minor be asked for consent?

Could a child sue his parents later in life for involving him in an experiment without his consent?

THE ABORTION ISSUE   The abortion discussion had almost (but not quite) become a "tame" subject by the third year of the course. We livened it up considerably one year by having as a guest discussion leader an obstetrician who had helped lead the fight in Maryland for abortion law reform. Some questions that held up well from year to year in this session were the following:

Does the ready availability of legal abortions put the "criminal" abortionist out of business? Should society accept the legal abortionist as a necessary part of life, like the professional call girl?

In countries where abortion has been legalized, what have been the results?

Is forced marriage or a foster home for the illegitimate child an answer to the unwanted pregnancy?

Is it bad for the ethical and legal fabric of society to have laws which people disregard?

When does a human being first "exist"? Is there some stage of development at which you can clearly state that to destroy a fetus after that time is murder? Is the decision a scientific one, a religious one, or what? Does historical precedent help us in analyzing the issue?

Dr. Robert E. Hall has said, "Doctors should not be asked to determine which women qualify for abortions. We are no more qualified to do so than accountants or street cleaners." Do you agree?

If your 19-year-old unwed daughter became pregnant as the result of intercourse with a man whom she met at a college dance, would you try to arrange an abortion?

OTHER CLASSES

THE DYING PATIENT   This session was always stimulating. It is not only intrinsically fascinating, but has special appeal for students who can easily imagine their own plight someday when faced with the need to care for such patients. Here is a sample of some of the questions used:

How would you decide what to tell a patient who has a fatal disease? Will a Golden Rule approach work? Would your approach to children be basically different from your approach to adults? Is this general question a researchable one?

What should the criteria for death be? Will the growing interest in "spare-parts surgery" require a change in the definitions of death? Should the law or medicine define the moment of death?

Do you favor euthanasia? "Active" or "passive"? Under what circumstances? Would you be willing to run the risk of prosecution for homicide by injecting a lethal dose of morphine into a child born with multiple congenital anomalies affecting brain, spinal cord, and heart?

Should a person be able to leave a request for euthanasia in his will? If so, how should the request be handled in actual practice?

On what grounds would you decide when,

and with how much vigor, to apply resuscitative techniques to someone whose circulation and respiration had ceased to function? Would you share the responsibility for the decision with one or more colleagues?

THE AMA   Another good class was one called "The Image of the AMA." To my surprise and pleasure, each class on this topic seemed to end with a fairly balanced appreciation by the students of the merits and deficiencies of professional "trade unions." This was achieved by the use of such questions as:

Is it fair to describe the AMA as a "trade union for doctors"? What does the term imply? Is there anything intrinsically undesirable about the medical profession having a powerful and effective lobby?

Has the AMA tried to limit the number of doctors? For what purpose? If there were an economic depression and doctors began to suffer serious difficulty in earning a living, would you favor cutting enrollment in medical schools? How would you decide how many doctors were needed?

What merits and demerits do you see in the AMA's belief that the less the federal government intervenes in medicine the better? Is medical care of high quality the "right" of every citizen? How high is "high"? If such care were possible only by tripling taxes, would your answer be any different?

Are there parallels between the factors affecting the quality of our national, state, and civic political leaders and those affecting the quality of our medical politicians?

EUGENICS   As the father of a mongoloid child, I found it especially challenging to lead the discussion on "Eugenics and Defectives," and I believe that the students benefited from my recounting the problem as it affected our own family. A sample of the questions employed follows:

You are a general practitioner. One of your patients gives birth to a child that looks mongoloid. What should you do? Should you call in other doctors to corroborate your diagnosis? What would you tell the family? What might suggest the need for institutionalization? Should institutionalization be delayed? If so, for how long?

Is forced sterilization morally defensible? Is it defensible as "expedient"? For what people? Who should decide whether someone is to be sterilized? Would you, as a parent, have your sexually promiscuous retarded daughter sterilized?

Are we on the way to "making the world a hospital" by saving "defectives" through medical advances?

What should we do to "guide" human evolution? To whom shall we entrust large-scale eugenic decisions? Can these be voluntary? Should they be? Is the Fore tribe quarantine justifiable?

MENTAL ILLNESS   Professor Thomas Szasz has been a fervent proponent of "The Myth of Mental Illness." I find much of his writing persuasive, but he loses me eventually by his unyielding simplistic theories. Nevertheless, his writings (plus those of some of his critics) helped considerably to pep up the treatment of such problems as:

Is mental illness a "myth"? Could you construct a definition that would satisfy both patient and society?

Does society use the diagnosis of "insanity" to control dissidents?

When is alcoholism a "disease"?

Was Ezra Pound a "martyr"?

Is mental illness an excuse for crime? For tort?

Is commitment to a mental institution a form of imprisonment?

Do inmates of mental institutions have a "right" to adequate care and treatment?

Who should decide about the custody of "dangerous offenders"?

Should sexually "deviant" offenders be sentenced to drugs that "control" their socially intolerable behavior?

Should an extra Y chromosome be taken into account in sentencing a criminal?

What role should the psychiatrist play in criminal proceedings?

MINORITIES IN MEDICINE Although one of my black students informed me that Jews and women—despite handicaps once or presently suffered in pursuing a medical career—cannot possibly be talked about in the same breath as blacks, I still found it convenient to have one session devoted to "Disadvantaged Minorities in Medicine." (Incidentally, one of the readings that I found helpful here was the "Soul Folk Chitling Test," which makes the point that whites are no better at answering questions dealing with ghetto experiences or language than ghetto blacks are at taking IQ tests geared toward white children.) Here are a few of the questions used:

Should a medical school adopt a quota system for blacks? For Puerto Ricans? For women? What criteria should determine preferential status (either permissive or restrictive status)?

Should there be more "black medical schools"?

Should MCAT scores be used to select medical students? Should the "Soul Folk Chitling Test" be used for this purpose? Should interviews be held?

Do you oppose ethnic labels in medical records?

If you were a black doctor, would you join the NMA, AMA, both, or neither? Why?

Would you object to a lady physician taking care of you? What would you do if a patient vehemently objected to a female intern, and you were chief resident physician on the service? What if the objection were made to a black male intern by a wealthy lady from Mississippi who has expressed a desire to donate money to the school?

Is the plight of the woman in medicine only a reflection of the general treatment accorded the woman in our society? Can these biases and inconveniences be changed?

DOCTORS IN THE ARMY Having once testified on behalf of Captain Howard Levy at his court-martial, I was able to convey a little extra drama in the session devoted to his trial and to the more general treatment of "Doctors and the Army." Some questions used with success were:

What do you believe Levy's chief motivations were for disobeying orders?

Were the war crimes and medical ethics issues real ones, or merely dragged in post hoc as rationalization for the anti-Vietnam War position of Levy and his defense witnesses?

Would the Army have court-martialed Levy if he were not such an "unmilitary" officer?

Was the Levy conviction inevitable? Was it justifiable? Would you have acted as Levy did in the circumstances? Is the last question relevant?

Should doctors be forced to serve in the armed forces in peace time? Should there be a specific "doctor draft" when no other U.S. group is subject to a special draft? Should medical students be deferred from army service?

Is it ethical not to provide medical care for wounded soldiers? Should a medical school penalize students or faculty members who sign proclamations indicating their intention not to serve in Vietnam and to break the law, if necessary?

Should professors take pains to hide their university affiliations when they take public positions on controversial topics? On any topic? When should a doctor identify himself as a physician in public utterances (such as letters to newspapers)?

Do psychology and psychiatry have legitimate roles to play in preventing war or in the formulation of foreign policy?

CONCLUSION

So much for the sessions. One final problem arose: how to grade such a course. (The university at which I was then teaching required that I hand in marks.) Grading on the basis of class discussions would tend to reward the verbal and punish the shy or the silent, yet participation was at least a partial reflection of time spent preparing for class and "mastering" the material. I decided to ask every student to hand in a brief term paper (giving a final exam would have been ludicrous, I thought). If a student did well on the paper, he could get a B or better despite a "poor" class performance. A student who did poorly on the paper, but had performed well in class, could also get a good mark. Not a perfect solution, but one I could live with. (The students were never told my marking strategy, since I felt embarrassed even to mention grades.)

The term papers were often interesting and at times exciting. I encouraged papers based on "research" rather than library work, and convinced a few students to conduct surveys or collect facts that proved fascinating both to them and to me. One student canvassed the faculty on their knowledge about chiropractic. Another studied the techniques at different hospitals in town for deciding on which women qualified for legal abortions. Still another reported on the successes and failures of local "methadone clinics" for heroin addicts. Rarely were the papers poor; my main complaint was that spelling seemed low on the list of achievements of the students.

The experience, then, was rewarding for me and for the students as well, gauging by their responses to a reporter who did a story on the course and by their responses to questionnaires dealing with the curriculum in general. I have no doubt at all about the value of such a course, if only to start students (and future doctors) thinking about these crucial socio-medical issues and about ways to deal with them.

"Can one teach medical ethics?" In the sense described above, I think the answer is yes. Is one course enough? Of course not. Ethical and humanistic approaches will have to be taught by precept and practice and reinforced by an appropriate system of rewards and penalties throughout the lifetime of the doctor if he is to be an ethical physician and an effective citizen. I submit that the question is not "can we teach medical ethics"—since we must—but rather "how can we best teach it"?

Epilogue

Despite the large number of contributing essayists to this volume, there is a surprising consistency with which certain themes have recurred.

In various ways, several authors called for a new corporate and social ethic among physicians, both to guarantee quality to the patient and to encourage a better distribution of health care. It was surprising how often the subjects of war, pollution, and population arose. There is a need for rational voices from the medical and scientific arenas to address themselves to the problem of finding solutions to these broad ethical and social issues. With ethics at the individual level, the Golden Rule still appears to have strong supporters.

Rewards from careers in medicine were dealt with explicitly and implicitly by most of the contributors and the emphases seemed to be on personal, psychological, scientific, and intellectual development. Although a few commented that medicine provides a good living, finances and income appeared to be relatively unimportant to this collection of authors in considering the goals and rewards of a medical career. A special point was made that medicine should be fun, and that each step along the path should be enjoyable rather than something to be endured in order to reach some future position. In part because of considerations such as these, some people indicated a need to expand the educational horizons of the medical curriculum to include more of the humanities and the social sciences.

One last point is noteworthy. Recently a young friend of mine praised some concepts of mine by referring to them as "radical" ideas. I was taken aback somewhat by the label because I don't regard myself as "radical" and because the concepts in question were ideas that I have been expressing for almost ten years. Looking at the essays in this volume from my friend's point of view, however, two things are apparent: lots of "radical" things are stated and in large measure they are stated by men of "established" medicine. It strikes me that many of our contributors, whether we call them radical or simply honest and candid, have shown themselves to be cut from the same mould as was Hippocrates, at least as Dickinson Richards described him. If, in a sense, our authors have revisited

Hippocrates through this volume, and if he were able to listen to their words, I suspect the experience has left him both anxious and proud: anxious because of the turbulence and troubles surrounding modern medicine and the society it serves; and proud because there seem to be so many incisive and concerned intellectual descendants of his who are attempting to diagnose and treat our diseases.

Roger J. Bulger, MD